D1014176

You Can Conquer Cancer

You Can Conquer Cancer

A New Way of Living

IAN GAWLER

JEREMY P. TARCHER/PENGUIN
a member of Penguin Group (USA)
New York

56788714

616.994
GAW

JEREMY P. TARCHER/PENGUIN
Published by the Penguin Group
Penguin Group (USA) LLC
375 Hudson Street
New York, New York 10014

USA • Canada • UK • Ireland • Australia
New Zealand • India • South Africa • China

penguin.com
A Penguin Random House Company

First edition published in Australia 1984
Revised edition published 2001
Second revised edition published 2004
Third revised edition published 2013
First published in the United States by Tarcher/Penguin 2015
Copyright © 1984, 2001, 2004, 2013 by Ian Gawler

Penguin supports copyright. Copyright fuels creativity, encourages diverse voices, promotes
free speech, and creates a vibrant culture. Thank you for buying an authorized edition of this book
and for complying with copyright laws by not reproducing, scanning, or distributing any part
of it in any form without permission. You are supporting writers and allowing
Penguin to continue to publish books for every reader.

Most Tarcher/Penguin books are available at special quantity discounts for bulk purchase for sales
promotions, premiums, fund-raising, and educational needs. Special books or book excerpts also
can be created to fit specific needs. For details, write: Special.Markets@us.penguingroup.com.

Library of Congress Cataloging-in-Publication Data

Gawler, Ian.
You can conquer cancer : a new way of living / Ian Gawler.
p.   cm.
ISBN 978-0-399-17263-2 (paperback)
1. Cancer—Treatment.   2. Cancer—Diet therapy.   3. Cancer—Psychological aspects.
4. Relaxation.   5. Meditation.   I. Title.
RC270.8.G39   2015   2014035591
616.99'4—dc23

Printed in the United States of America
1   3   5   7   9   10   8   6   4   2

BOOK DESIGN BY TANYA MAIBORODA

Neither the publisher nor the author is engaged in rendering professional advice or services
to the individual reader. The ideas, procedures, and suggestions contained in this book are not
intended as a substitute for consulting with your physician. All matters regarding your health require
medical supervision. Neither the author nor the publisher shall be liable or responsible for
any loss or damage allegedly arising from any information or suggestion in this book.

Through arrangement with the Mendel Media Group LLC of New York

*This edition is dedicated
to the health, healing and well-being
of all who read it.
May you all live long and happy lives!*

Contents

The Big Picture

What Is Possible and How

IT IS A GREAT FEELING TO HAVE RECOVERED FROM CANCER—TO HAVE BEEN through it all and to be living a full, happy life again. I have done it. I have seen others do it and know many more will repeat the process in the future. This book, then, is offered with a sense of excitement and joy—the joy in having done it and the excitement of being able to help others to do it.

We all share a common goal. We all want to enjoy good health along with long, happy and meaningful lives. And we can. However, when a diagnosis of cancer comes into a family, all this is severely threatened. There is the real threat of life cut short, along with fear, distress and potential suffering.

Good news. We can turn all of this around. I have done it myself and I have seen many, many others do it as well. You can conquer cancer. That is a fact. It is possible. There is a process by which you can combine your own resources with those of the medical and allied health professions so that you can transform the experience of cancer and recover. This book examines the patient's role in disease and healing. It is intended as a self-help manual that provides the signposts along the path to well-being and long-term health.

Currently, of all the people diagnosed with cancer, Western medicine helps around 65 percent to be alive five years later. For someone whose prognosis predicts they are likely to be in that 65 percent, this approach will mobilize your own inner resources, along with those who support you, and give you every chance of becoming a long-term survivor.

For those with a poor prognosis from the medical point of view, take heart. You too can do it. I did. At my lowest point in 1976 my surgeon thought I would only live for a few weeks. So it is wonderful not only to still be alive, but to have raised a family, had the good fortune to be able to help many thousands of others and, importantly, to have seen many, many others recover using these methods.

For more than thirty years now, people have continued to ask me the same question. It is a good question and it is as relevant to the start of this book as it is to every person who asks it.

"When it comes to cancer, what is the most important thing that will help me, or the person I love, to recover?"

I never tire of this question. Is it the food? Is it all in the mind? Is it some new medical breakthrough or some ancient herb? Is it the meditation? What is it? What is *the* thing that helps the most?

Well, in my experience it is a combination of things. You need the best of all that is available.

You can conquer cancer. But you do need to work at it. This is not a casual business. You need to learn what to do and you need to do it. And when you do, you are bound to feel better in ways that right now you may not even imagine. There is the real prospect of becoming cancer free and enjoying a whole new phase of your life.

WHERE THERE IS A RHYME, THERE IS A REASON

My right leg was amputated with osteogenic sarcoma (bone cancer) in January 1975. While there were no signs of the cancer anywhere else in my body at that time, I was told that only 5 percent of patients could expect to be alive five years after such surgery. If my cancer reappeared, it would be expected to be rapidly fatal. In those days, most people died within three to six months of developing secondary growths of this form of bone cancer.

In fact, my cancer did reappear in November 1975. By March 1976, my specialist thought that I would live for only two more weeks. My subsequent recovery ran the full gamut of available treatments and, in June 1978, I was declared free of active cancer.

Over the next few years, my former wife, Gail (who later changed her name to Gayle and then Grace), and I had four children. I began a new veterinary practice, took up a thirty-seven-acre farm, developed vegetable gardens and orchards, and built a new house.

In 1981, Grace and I initiated the Melbourne Cancer Support Group. This lifestyle-based support group was one of the very first of its kind anywhere in the world. It began with an initial urge to pass on the benefits of my own rather extraordinary experience of recovering against the odds. Having been through it all myself, I understood the problems cancer patients face. Furthermore, being a rather pragmatic veterinarian, I had enough medical knowledge to understand my own position at the outset, evaluate my progress, and assess critically the wide range of treatments considered. Fortunately, I was blessed with an open mind, so I was ready to consider anything that worked toward my aim. That aim was to create the right environment in which my body would heal itself. To think that the body can play a major part in healing itself was a novel approach way back in the mid-seventies, but is one that we now know to be full of possibilities.

When my cancer had recurred and the situation looked hopeless from the medical viewpoint, I remained confident that there *was* another way. Already I had been introduced to the idea that cancer involved a state of immune deficiency, a weakness in the body's healing defense system. To explain: it is known that throughout the lifetime of every healthy person, cancerous cells develop in their body. This is a medically accepted fact. It also is accepted that the body normally recognizes these abnormal cells as a potential threat to its health and acts quickly to isolate and destroy them. It does so before any physical symptoms become apparent. However, in people who go on to develop cancer this does not happen and the growths continue unopposed. The body offers no resistance and symptoms of cancer are the result.

So I began with the attitude that it was possible to restimulate the body's natural defenses—in particular, the immune system. This being so, it followed that the body itself could destroy and remove all traces of the cancer. As an extension, if the immune system remained intact and functioning properly, there should be no worry about the cancer reappearing. An exciting prospect!

That attitude was my starting point, my basic premise. All I did was directed toward that end. So, while I explored many avenues of treatment, every one was a part of the process of finding the right balance for me. Now more than thirty years later, and having worked with many thousands of people intent on dealing with their own cancer challenges, what this book is able to present are the key principles that will be helpful, as well as exploring some of the more peripheral options.

This attitude of being empowered and learning how to overcome the many challenges cancer can present is so very different to the fear that normally surrounds the word.

FEAR AND THE FOUR MISCONCEPTIONS OF CANCER

Probably no other word strikes as much emotional fear in the community today as does *cancer*. While over the years the intensity of this fear may have lessened to some degree as more people have come to realize there is something constructive they can do in response to cancer, for most the fear is still very real.

When *You Can Conquer Cancer* was first published in 1984, it was regarded as somewhat provocative and revolutionary. First, there was the title, *You Can Conquer Cancer*. Conquer? Maybe "get help with," maybe "manage," maybe "live with" would have fitted the expectations of the day better. But "conquer" and "you can" in the same sentence? You can conquer cancer? Is that for real?

Actually the title was quite deliberately chosen to confront what many people believed back then and what some people still do believe: you get cancer and you die. This of course is the primary fear cancer engenders. But there is more to it. The fear of cancer is based on four basic misconceptions:

1. The cause of cancer is unknown.
2. Cancer is generally associated with pain and an untimely death.
3. There is nothing patients can do to help themselves except hand over responsibility for their well-being, and indeed their lives, to a doctor.
4. Treatments are unpleasant and probably will not work anyway.

It is the work of this book, of the Gawler Foundation and of other likeminded practitioners and groups to dispel these fears, to replace them with a positive attitude, and then to show how people can make a decisive contribution toward restoring their own health.

GOOD NEWS • Cancer Is a Process That Can Be Reversed

This book presents the good news on cancer. It is not a book about dying gracefully with cancer. It is about a process of living—living to the fullest.

The starting point is seeing cancer as a process. We must realize that most of the causes of cancer are now known and that cancer is not a chance happening of random fate. Once the causes are identified it becomes possible to plan appropriate action. To do this satisfactorily we need to expand our horizons. We need to consider the roles of those three aspects of our human condition that we know as *physical, psychological* and *spiritual.*

While personally I recognize the overriding importance of spiritual factors, I do not confuse these with religious issues. Religious preference is something different and personal to the individual, and therefore I talk little of this. Some prefer to leave religion alone, others take their religion seriously indeed, and it is my experience that whatever their choice, people explore that avenue for themselves. The techniques talked about in this book have no religious loadings, nor do they interfere or impose on patients' preferences in any way. However, the majority of people do find the techniques an aid in their search for their own spiritual reality.

Most people, and people diagnosed with cancer in particular, are concerned with the basic questions: Who am I? Where did I come from? Where am I going? These fundamental spiritual questions are often prominent in the mind of someone diagnosed with cancer and are certainly worth exploring later in the book.

In these pages we shall consider also the role environmental and psychological factors play in the causation and treatment of cancer; for herein lies the key to success. We can identify the majority of the causes of cancer. I contend that there are techniques which provide effective antidotes to those causes. The techniques center on appropriate diet, exercise, positive thinking, stress management and meditation—all in conjunction with suitable specific therapies. By utilizing all these means, the body's natural healing urge can be helped to reassert itself.

A body with properly functioning defenses cannot have cancer.

WHAT IS POSSIBLE?

I have experienced the pleasure of working with other people who have been able to repeat the process I went through and become free of a supposedly terminal illness. But just as exciting and pleasing is the fact that these techniques have consistently produced a deeper love for life coupled with a profound acceptance of the outcome of that life.

So, while I have seen and continue to see many recoveries, I accept that not everyone is going to become free of their physical problems. Sadly, some may die of their illness. But it has been part of my joy to know that the great majority of those who used these same techniques and did not recover were able to die with great dignity, and a poise that often surprised and always impressed themselves and their families. In this way, too, cancer was truly conquered. So, although the aim is always first and foremost to help people back to full health, this approach is of great value to those who face dying.

While in general the earlier in the course of the illness a person begins using this approach, the easier they will find it and the better their result, for those making a later start there is still the real prospect of overcoming cancer. There are always genuine grounds for hope, plus the bonus of overcoming fear and the problems associated with the disease. For many others there is the exciting prospect of using this approach to prevent cancer. I have found that, indeed, you can conquer cancer.

A COMMITMENT TO WHAT WORKS

This is a book about what works. The essence of this book has been distilled in the cauldron of major disease. People faced with cancer take life seriously— very seriously. They want answers. They want to know what works. They need to know what works.

What you are reading in *You Can Conquer Cancer* represents the accumulated wisdom of thousands of people over several decades who were all focused on these question: What are the best things to do? How best to respond to the many challenges cancer presents? How to recover physically? How to transform what for many at first diagnosis was shock and fear? How to transform the potential suffering of this illness into good health and long-lasting well-being?

The reality is that between the thousands of people I have worked closely with, we have tried many things. In fact, between us, we have tried most, if not all, the things you could think of, and probably quite a few you could not! My job has been to collect, distill and communicate the lessons learned from all this experience—this experience of what works. It is presented here in the hope that you too will benefit from the experience of so many others, and from the knowledge that comes out of it.

Of course, both myself and the many people I have worked with as group participants and colleagues value science and its evidence base. I love research, read lots of it, take it into account, and highly value it. But then science needs to be tested in the real world. So in this book, the focus is on what works in practice, what I can share with you based on so much practical experience. As such, I have deliberately chosen not to attempt to document what I present with more than rudimentary research evidence. This book is not intended for research scholars it is intended for practical use.

I first wrote this book back in 1984, and have thoroughly rewritten it in 2012. On both occasions I had in mind what I would say if I was speaking personally to the most valued person in my life. What follows is the best I can offer. It is informed by research; much of the book is validated by research. But unashamedly I suggest its real strength is that it is the product of shared human experience.

The accumulated experience of all the people I have been blessed to work with, gathered together here in this one book, can save you a lot of time. It may even save your life!

This book, then, focuses upon the principles of self-healing. What you can do to restore natural health, what you can do to help someone you love and care for. As a bonus, for those still well, the book can guide you directly with how you can prevent illness and experience lasting good health.

You Can Conquer Cancer presents an integrated approach, a guide to health and well-being.

GRATITUDE

There is nothing like sitting and talking with a room full of people whose lives are on the line to clarify what is important and what works. This book is a tribute to all the thousands of people affected by cancer who over three decades have helped to test, trial and debate the possibilities. The strength of the book resides in the fact that what it presents has been tested in the crucible of human experience, intense human experience, the intensity of aiming to overcome cancer and all the challenges it presents. So my gratitude, and respectfully I would suggest, your gratitude as the reader, needs to go to those people whose experiences the book reflects. This book stands as testament to their commitment and achievements.

There is a need to acknowledge and thank my two main meditation teachers, Dr. Ainslie Meares and Sogyal Rinpoche. It is useful to be aware that it was only a few decades ago that medical innovators like Dr. Meares began to identify the health-promoting possibilities of the ageless forms of meditation and adapt them to modern, everyday problems. Dr. Meares' first major contribution in this area was popularized in his international best seller *Relief Without Drugs,* first published in 1967.[1] I was fortunate indeed that at the time when my cancer recurred in 1975, Dr. Meares was putting forward his hypothesis that intensive meditation may help people with advanced cancer to recover. I was then equally fortunate to meet the great Tibetan lama Sogyal Rinpoche in 1985 and I continue to learn from him. Rinpoche, as he is known, is the author of the international classic *The Tibetan Book of Living and Dying*[2] and has been at the forefront of bringing the ancient wisdom of the Tibetans into a vibrant, modern context. What I can offer regarding meditation stems largely from these two great teachers, Dr. Meares and Sogyal Rinpoche, along with the many people who have taught me as I attempted to teach them.

You may be able to imagine that working in this field has its challenges. I have so much gratitude to my wife, Ruth Gawler, for all that she does to support me both professionally and personally. Ruth is an extraordinary doctor, a wonderful meditation and yoga teacher, and she has had a profoundly positive impact on so many people she has counseled. She has taught me what real love is and it is a delight to be married to her.

I have also been fortunate to work with many extraordinarily talented and compassionate colleagues. I think of the many people who volunteered to sit on the Gawler Foundation's board and the many staff I have worked with. Of course things go up and down a little when you work with lots of people, but one thing that has been a constant is the clarity of purpose all the staff have taken to their work which manifests as their unfailing capacity to work together for the interests of those attending programs and to create a caring, nurturing, transformative environment. This capacity is truly wonderful.

As to the book itself, I am deeply grateful to the Brady Foundation for supporting me in a very direct way and providing the opportunity to concentrate on the writing. Particular thanks is due to Ross Taylor, himself a long-term remarkable cancer survivor, who has encouraged and inspired me personally, as well as a multitude of other people dealing with cancer.

Then to thank my publisher, Michelle Anderson, who has been a tireless advocate for the book and become a very supportive friend in the process. Robina Courtin brought her formidable skills as an editor to bear on the book and contributed significantly to the end result. Pam Cossins did great work transferring my handwriting into type, while David Johns did his best with his photography to make me look good for the front cover. Great photography at least! Ruth also made a significant contribution reading and assisting with many drafts, and thanks to Maia Bedson, Michelle Anderson, Professor Gabriel Kune and Rohan Erm for reading some or all of the book and offering useful feedback and suggestions. As with the first edition, John Simkin contributed the index.

Finally, a thank-you to the critics. Criticism provides the opportunity to reexamine what you take to be correct, to reconsider how you can express things more clearly or in a more accessible way, and to check how what you say resonates with others. While destructive skepticism has little merit, constructive criticism is always welcome.

THE BENEFIT OF THE YEARS

Given the years since the first edition back in 1984, I now have even more confidence in these principles because I have observed them at work for so long. They can transform your life! For many people, they have been life-saving. For others they have sustained and prolonged life, then helped them with a dignified, honorable death. For all who do use them, these principles bring more inner peace, more joy, more happiness.

One of the personal delights in writing this new edition has been to reaffirm that the essence of what worked over thirty years ago is very similar to what it is today. While this new edition represents a very thorough rewrite when compared to the original, there is a fundamental truth here. Your lifestyle affects your health. Your lifestyle can produce disease and your lifestyle can produce healing. So while this new edition is updated, the language more current, the stories often more recent, the basic principles have stood the test of time and remain constant. The reason for this? What is presented here is how you can use your own resources to get the best from your body's potential to heal. These things are constants: good nutrition, exercise, sunlight, healthy emotions, the power of the mind, meditation—your lifestyle.

Do not be confused by the simplicity of the theory. What we will be talking of here are things you can control for yourself and apply in your own healing journey. They can be highly therapeutic. The book will explain how!

A FINAL WORD

There is no magic bullet in this book. No wonder drug or herb that can be taken three times daily and which, leaving all else unchanged, will offer you a cure.

You *can* conquer cancer using a process—a healing process that takes effort, perseverance and does require changes to be made. It is a process through which our natural state of health can be regained. For those prepared to walk this road, I know that cancer can be prevented or overcome. My wish is that more and more people will do it.

For the benefit of others, I offer this book.

Ian Gawler
The Yarra Valley, 2013

CHAPTER 1

The First Step

How to Begin

WHAT YOU DO WILL MAKE A DIFFERENCE. THERE IS A COMPELLING LOGIC TO this. If you, or someone you love, have been diagnosed with cancer, it makes good sense to get all the outside help you can. But then, as with everything else in life, how you respond, how you react, what you actually do—all this will affect the outcome significantly.

For those willing to take up the challenge that cancer has put to them, there is a road back to health.

What to do? There is so much information available these days. Advice from friends, opinions from medical and other health professionals, lots of great books and so much information on the Internet. This book will distill the benefits of years of experience and gathered knowledge, present it in logical, sequential form, help you to evaluate the many choices available, and then support and guide you along the way.

We will begin in the first two chapters by working through the options, from first diagnosis to long-term survival. Then come the details you will need to convert a good idea into a practical reality. You can conquer cancer. What follows spells out the process of how to do it.

HOPE IS REAL

The starting point is having hope. And hope has a compelling logic to it. No matter how dark it may seem as you start on this road, you need to be assured recovery is possible. It may not always be easy, it may well take a good deal of planning and commitment, but it definitely is possible.

At my worst I was expected to live for only a few weeks. That was early in 1976! After I recovered, Dr. Ainslie Meares said a very important thing: "It only has to be done once to show that it is possible." But these days there are many documented cases of people who have recovered against the odds. I have helped to publish two books recounting the lives, the methods and the recoveries of some of these people. The first, *Inspiring People*,[3] gathered the stories of forty-four people who had attended groups I ran in the early years and went on to become long-term survivors. Out of print now, that book was replaced by *Surviving Cancer*,[4] which recounts the remarkable journeys of twenty-eight people. Written by Paul Kraus, himself one of the longest-known survivors of mesothelioma, his is a wonderful book to read and then dip into from time to time whenever inspiration is needed.

FEATURES OF LONG-TERM SURVIVORS

There are two important features I observe in the many long-term survivors I have worked with and come to know well. First, they really applied themselves—they did many things. Second, the main things that they did they had in common, while many varied some of the minor details.

Let me explain. Some years back, I surveyed thirty-five long-term survivors. These were all people who had been given short-term prognoses by good medical people. But they went on to turn their difficulties around and were alive many years later. In the survey, they were asked to consider all the things that may have helped them to recover and to rank their importance on a sliding scale. They were asked to reflect on the importance any medical treatment had played, any natural therapies, overcoming fear of dying, forgiveness, nutrition, meditation—all the options you could think of.

The first thing that stood out in this survey was that most people valued most things highly. What this indicated was they did do a lot. Turning around a major illness is not a casual affair. It does take work. These people were committed. They did a lot, and they rated highly the value of many things that they did do.

These people were then asked to think back over their recovery and to identify what they considered to be the three most helpful things they did. Interestingly, quite a number took the trouble to write on the survey that they did not like the question! They had done so much, and found so many things to be helpful, that choosing just three was quite challenging.

Anyway, they did choose three, and the results were fascinating and important. Three things stood out way and above the others. They were the diet, the meditation and the development of their spiritual life.

Now, many of these people were alive ten years after they had initially been predicted to die. So next I asked them what they would recommend to people newly diagnosed. Here four things stood out. The diet and meditation again, but then the advice was to attend a well-run, lifestyle-based self-help group (presumably to learn these techniques and be supported in applying them) and to aim to find meaning and purpose in life.

So what is it with the spiritual life and the meaning and purpose? What our survivors are pointing out is the importance of the mind and its key role in all we do. What inspires you? What motivates you? Why do you want to get well? How important is getting well to you? How much are you prepared to do? How much effort do you want to make? What can you learn through this illness? What meaning and purpose does it clarify for your life? What will you do with your good health? What will you do with your life once you are well again?

These are all questions for our mind. They come under the heading of spirituality, meaning and purpose. It is well said that if you have a "reason" to do something, you will find a "how." If the desire to live is strong and you follow a logical approach, there is every reason to expect a good outcome.

Have enough courage to believe in the possibilities. Then take the next step.

THE FIRST BIG QUESTION • Do I Really Want to Get Well Again?

You may say I am crazy to ask a question like this. However, the fact is some people diagnosed with cancer do accept their condition as terminal and cannot imagine themselves getting well again. For many of these people, this reflects their lack of any real hope. In some cultures there is still a pervading belief that you get cancer and you die. Some families, some individuals still hold this view, either as a result of some morbid fear or maybe as the product of experiences they have had with people they knew who did not do so well.

The antidote? Hope. People in this situation need inspiration—they need to realize the possibilities. This is where groups can be helpful, especially if they contain long-term survivors who can be met, seen, and touched! Even hearing stories of recovery or reading of them in *Inspiring People* or *Surviving Cancer* can help reawaken lost hope and help people to move forward.

However, there is a deeper issue. Some of the people whom I have known had given up on life itself. Some of these people had enough clarity to tell me that life was just too hard. We will examine this possibility in more detail in the chapter on the causes of cancer, but some people, when you come to know them really well, confide that they have lost their zest for life. Perhaps through past trauma, maybe through a variety of accumulated reasons, the future just seems too difficult. It is almost as if they have had enough of life and if cancer is the way to go, then they are not going to fight it.

The antidote? Like our survivors said, find the meaning and purpose in life. What ignites your passion? What inspires you? What have you got to live for? Is there something from years gone by that you put aside that now can be rekindled? Could you change your circumstances to make life seem worth living again? It is so extraordinary to be a living human being. Even the tough times are extraordinary. When we reflect on it, there really is so much to live for.

But what to do right now? If you are clear you want to recover, then no problem, go for it. Move on to the next step, the next question. If you have doubt, if you are unsure about survival, first examine the question of hope and seek inspiration. If there are deeper doubts or fears, or a lack of motivation, look into your heart, seek inspiration, and seek solutions. This may well be the time to talk to a trusted friend or an experienced counselor who can assist you to reach a point of clarity.

So while there is nobility in a good death and while the prospect of a good death is important for all of us as certainly we will all face it one day, the majority of *You Can Conquer Cancer* focuses on the process of getting well and being well.

THE SECOND BIG QUESTION • Who Is Responsible for My Decisions?

This question is best characterized by imagining a visit to your doctor. Do you go to them and say, "Here is my diseased body. You fix it. You tell me what is wrong. You decide what treatment I will have. I will accept whatever you say. The responsibility is yours."

Or, do you go to them and say, "Here is my diseased body. What can we do to get it better again?" With this latter approach, the relationship becomes a more equal one. Instead of handing responsibility for your well-being— and your life—to someone else, you are embarking upon a shared quest for health, a collaborative venture.

Now, in all probability, as time goes on, you are likely to work with a range of health professionals. Their technical skills and their communication skills are bound to vary. Some will be excellent; however, whether through lack of time, lack of aptitude, interest or training, some may well be poor communicators. For the same reasons, some may have a narrow range of expertise. Being practical, it may well serve you best to use some doctors and other health professionals almost mechanically. You take advantage of their technical skills, you take their treatment while accepting that to attempt a deep and meaningful discussion may be rather futile.

What is paramount is to identify the key person in your healing team. I suggest the ideal person for this could well be a general practitioner (GP) or family physician. This implies the need to find and work with a broadly trained, open-minded doctor you can respect and trust. Someone you can talk with freely. Someone who is interested in and takes account of your own, unique situation. Your hopes and your beliefs. Someone who is prepared to set out your options, explain the possibilities and the risks and then give time for questions. Someone who is not afraid to offer a considered opinion, to tell you what they would recommend if you were their own partner, parent or child. And then encourages you to make your own choices and supports you in them.

Currently, many hospitals are working in a more integrated way. They are setting up teams of doctors and allied health professionals who can come together to discuss individual cases and make specific recommendations. This is all to the good, but the questions still remain, who do you talk to? Who coordinates your management? Who is the focal point?

While encouraging you to take ultimate responsibility for your own decisions, the key question remains, who will be your chief adviser?

You may be fortunate and find a cancer specialist who can fill this role. However, experience tells us this is not so common. While I regard the role of doctors as pivotal, it is a sad fact that many patients and their families bemoan the communication skills of their specialists. This criticism has been around for many years and while it does take good training and committed practice to be able to give bad news well, one would hope the quality of communication improves soon.

In some hospitals, nurse-practitioners fill this coordinating confidante role. However, maybe a GP who is trained in and enthusiastic about the integrative approach remains the best choice.

Statistics tell us the average GP sees around three new people diagnosed with cancer each year. Only three. So it is a big thing for them when it happens. However, GPs are very well placed to understand both the medical treatments and your other options. They can provide time for discussion, and they may be specifically trained and experienced in counseling.

You may well have a long-standing relationship with a GP who can fill this role. Unfortunately, what often happens for many people is that they go to the GP with the initial complaint and have their help during diagnosis. Then often they will be referred to specialists, spend plenty of time with them and not revisit the GP. So you may need to remember to go back to your GP for this coordinating role, or you may need to seek a doctor who is more suitable for your current needs, and make ongoing appointments.

Do make it a priority to identify the coordinator of your healing team. Then tell them everything. Tell them about any other treatments you are having. Any and all the supplements or herbs you are considering or taking. Seek their advice to ensure you avoid doubling up or using things that conflict with each other. And seek their support and encouragement. A good GP in this situation can be invaluable, providing clarity, confidence and stability. They can be like a life coach, a healing coach. It is well worth keeping in regular touch with them.

So assemble a good team, seek their advice and support, and make your own decisions.

THE THIRD BIG QUESTION • What Is Most Likely to Heal Me?

Essentially there are three main sources of healing: conventional medicine, natural medicine, which has three components, and your own resources, best expressed here as lifestyle medicine.

Conventional or Orthodox Medicine

Conventional medicine generally describes medical interventions that are taught at medical schools, generally provided at hospitals and meet the requirement of peer-accepted mainstream medicine and standards of care.

Natural Medicine—Made Up Of:

COMPLEMENTARY MEDICINE

Complementary medicine refers to a medicine or therapy that is used in addition to, or complements, conventional medicine. Complementary medicine is increasingly taught in medical schools and practiced in hospitals and is steadily gaining widespread support. More research is needed to better evaluate it.

TRADITIONAL MEDICINE

Traditional medicine includes well-documented or otherwise established medicine or therapies that are based upon the accumulated experience of many traditional health care practitioners over an extended period of time.

Traditional therapies include traditional Chinese medicine, traditional Ayurvedic medicine, Western herbal medicine and homeopathic medicine. These traditional medical systems represent a different paradigm of health care when compared to conventional Western medicine.

ALTERNATIVE MEDICINE

Alternative medicine is the term widely used by many medical authorities to describe modalities that they regard as being on the periphery, being unproven and unwelcome. We will investigate what all these different modalities have to offer in the later chapter on healing.

What is helpful to understand now is that all four—conventional, complementary, traditional and alternative medicine—generally involve seeking help from the outside and having things done to or for you. This makes good sense. You go to a surgeon, massage therapist or acupuncturist for the help they can provide. You take the drugs, herbs or supplements recommended for you and receive their benefits. You have things done to or for you. But then there is another completely different possibility—what you can do for yourself.

Lifestyle Medicine

Lifestyle medicine focuses on what you can do for yourself in the context of your daily life. This is what we focus upon in this book. Lifestyle medicine can be highly therapeutic. It can improve your quality of life and increase your chances of long-term survival dramatically.

Lifestyle medicine involves attending to physical, psychological, social and spiritual factors. The actual techniques include nutrition, exercise, sunlight, stress management, social support, emotional health, the power of the mind, relaxation, imagery, mindfulness and meditation.

It is strongly recommended that anyone diagnosed with cancer attend to their lifestyle right from the start. If you have conventional treatment, lifestyle medicine is likely to minimize any side effects and maximize the benefits. If no curative conventional medical treatment is available, then lifestyle medicine still offers real hope.

INTEGRATIVE MEDICINE • Finding a Suitable Doctor

It is worth emphasizing one more term: integrative medicine.

Integrative medicine refers to a style of medical practice that is holistic and integrates the best and safest of conventional medical care with lifestyle advice and evidence-based complementary medicines and/or therapies. It aims to use the most appropriate of all available modalities and to help each individual patient make informed choices. Integrative medicine is an umbrella term that aptly embraces all styles of medical practice, including lifestyle medicine.

Integrative medicine is becoming a major specialty and many doctors now describe their approach to health, healing and well-being as being integrative. Simply put, perhaps this is what good medicine has always been— taking full regard of the patient as a whole and working collaboratively with a comprehensive range of allied health professionals.

When seeking a medical practitioner to head your healing team, a good starting point would be a doctor who is an advocate of integrative medicine, and preferably a member of an integrative medical association.

Most people start their cancer journey by consulting a doctor. So now, let us take a logical approach and consider how to manage diagnosis, prognosis and treatment options.

START AT THE BEGINNING • Seek an Accurate Diagnosis

Diagnosis is something modern medicine is very good at. Establishing whether you have cancer or not, what type it is, where it is, how extensive it is—all these facts modern medicine generally gets right. Sure, as in anything, mistakes sometimes are made, and particularly in unusual cases second opinions may be worthwhile, but generally the diagnosis can be taken as a fact and as such warrants being accepted.

The Reaction to a Diagnosis of Cancer

Some people accept a cancer diagnosis quite calmly, but I have seen people of all ages and from all walks of life go into deep shock on hearing the fateful words: "You have cancer." A strong emotional reaction is common, completely understandable and needs to be taken in context. Quite often the reaction is one of disbelief and numbness. Sometimes an outpouring of grief. Often confusion, uncertainty and fear. While any or all of these are understandable and common, none of them are good states of mind to be in when making important decisions.

A strong word of advice: Following a diagnosis, give time to adjust emotionally and take your time before making any major decisions. Contrary to common belief, there are very few decisions in cancer medicine where waiting to make them, waiting to act for a week or two, will affect the overall outcome. Many people think that the need to receive treatment for cancer is like when you are hemorrhaging—it needs to be done now, as soon as possible. While it is sometimes true that there can be medical emergencies involved that do demand urgent attention, in the main, a short delay of a week or two will not affect the long-term outcome. Taking your time could have you in a far better state of mind to make crucial decisions and to work well with the treatments you do accept.

This then is a time to be close to family and good friends, particularly those who have the capacity to stay present and offer their stability amid turbulent emotions. Here it is important not to be confused. Many people think the need is to be "positive," which is true, but some think to be "positive" is to be unemotional, which is not true. I have met people who were so afraid of their emotions that they thought it was almost as if they were to cry even once, it would take a week or two off their lives. Of course if one were to cry all day, every day, that may well be a problem, but it would be perfectly natural and normal to have a few, tough emotional days as you take in a cancer diagnosis and what it means for your life and the lives of those around you.

What to Do with the Emotions

Healthy emotions are natural emotions. Unhealthy emotions are when wild emotions control you, or, as is often the case with people affected by cancer, when emotions are suppressed.

Everyone feels emotions. It is how we express them that is the issue. The observable fact is that people vary quite naturally in their range of emotional expression. Some are naturally very expressive, some quite reserved. This is influenced by a variety of factors. Some cultures are very emotionally expressive—Italians often come to mind in this regard. Some keep their emotions under pretty tight control—my culture of origin, the English, seem pretty good at this.

The point is, with emotions, as with all else, individuals do vary. Your aim is to be authentic. To allow yourself to be natural and to be comfortable with your own emotional expression.

Emotions are so important we have two specific chapters on them later, but for now, recognize that allowing your natural emotions to flow is natural, normal and healthy. While the emotions that result from a cancer diagnosis may be painful, do what you can to let them out, either on your own or in the company of those you trust. Once they have been released, it will feel like a real weight has lifted and you will be in a much better place to move on with treatment, using your own resources and taking the steps to recovery.

If you are in doubt about your emotions, if none come or if they seem to be going on forever, do be brave. This is a time to seek help, talk with a professional counselor or an experienced, trusted friend and check your situation out.

Experience says it is very difficult to think clearly, to make good decisions, to really commit to what you need to be doing, if your emotions are all over the place. Once the immediate emotional response to a diagnosis is felt, expressed, and showed, usually the intensity goes out of it. Maybe emotions will arise again in the future. Again that would be natural and normal. But be authentic. Be comfortable with your own degree of emotional expression and realize emotions are another natural part of a healthy life.

So do take time. Sit with those you are close to. Be with them. Maybe in silence. Maybe with tears. Maybe with talking and discussion. Take it in. Let it out. Allow yourself to settle. And then begin to plan. To move forward again.

CHAPTER 2

Keeping Hope Alive

Prognosis and Looking into the Crystal Ball

WHILE DIAGNOSIS IS BASED ON FACT, PROGNOSIS IS BASED ON SPECULA-
tion. With a prognosis comes an attempt to predict the future, to give an
informed estimate of what the diagnosis, along with any treatment, is likely
to lead to.

The problem with a prognosis is that it can have power in its own right.

In the ancient culture of the indigenous Australian Aborigines there is a
phenomenon called the "pointing of the bone." This culture is the oldest
continuous culture on the planet and its roots stretch back in time for at least
forty thousand years. Many of the Aboriginal tribes lived in small nomadic
groups that thrived amid extremely harsh environments. To survive and
flourish they had quite strict laws that everyone recognized and generally
adhered to. One of the ultimate penalties for transgressing these laws was the
pointing of the bone. Here is how it works.

If a person broke a major law, they would be very aware of it themselves.
They would know something serious was wrong and they would be aware
of the likely consequences. Once the transgression was recognized by the
tribe, the senior people would confer, and if all agreed, the punishment of
pointing the bone would be carried out by the senior law holder. This person, often referred to as a man of high degree, would dress up in ceremonial
garb and the instrument of the punishment literally would be a bone—a
human thigh bone.

But there was no beating or physical assault with the bone. It was "pointed."
Amidst the ritual of the process, the bone was pointed at the transgressor

along with the words—the curse, if you like—the threat, the promise, that the person would die.

Interesting things would begin to happen immediately. First, the law-breaker, the person who had been pointed, would go into a rapid decline. Then, all of the tribe would withdraw and avoid contact with them. The person would become depressed, lose all interest in life, then they themselves would withdraw and become listless, apathetic.

At this point there are frequent records of Western medicine attempting to intervene. No conventional treatment has been shown to prevent the ongoing decline toward death.

As death approaches, another significant observation. The tribe members, sensing the closeness of the end, gather around again. This time they go into pre-mourning rituals and, in the process, seal the fate of the wretched victim of this extraordinary punishment.

So the pointing of the bone is invariably fatal in this Aboriginal context.

Now let us make some unnerving comparisons. A person knows they are not well, that something serious is wrong. They go for help. Senior people confer. Then comes the consultation where the key figure dresses up in ritual garb, with white coat and stethoscope, and makes a pronouncement.

When bad news is given badly, there are all the hallmarks of the pointing of the bone.

"You have only three months to live and there is nothing we can do about it."

In days gone by the message was often given this bluntly. These days, many doctors attempt to be more subtle and compassionate, but even so, many people get the take-home message: you have cancer, you will die.

All too often what happens next is that they go home in shock, they withdraw and then so do their friends. Often friends, even family, are unsure of what to do, how to respond, how to help. Many of these people, well-meaning, kind and considerate in their nature, have told me how they were deeply concerned about doing or saying the wrong thing and so they thought it safer to do nothing, to stay away.

However, if a person with cancer does decline and seems close to death, it is common for people to gather around to say their good-byes. This is natural and we will discuss how to do this in a healthy, constructive way in the chapter on death and dying, but here again, done badly it can fit exactly into the pointing of the bone process.

The message is simple. If bad news is given badly, if a prognosis is given bluntly and taken to heart, the person affected may well have two life-threatening conditions to deal with. The first is the actual illness. The second is the "pointing of the bone." And we know both have the potential to be fatal.

Traditional Aborigines have survived the pointing of the bone. There are accounts where Aboriginal elders or today's doctors have used their own rituals to persuade the person who has been pointed that the punishment has been countered or reversed. No medicine will do this. It all needs to come through the mind of the individual who has been pointed.

Therefore, we need to take heed of all this. For a start, let us use our logic again. In reality, offering a prognosis is a bit like setting the odds on a horse race. While in cancer medicine this process will involve high levels of technical skill and clinical expertise, setting a prognosis remains a process of making an informed guess. One takes into account all the factors one can and then makes the best estimate possible.

Now, we know that in horse racing the reality is that favorites win quite often. Yet we all know long shots get up from time to time. The only way to find out the result of a horse race is to wait until the race is run. Just the same in life. Just the same with cancer.

A prognosis is a bit like setting the odds. It can be helpful in giving all involved a sense of the degree of difficulty the diagnosis implies. Obviously, the odds of recovering from a cold are very high. No one who develops a cold takes it too seriously and fears dramatically for their future. The prognosis with a cold is usually pretty good and we can afford to treat it rather casually. If someone is diagnosed with a widespread aggressive cancer, obviously that is a vastly different matter and makes for a situation that requires the focused attention of everyone concerned.

YOU ARE A STATISTICALLY UNIQUE INDIVIDUAL

But let us go a little deeper. Here is some more good news. Human beings are statistically unique events. What does this mean and why is it so important?

Easy to explain. Consider a game of chance like Two-up. Two-up is where you take two coins, each with heads and tails on either side, throw them into the air, and bet on whether they land with two heads up or two tails. If they land with one head and one tail, you throw them again. Imagine now that two heads have come up five times in a row. Most people instinctively feel the next throw is now more likely to produce two tails. Surely, the odds predict this, we think. Not so. Each time you throw two coins, you have a statistically unique event. There is no connection, no link between one throw and the next! Statistically unique. Sure, if you throw two coins one thousand times you are highly likely to have around five hundred heads and five hundred tails. On average, over large numbers, statistics are relevant and work well. But individual events like tossing coins are unique.

So too with people. People diagnosed with cancer are statistically unique. On average, statistics are useful to predict what might happen, to set the odds. That has some validity and some use, but you will never know the outcome for a unique individual until time moves on and the race is run.

Before my own secondaries were diagnosed, I had been into the medical libraries and had not been able to find a record of anyone surviving my type of metastasized cancer (osteogenic sarcoma) for more than six months. If I had accepted this fact, accepted my prognosis, I could very easily have withdrawn, become passive, and died on time. What a blessing in retrospect that I was "crazy" enough to believe it was possible to recover—"crazy" in that to aspire to recovering I went against all the prevailing evidence of the day. However, there is real logic to what I did and how any other person with cancer needs to approach their prognosis.

When one looks at the range of outcomes for nearly all situations in life, they commonly vary quite a deal. In cancer it is just the same. The evidence is clear that faced with similar diagnoses, some people will live a long time and some not so long at all. This is often referred to as normal distribution and expressed graphically via the bell curve. The bell curve records how, if, say, a thousand people were diagnosed with a similar cancer, as time goes on, some die soon, most die in average time, and some do live on for a much longer time.

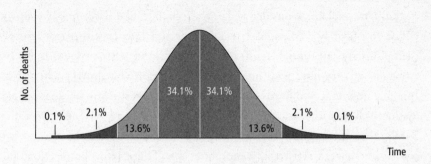

The Bell Curve or Normal Distribution
Where the numbers shown represent the percentage of the whole

The time factors will differ for different cancers and the exact shape of the curve may vary too. But the idea is clear. When a large number of people with a given cancer are tracked, most die around the same time. This is the statistic most prognoses are based upon. Maybe if the doctor is optimistic, it is pushed a little to the right; pessimistic, a little to the left. But the message is clear. This represents statistics.

If you or someone you love have been diagnosed with the same cancer as many other people, their history is interesting and points to what is possible, but not to what is certain. You are a statistically unique event. You could fall anywhere on the curve. That is a statistical fact. That is reality.

The big question then is, what affects where you end up on the graph? Is it simply a matter of statistics and random chance, or will what you do influence the outcome?

Back to horse racing again. If you were interested to back a horse in a race and you knew it was not being fed well, how would you feel? What if it was not well trained? How about if it was one of those horses that did not enjoy racing? Surely, these factors affect the outcome.

So too with cancer. If you embrace a good treatment, what direction will that head you in? If you eat well, will that take you right or left on the graph? Eat badly? If you remain filled with fear and dread, or if you develop a positive, committed approach, what is likely?

Given that everyone is a statistically unique event, everyone therefore deserves to be treated uniquely, to be regarded uniquely. Whether you have been diagnosed with cancer or are helping someone through cancer, your situation is unique. No one else has exactly the same situation as you. No one else has exactly the same body. Your emotions will be different, the state of your mind is bound to vary, and your spiritual realities differ. You are unique.

So two women diagnosed with breast cancer may be described as having the same disease, breast cancer. Just as two men with prostate cancer may both be said to have prostate cancer. Same label, very different situations, very different possibilities. Maybe it is more useful to say one woman by the name of Jane who is diagnosed with breast cancer has Jane's disease, another Mary's disease—they could well be that different.

Again, while statistics are useful to generalize, you need a large group for statistics to be useful. The key point is this:

Individuals do not behave statistically. Individuals behave individually.

We are all individuals. If you want an average outcome, do what the average does. If you want a unique outcome, an extraordinary outcome, be logical, regard yourself as you are, unique, and do something extraordinary!

CHAPTER 3

What Treatments Will I Use?

Attending to Individual Needs

MOVING ON FROM DIAGNOSIS AND PROGNOSIS, WHAT ABOUT THE TREAT-
ment options? How do you develop a comprehensive treatment plan that is
most likely to work and take account of your individuality, your personally
unique situation? How to move beyond generalizations and standard treatments, to taking account of individual needs? How do you personalize the
appropriate response for your particular situation?

Again, we rely on logic for the framework and then aim to draw on experience, wisdom and insight for the details.

Nearly everyone in the Western world will be diagnosed and consider
initial treatment within the conventional Western medical framework. This
makes good sense and is as it should be.

Given that the diagnosis and prognosis will be provided by the best medical people available, it is they who will recommend an initial treatment
plan. This too makes good sense. Certainly if there were a simple, medical
solution to cancer, one piece of surgery, one pill we could take that ensured a
cure, we would all do it. You would be a fool not to. But it is not so simple.

DEFINITIONS • Curative Treatment, Palliative Care
or Living with Cancer?

While the medical treatment of cancer tends to focus on one of two outcomes, to be curative or to be palliative, there is a third option. Let us be
clear with the definitions.

Curative Treatment

Curative treatment involves more than what many people imagine it to be, which is to be free of cancer after five years. Actually, curative treatment aims to render the person clinically free of detectable cancer and restore the person to their normal life expectancy.

Palliative Care

On the other hand, palliative care is an umbrella term for assisting those approaching death—a fundamental need and right. It is generally used in the context that death is imminent and inevitable and aims to make dying as easy and comfortable as possible.

PALLIATIVE TREATMENT—LIVING WITH CANCER

Palliative treatment is a specific but integral part of palliative care. Palliative treatment can be more interventionist. It is noncurative by definition but aims to extend life, ameliorate symptoms, and increase quality of life in situations where a cure is not medically feasible.

The lines between palliative care and palliative treatment can often be blurred, but these days, palliative treatment is often called living with cancer.

While overall survival rates in the conventional management of cancer may not have improved all that much, in recent years many people are living longer with cancer. This can involve significantly slowing the progression of the disease, minimizing any side effects and maximizing all the quality of life issues. Palliative chemotherapy often plays a significant part in conventional medicine's management of palliative treatment.

WHAT TO DO WHEN A MEDICAL CURE IS LIKELY

Now the logic. If a person is offered medical treatment for cancer where there is a high probability of a cure, then, in my view, what to do is fairly straightforward. Embrace that treatment as your main focus while you go through whatever it entails. The common treatment options are surgery—which often comes first—then maybe chemotherapy and/or radiotherapy.

However, right at the start or even better still, before you start your treatment there is more to do. As soon as possible, review your lifestyle and do whatever you can to complement and support the treatment with your own efforts. The details of what this entails follow in the subsequent chapters. Lifestyle medicine will have your body and your mind in the optimal state to get the best out of any treatments and to minimize the potential for any side effects.

When it comes to the complementary, traditional and alternative options, there may well be useful things to consider that will support your body's healing capacity, minimize or manage side effects and have other useful benefits. These options will be discussed in later chapters as well.

THE CHOICES WHEN A MEDICAL CURE IS NOT SO LIKELY

However, what if a cure is not so likely from the medical point of view? What if at first diagnosis, or further down the track, it becomes clear that a medically based cure is improbable? What if palliative care or living with cancer is all that remains medically? There are three options.

1. Acknowledge Death as the Likely Outcome

This is probably not the option you are opting for if reading this book. However, we do need to recognize and accept that some people do accept their prognosis and do acknowledge death as the likely outcome. They then may choose to focus on what can be done to garner the best from whatever time remains, to live with cancer as long as possible and to prepare for a good death.

Yes, prepare for a good death. Death is like everything else in life. We can stumble into it, hoping for the best, or we can prepare for it and, in all likelihood, have a good death. To be open about this, when I started working in the early eighties with others affected by cancer, I knew little of death and I was preoccupied with the desire to help people to recover. I admit to being apprehensive about what would happen if and when people died of their cancer. While many did recover, others did go on to die of their disease. Over the years I have worked closely with many of these people and it has been incredibly heartening to observe how consistently the people I have known who prepared for death were able to die well. What they learned and what they did stood them in good stead, and the quality of their deaths was exceptionally high. We will speak more of this in a later chapter.

For now, it needs to be said that some people faced with the situation where there is no medical cure on offer do accept death. Some are content to focus on living with cancer and are keen to utilize palliative care when the time comes. Again, that is a perfectly reasonable and logical choice. However, if for whatever reason you are not ready, if you do not accept death, and if you are still intent on getting well, you need to be logical. If medicine cannot cure you, what will? Can anything?

2. Seek a Cure from the Nonconventional Medical Options

Remember the different styles of medicine: conventional, traditional (TM), complementary and alternative (CAM). If conventional medicine says a cure is beyond them, do any of the others have a solution? I have the personal knowledge of many individuals telling me that individual TM or CAM therapies were very significant in their recoveries. But I do not have the experience of consistency in this. It seems that from time to time, for some individuals, individual TM and CAM modalities fit really well with that particular person and are highly effective. But I am not aware of a TM or CAM therapy that reliably will be of major benefit to a wide range of people. I do not know of a magic bullet in the realms of traditional, complementary or alternative medicine.

3. Seek a Cure Within—Recovering Against the Odds

Even when conventional medicine says there is nothing more we can do toward a cure, I do believe there still is real hope on offer. Where the "magic bullet" actually does reside is within you. In the face of difficult odds, a cure may be much more likely through mobilizing your own inner healing than through chasing after some elusive external TM or CAM treatment.

Remember, it only has to be done once to show that it is possible. You only need one person to use their own inner resources to recover without the aid of external, curative medical treatments and you know that it is possible. Just one case demonstrates that there is the potential for the body to react, to reject the cancer within it, and to heal. And if it can be done once, it can be done again. And the truth is it has been done many more times than once. What I have been studying and teaching for over thirty years is what makes this most likely to happen.

Clearly, if you aim to recover against the odds, it is not likely to be easy. There is no point misleading anyone here. If it was easy, everyone would be doing it and no one would be dying. My experience is, as we have discussed already, those who do become remarkable survivors make a good deal of effort. They dare to hope, they seek out good information, they rally support, and they put good intentions into action. Then they persevere. They deal with the ups and downs. They learn from what others might judge to be mistakes, are prepared to experiment, try new things, and in doing so, develop an inner confidence. They learn through their process, often see it as a journey and commonly come to enjoy the challenge and reflect warmly on their achievements. And in all probability, they have a little good luck as well!

Recovering against the odds is not a casual business. It takes focus, energy and commitment. What then is the main thing to focus upon? Clearly if conventional medicine has said it cannot cure you, it is not that. In my view TM or CAM therapies cannot do it reliably either. The focus in this situation needs to be on inner healing, and to support this inner healing with the best of what conventional medicine, TM and CAM have to offer. Maybe more surgery or chemotherapy is useful to minimize the amount of cancer your body needs to attend to. Maybe you use medical, TM or CAM treatments to boost your immunity and your healing capacity, or to minimize symptoms. But in the situation where no medical cure is on offer, you may be wise to focus on your potential, the lifestyle medicine as we call it, and support that with all else.

HOW TO COMBINE THE BEST OF WHAT IS AVAILABLE • A Summary

When Curative Treatment Is a Real Prospect

Focus on the medical treatment, and support that with all the other options available to you. Lifestyle medicine will always be useful; use TM and CAM judiciously.

When No Curative Conventional Medical Cure Is on Offer

The choices are

i) Palliative care—accept the diagnosis and the prognosis, and plan for a good death. Lifestyle medicine is likely to be of great benefit for extending life as well as preparing for a good death. Use conventional medical treatments and CAM judiciously.

ii) Living with cancer—accept the diagnosis and the prognosis, then accept that your real goal is to live as long as possible, as well as possible. Quality of life becomes the focus—along with whatever is likely to extend your life. So again, the lifestyle factors set out in this book warrant being the focus of your plans, supported by good medicine and whatever TM and CAM therapies may be helpful.

iii) Accept the diagnosis and reject the prognosis. Dare to recover. Focus on developing healing within by employing lifestyle medicine—and support that with all else. Use conventional medicine, TM and CAM judiciously.

WHAT SPECIFIC TREATMENTS WILL YOU ACCEPT?
HOW TO DECIDE WHAT TO DO

Before we examine in detail how to activate the healer within, let us pause to investigate what external forms of treatment, if any, to which you will be wise to commit. Let us begin with the medical options.

The logical way to assess any proposed form of medical treatment would be to ask your doctor the following questions:

(a) What does the future hold for you if no treatment is given, and in such circumstances what range of life expectancy would you have? The best way to ask this question is statistically. Ask if there were one hundred patients just like you and they had no treatment, what would be a reasonable estimate for the following:

  i) How many people would be alive after one year and what would their health be like?

  ii) How many people would be alive after five years and what would their health be like?

(b) What range of life expectancy would you have if given the proposed form of treatment? Again, ask for the answer to this question in statistical terms. If there were one hundred people like you who had the same condition and they received the proposed treatment, what would be a reasonable estimate for the following:

  i) After one year, how many people would be alive and what would their health be like?

ii) After five years, how many people would be alive and what would their health be like?

Note: These statistical ranges should be available in virtually all medical situations, barring those that involve very rare cancers or experimental treatments including chemotherapy trials. If they are not provided upon request, I would seek another opinion. If you are considering an experimental treatment or a trial, you can only assess it on its possible merits.

In other words, through these first questions you are aiming to find out the anticipated benefits of the treatment, expressed in statistical terms.

(c) What are the side effects of the treatment? It will be most useful to obtain the answer to this question in statistical terms as well so that you obtain a real sense of any potential risks. So again, ask:

  i) If there were one hundred people like you who had this treatment, what side effects are possible and how many people are likely to be affected by those side effects? Do 5 percent or 95 percent have nausea? Do 5 percent or 95 percent lose their hair?

  ii) And how long are those side effects likely to persist? For a few minutes, weeks, years? Will they be permanent?

  iii) How might they be managed if they do occur? For example, there are many good treatments available these days for the side effects of chemotherapy, and hair that falls out because of chemotherapy commonly grows back fairly quickly.

(d) What impact will my own response to the treatment have on the outcome? In truth, the answer to this question may be harder to define than the previous three. The medical system is very good at evaluating its results. This is made easier by the fact that a single intervention, such as a drug therapy, is relatively easy to study and accurately evaluate. By contrast, the human being is incredibly complex—the role of emotions, mind and spirit are extremely interwoven. They are not so amenable to the standard double-blind, crossover trials used to research and evaluate so many drugs.

What does seem clear, however, is that how you respond has the potential to affect the outcome of anything you do. If in cancer treatment you are treated with chemotherapy, full of fear and loathing, preoccupied with potential side effects and the possibilities of damaging your immune system, you are highly likely to undermine the potential benefits of that treatment. If, on the other hand, you think it through and decide to accept the treatment, regard it as in your best interest and do all you can to work with it, you are likely to get the very best from that treatment.

THE KEY TO GREAT OUTCOMES • Embrace Everything You Do

This is why you are strongly advised to make conscious decisions about all you do. Nearly always, there are pluses and minuses to consider when making medical decisions. Take your time and think things through. If you need help with this, a very useful decision-making technique that draws on both the intellect and intuition is presented soon in the first chapter on mind training (chapter 7).

Once you do come to a decision, the strong recommendation is to embrace all that you do. Embrace! Not just put up with, not just tolerate, nor even just accept it. Embrace it! Understand that this is what you have chosen to do. It is in your best interest—like when you would take antibiotics for pneumonia. Know that whether it be having chemotherapy, changing your diet or practicing meditation, the more you welcome it into your life, the better you feel about doing it, the more you support your choice, the more you embrace it—the better it will work.

When you embrace what you do, you release all the positive potentials of your mind, emotions and spirit. My belief is that when you embrace a treatment and really work with it in positive expectation, then you can reasonably hope to get the best possible results with the least side effects.

However, given all this, you may still have a very difficult decision to make.

The reality is that most current treatments for cancer are hard on the patients—sometimes very hard. It is a fact that most of the conventional therapies are toxic to the body. Radiation and chemotherapy frequently impair the body's own immune system along with other components of its defense mechanism. This reduces the body's ability to heal itself. Often this impairment is severe and side effects can be marked. Radiation burns, vomiting and loss of hair are obvious problems that can follow. Tiredness, lethargy, "foggy" thinking, depression and loss of memory are all observed as regular consequences of cancer treatments.

The impact of many medical treatments upon the rest of the body can be less obvious, but nevertheless more drastic in nature. Minor infections that previously would have been of no consequence can assume major proportions. Most important, the body's own ability to fight the cancer is frequently lessened.

However, while the side effects of conventional treatment require careful consideration, chemotherapy or radiotherapy may still be the best medical treatments that are available at present. It may well be that it is in your best interest to use them. If this is the case and if you are having a toxic form of therapy, it is all the more important to concentrate on those self-help techniques that aim to boost the immune system and help the body to help itself. These techniques are discussed in later chapters.

Be Brave—Communicate!

Here again, good communication with your doctor is essential. The ideal is to be able to discuss all your concerns freely and easily with your main doctor. If this is not the case, talk with that doctor about the communication problem. We all know how some personalities clash and there are some people we just do not seem able to get along with. If you cannot find a way to correct the situation and communicate well, then request a referral to someone more suited to your temperament. No one should be offended by this. It will make life easier and more constructive for everyone. (For more detailed recommendations, see Appendix A.)

The final choice regarding what conventional treatment to accept may still be difficult. Again recognize the value of making this decision with clarity and confidence and the imperative of committing to what you do decide to do. A reminder then of the value of taking your time. Better to avoid a rushed, hasty decision that may later cause you doubt or regret. Best to take your time, seek expert opinion, discuss the options with those you value, contemplate, give due regard to your intuition and then commit.

Maybe in the final analysis it is the level of confidence and trust you place in the doctor(s) involved that decide it for you.

If surgery is what seems necessary, it seems wise to leave the details of the surgery to your surgeon. If chemotherapy is something else that you decide to commit to, again it would seem wise to leave the choice of agents to your chemotherapist.

You may desire, however, to know more or less of the details of your treatment and you can reasonably expect to have your questions answered in an open, cooperative manner.

Whatever the final choices you make, the next step is to do all that you possibly can to make sure the treatment works to full effect. We will discuss the means to achieve this throughout the book.

How to Enhance Surgery, Chemotherapy or Radiotherapy

The majority of people diagnosed with cancer will have one or more of the conventional treatments recommended to them, and decide to commit to the treatment. With the intention of minimizing any side effects and maximizing the benefits, it is important to be well prepared and to do the best possible to work with any treatments. While the details of what to do unfold in the coming chapters, a quick summary of the recommendations regarding how to prepare for medical treatments forms Appendix B.

Activating Your Inner Healer

Based upon many years of clinical experience and supported by the most recent research, the way to activate healing through your own efforts is easy to define. Your body's capacity to heal is directly affected by what you eat, what you drink, and whether or not you smoke. Sunlight, vitamin D and exercise all play important roles, as does your emotional life and state of mind. How you manage stress, your capacity to relax, to be mindful and to meditate—along with the way your spiritual view impacts on your life and those around you; all these factors impact on the inner healer.

While I have to say it strikes me as a somewhat bland term, all these elements are best described as being under the banner of lifestyle medicine— they are to do with the things you can control and do in the course of your daily life. And the key? It is your mind. Again, it is your mind that decides what you eat and drink. It is the mind that helps you to adopt a healthy, healing lifestyle or remain stuck in old unhelpful habits. Truly, it is the mind that changes everything and so we will begin the road to recovery with the mind.

To embark on the healing journey, to embrace outer help with conventional medicine, TM and CAM, to begin to activate the inner healer—all this is best achieved by being in a stable state of mind, clear and confident. What meditation promises and reliably delivers is a stable, clear mind. As stability becomes more constant, clarity more natural, and confidence more assured, it becomes easier to go from the broad recommendations regarding what to eat, how much to exercise and so on, and to be able to personalize those recommendations. Therefore, in seeking a stable, calm and clear mind, we begin with meditation.

To Those Interested in Prevention

If you are well, just how well are you? Are you just symptom free or are you as fit as your true potential allows?

When this book was first written in 1984, the statistic quoted was that "one in three people alive in the United States today will get cancer during their lifetime. One in five in Australia will die from it." Now the figure is closer to one in two people alive today will develop cancer and currently one in four Australians dies of cancer. This is not scare-mongering. This is fact. Cancer is a lifestyle disease. Are you prepared to learn the lesson of this disease and take up on a lifestyle aimed for optimal health? A lifestyle that is highly likely to prevent the majority of cancers?

These techniques we talk of can save the lives of people affected by cancer. We have seen them work for many other disease conditions as well. Also they can make a basically well person a picture of health. Back in 1981, in his landmark work, *The Causes of Cancer*,[5] Professor R. Doll gave the medical evidence that 85 percent of all cancers could be prevented by changes in lifestyle! The challenge is there. It takes effort; it requires commitment and an ability to be open to change. Again, it can be done. Our natural state *is* health. Please take up that challenge. It would be wonderful to see people learning from the difficulties of others and not having the need for change forced upon them by physical disease. While it is wonderful to help people to recover from cancer, how much better—and wiser—not to get sick in the first place.

Four Features of Long-Term Survivors with Advanced Malignancy

Throughout this book you will pick up many features of long-term survivors and gain insights into what they did to recover. However, reflecting on a long and illustrious career as a cancer surgeon, Professor Gabriel Kune highlighted special characteristics of a particular group—people with advanced malignancy who became unexpectedly long-term survivors, and I quote:

1. They seek a wide exposure to conventional medical opinion and treatment.

   They take "control" of their health. They will decide for themselves what advised treatment to have and what treatment not to have. They are often critical of their medical management.
2. They seek a wide exposure to nonconventional opinion and treatment. Again, they will decide for themselves what they will choose to have and they are often critical of nonconventional management.
3. They operate at an intuitive level.
   They are usually not "thinkers" or intellectuals. They tend not to operate at a rational level as their main guide for making decisions and appear to make decisions "intuitively."
4. They are at peace with themselves.
   One often gets a sense of tranquility, peace and spirituality while in their presence. They are not at all fearful.[6]

Now, in my own experience I would agree with all this generally, and while I certainly recognize the importance of the intuition in decision making, many of the long-term survivors I have known have also been very smart and drawn on their intellects well. Where people can get into trouble is when they think too much, get lost in the range of options, lost in doubt and worry, and as such do not access their intuition, do not make clear and confident decisions, do not commit to what they are doing.

Maybe we can summarize Professor Kune's four points by saying that long-term survivors have a calm and clear mind. This enables them to think clearly, to make good decisions and to be at peace with the world and themselves. Given all the challenges cancer can present, how do we avoid fear and even panic? How do we develop a calm and clear mind? Meditation provides a well-proven solution, plus it has real healing benefits in its own right. In the next chapter we will begin to unlock meditation's secrets.

CHAPTER 4

Meditation

The Principles Behind the Silent Healer

MEDITATION IS THE SINGLE MOST POWERFUL SELF-HELP TOOL THAT ASSISTS recovery from disease and leads to a life of maximum health. It provides all the basic ingredients. It has direct physical effects ranging from relief of physical tension to reactivation of the immune system. Meditation reliably leads to a calm and clear mind, the ability to think clearly, to make good decisions, and to see them through to completion. On top of this, meditation aids the development of emotional and mental poise, generates a positive attitude, and most important, leads automatically and effortlessly to a heightened level of well-being.

Currently, more than six thousand scientific studies published in the medical and scientific literature around the world attest to meditation's capacity to positively affect physical and psychological health and well-being. Little wonder then that it has enjoyed such a rise in popularity as a self-help technique! When coupled with dietary considerations and active efforts to utilize the benefits of positive thinking, it forms the pillars upon which to build our capacity for healing and total health.

In the past, meditation has been used by most major religions as one part of a complex process intended for developing a heightened level of consciousness. Today the word "meditation" is used to describe many different processes. The specific form of meditation that interests us here, with its emphasis on being used as a therapy, relies on learning how to relax profoundly in body and mind. We call it mindfulness-based stillness meditation (MBSM). This form of meditation is disarmingly simple to learn and apply in our daily life, and has played a major part in transforming the health and lives of many people I have known.

My initial introduction to this form of meditation, and its therapeutic application, came through the great Australian psychiatrist Dr. Ainslie Meares. Interested in pain management, Dr. Meares first became interested in meditation as a means to relieve pain. However, he soon realized meditation had much more to offer and he began to experiment with meditation as a means for helping people to cope with anxiety and stress-related symptoms such as phobias, high blood pressure, allergies, nervous tension and pain intolerance. Then he wrote the world's first book on the therapeutic benefits of meditation, *Relief Without Drugs*, in 1967.

One of Dr. Meares' major contributions has been that he recognized the importance of stillness. A still mind, in a still body. He suggested that in this stillness, the body has the opportunity to return to its natural state of balance. He also observed that when meditation was practiced regularly, this refound state of balance persists throughout the day, helping the person to return automatically to that condition of balance we call health! Just as a cut finger heals itself automatically without us dwelling upon it, so meditation can reactivate natural healing mechanisms that operate automatically and have profound effects. It is to his great credit that Dr. Meares was able to perceive this and then devise a simple and quick technique that leads to that point of stillness and balance without, say, twenty years of rigorous concentrated study and practice of Zen discipline.

To understand why meditation is so helpful for so many health conditions, and for cancer specifically, we need to understand the role stress plays in our lives, in our health, and in our capacity to heal. This will then provide us with vital clues as we plan our self-help program.

MEDITATION, STRESS, ANXIETY AND RELIEF

To understand how stress does affect us, let us look at the simple case of what happens when we get a sudden fright. Suppose that a bolt of lightning were to hit the ground near where you were standing. Your body would react very quickly, almost instantaneously. With a gasped "Oh!" you instinctively would take a sharp breath in and your muscles would contract with a jerk. Your body chemistry would change almost immediately as an array of hormones was released. Adrenaline would flow and cortisol levels rise. Your heart would race, your blood pressure would increase, and your blood would be diverted to the muscles of action. You would have been readied for immediate action, thanks to the automatic changes produced by what is called the fight-or-flight response. In our example, if you were quick, you may have dove under cover. But then, also quite quickly, you would have realized that the big bang really was just lightning, it had missed you, and everything was all right. "Ah!" would have come the response. The tension would be released and you would relax.

The events in this sequence are very important. The challenge gave rise to a bodily reaction that immediately prepared you for physical action. In the normal course of events, a period of physical activity would follow, which in turn would be completed and be followed by release. The sequence can be summarized:

1. Challenge
2. Bodily reaction with changes in body chemistry
3. Appropriate physical action with a clear beginning and end
4. Release and relax
5. Body chemistry returns to its usual, daily balance

This is a perfectly healthy sequence that was developed in earlier times when life was simpler and very physical in nature. The fight-or-flight response was then, and remains to this day, a vital aid for self-preservation. So if, for example, in older times, a saber-toothed tiger came charging over the hill toward you, intent upon making you dinner, the threat was very obvious! That threat produced rapid changes in your body chemistry and you were immediately prepared for action. This would lead to your doing the appropriate thing. If you felt you had a chance, you stood your ground and fought it out; if not, you ran. Either way, the challenge was resolved by a period of intense physical action that was followed through to a definite conclusion. You would then be free to relax, either licking your wounds or basking in success.

This sequence flowed with the rhythm of a simple life and it left no adverse aftereffects. Any fears that did remain were healthy ones based purely on instinct and self-preservation. Such fears did little to lessen the quality of life or lead to any physical symptoms. Animals in their natural state still demonstrate the appropriateness of this fight-or-flight response in a physically oriented world.

However, for us humans living in modern times, things are no longer so simple. The challenges we face now are rarely of a purely physical nature and frequently are complex indeed. Most, if not all, of our challenges nowadays are emotional or mental in their origins. However, an even greater problem is that frequently they are difficult to resolve.

So when the boss is overbearing and demanding, or the neighbor disturbs our sleep early on Sunday morning with his lawn mower, we react in the same old way. We take that short little gasp and tense our muscles. Our body chemistry changes rapidly, preparing us for action. But can we punch the boss's nose or wrap the neighbor's lawn mower around his ears? Not if we want the paycheck that we need to meet our commitments; not if we want to remain socially acceptable in our community! Often then, taking the action we might feel inclined to take instinctively is inappropriate and so our response is stifled. Worse still, we can have the situation where we do act reasonably, we do take what seems to be the appropriate action, and yet, even so, the challenges in our lives remain unresolved. We do all we can to reduce the mortgage, but it still remains, nagging away and causing us fear and worry.

When we do have an unresolved challenge, people tend to react in one of two general ways. The first is to accept the situation, let it go, and get on with life. No problem. The other is to stew on it, hang on to it, worry over it. Big problem! Common problem!

If we are one of the many people who do stew on things, then the problem is that every time we face that same situation or even think about it, the physical changes in our body chemistry are reinforced. Feeling that there is no obvious resolution or conclusion to our problems, having no way of finding an adequate release, there is no return to our basic, healthy body chemistry. We are locked into a situation where the fight-or-flight changes in our body chemistry persist.

A crucial point here is that the changes in body chemistry we are discussing and that are associated with the fight-or-flight response are fine in the short term. They are an appropriate preparation for a short period of intense activity. Where they are not appropriate is when they persist for long periods.

This brings us to another important point. Some people who are intent on de-stressing and getting well worry if they get an occasional fright or a even a brief moment or stress. Let us be really clear about this. In the short term, the fight-or-flight response is no problem and, in fact, can be quite helpful. It is when the biochemical changes that accompany the response become chronic and stay with us long term that we develop real problems.

If the changes in our body chemistry persist, we experience what is known as destructive stress. This type of stress is a challenge that leads to a prolonged untoward effect on a person. Stress occurs when there is an inability to take appropriate action in response to a challenge and so release it. Therefore, stress is an unresolved challenge.

It is easy to appreciate that stress is a very personal thing. It is really determined by how we respond to a challenge, rather than by the nature of the challenge itself. What may be an easily resolved challenge for one person may produce profound stress for another.

STRESS AND CANCER

The next key is that persistent stress affects the body chemistry in such a way that the body's immune system is depleted. It is the changes in hormonal levels particularly that reduce the body's immune function, along with its ability to maintain and repair itself. And so, with time and other factors such as poor diet, stress leaves the way open for many diseases to precipitate. The American Academy of Physicians states that stress-related symptoms lead to two-thirds of all visits to American family doctors. Stress is a major contributor, either directly or indirectly, to absenteeism, coronary heart disease, lung conditions, accident injuries, cirrhosis of the liver, suicide and a host of lesser ailments. I am convinced that stress is a major causative factor in cancer.

Virtually all the many thousands of cancer patients I have asked believe stress was a major factor in the development of their disease. Most recognize that first there was a chronic level of stress in their lives. But, more important, they generally identify readily with a psychological profile common to cancer patients. In about 95 percent of patients asked, this profile involves one particularly severely stressful experience precipitating a drastic drop in their well-being. The stressful event invariably occurred well before the cancer was diagnosed but its untoward effects continued. This highly significant factor will be discussed in detail in the chapter dealing with the causes of cancer (chapter 15).

RECOGNIZING STRESS

For the moment, though, how do you know when stress is a problem? If it is not patently obvious, as it often is, muscular tension is a good guide. If you suffer from stress, one of the body changes it will produce is physical tension. Your body can be your guide. If you are free of muscle tension, feeling relaxed and well, then you almost certainly have no problems! If your brow is knotted, your jaw clamped shut, if you have a persistent knot in your stomach, your shoulders are rigid or your hands clenched tightly, if you feel physical tension—beware! It is a warning signal. However, with appropriate action we can transform this, avoid future problems and generate healing.

RELIEVING STRESS WITH MEDITATION • The Theory

Understanding the stress cycle makes it easy to understand how to deal with stress. It is not necessary to avoid stress totally, just deal with it appropriately. What we need is a means to release it. All successful people who cope well with potentially stressful situations have their personal means of finding release, of relaxing, of letting go.

But based on more than thirty years of experience assisting people with cancer, the easiest, the safest and the most reliable method—the best method for relieving muscular tension and stress—is the specific meditation technique we call mindfulness-based stillness meditation (MBSM). Because this type of meditation concentrates on a profound relaxation of the body and mind, it provides the opportunity for release—it allows us to let go! It allows us to regain a healthy balance in our body chemistry.

To learn how to achieve this, we begin by meditating formally and learning how to relax body and mind. The release found in these initial periods of meditation soon flows on to become an integral part of our life. As we return to a more relaxed state, we return to that healthy balance of body chemistry that is essential for promoting healing and maintaining good health.

Moreover, once we understand the stress cycle, we can understand why meditation for healing needs to be so simple and so uncomplicated. We can understand why it needs to begin with the relaxation of body and mind, and advance to include the release that comes with inner stillness.

For it is by entering this state of simple stillness that we enter a state of profound rest. When we are still, everything comes to rest—profoundly! And in that state of deep rest, we return to a natural state of balance. It is this state of balance we call good health. Good health is a state where we are in balance—a state where balance involves body, emotions, mind and spirit.

For many people, then, meditation has been enough in their quest for sustainable good health. Practiced regularly, meditation frees them from the bondage of stress, allows them to relax, to regain balance, and so enjoy life to the fullest. Do use this basic self-help technique and make it a part of your life. The benefits will repay the initial effort.

THE TRADITIONAL ROLE OF MEDITATION

As we seek to adapt this ancient technique into a modern context, and apply it specifically in a therapeutic setting, it may well be helpful to understand meditation in its historical context, to consider and be informed by some of its traditional techniques.

Meditation has been practiced for thousands of years in all major cultures and traditions, primarily as a major tool on the spiritual path. It has been well said that meditation provides a reliable means through which we can come to know our own minds more fully. Meditation is an ideal technique to call upon when we are interested to examine the question of who we really are, and delightfully, history tells us that reliably it does lead to satisfying answers. Appendix C offers an insight into the traditional role of meditation and some of its key techniques. The book I cowrote with my colleague Paul Bedson, *Meditation—An In-depth Guide,*[7] is a good reference point.

Personally, I feel very grateful for having close contact with and learning from a wide range of extraordinary meditation teachers over many years. Initially there was Dr. Meares, and more recently Sogyal Rinpoche, an authentically trained Tibetan master of meditation who has provided me with the rare opportunity to access ancient and authentic wisdom teachings that marry so well with modern needs. Then, too, I have learned so much from the many thousands of people who I have taught to meditate over the years. What I can offer here is a testament to all these great teachers.

WHAT DOES MEDITATION OFFER TO THOSE WITH CANCER?

I had been fortunate to develop my cancer at a time when Dr. Ainslie Meares first contemplated the use of meditation for people affected by cancer. I had an emerging interest in the traditional forms of meditation and felt that these principles should be able to restore the inner harmony I felt I had lost. I believed if I could regain that inner harmony, it would be reflected on the outer physical level. Dr. Meares' idea was that the meditation would relieve anxiety and stress. This would lead to a reduction in the levels of cortisone in my body and so allow my immune system to operate normally. Then my body would remove the tumors itself. It would return to normal. Putting it all together sounded good to me!

As I have practiced meditation more and come to see others benefit from it too, there do appear to be two broad areas of benefit. Meditation increases quality of life and quantity of life. In my experience, people who meditate regularly do feel better, and they do live longer.

Considering quality of life first, we see benefits on all levels of human experience. There are physical, emotional, mental and spiritual gains.

Physical Benefits

Chronic physical tension is a symptom of stress that we know inhibits the body's natural function. Meditation relieves physical tension. Many people are struck by how good their body feels once this tension is removed. They realize just how much tension they had before learning to meditate in this way. While previously they had come to accept the tension as normal, now they realize just how unpleasant it really was.

Athletes have found meditation can increase their performance and certainly most people find their general efficiency in day-to-day tasks goes up extraordinarily once they begin to meditate. Consistently, heart rates go down, and even severely elevated blood pressure can return to normal. A typical example was Dr. Colin, who joined our group not with cancer but as an interested observer, and found much to his surprise that meditation and diet brought his severely elevated blood pressure back to normal within two months.

Emotional Benefits

Emotionally, our own level of ease is greatly improved through meditation. People find that they feel better about themselves. They feel more able to accept their limitations and to use their strengths positively. In so doing, they are more able to relate to other people in an open, honest and meaningful way.

Any cancer patient knows that being just that—a cancer patient—has its problems. Before cancer was diagnosed, you may have been a doctor, a teacher, a housewife, whatever. So often after diagnosis, to your friends you are now a cancer patient first and foremost, and everything else comes a poor second. This can cause much awkwardness and can become quite a cause for anxiety in itself. However, it is remarkable how meditation reliably leads to an acceptance of the situation and an openness that is infectious, putting everyone at ease.

Also, many people find meditation reduces any feelings of guilt and negative emotion they may have. As a consequence, they develop a greater capacity for loving. While this often results in an improved quality of sexual love, it also improves that more erudite, selfless love and compassion for all. People find they are able to feel good about themselves to a higher degree and, in doing so, give of themselves more safely and freely, and to be of more help to those around them.

Mental Benefits

Mental anxiety, if present, hinders all aspects of our being. Its causes are endless, often unidentifiable. Frequently, psychiatrists have spent long hours raking over the traumas of the past in a quest for the elusive cause of present anxieties. From the womb, to birth, the formative years, adolescence and beyond, all manner of incidents can be identified as potential causes for anxiety and stress. Even if the cause is identified, treatment often remains difficult.

Here is a vivid example. The Lancaster bombers of World War II had their rear ends protected by tail gunners. These men climbed into the tail section of the plane via a ladder. They lay down in the cramped fuselage and then had a Perspex bubble slammed tight around them. Their only communication with the rest of the crew was by headphone. They then set off on an incredibly rough ride with little to dwell upon except their solitary machine guns and the fact that on average they could expect to survive about two missions. An extreme and obvious cause for anxiety. It was not surprising then to find that after the war those who did survive frequently felt great tension when they were confined in small spaces. Many of these men found great difficulty in relaxing enough to urinate when in the narrow confines of a toilet! Frequently they knew the cause of their problem as did all who tried to relieve their anxiety. What happened? The problem remained and invariably they needed to leave the toilet door open!

There are two principles operating here. First, just knowing the cause of a problem is not necessarily enough to relieve it; an appropriate technique is also important. Second, if those men could not have related their inability to go to the toilet to their wartime experiences, they would have felt a great deal more anxiety and suffered greater distress.

Actually, it was with these very tail gunners that Dr. Meares began his foray into the realm of stress and anxiety. He found the standard psychiatric techniques of the postwar period were of little help to these men, but that hypnotherapy brought rapid relief. Dr. Meares went on to become a world authority in hypnotherapy and it was through this interest he came across meditation and pioneered its therapeutic use.

What he realized was that in seeking health, we need to understand as much about our situation as possible, as well as having appropriate techniques to deal with it. We benefit greatly from our own realization of what a constant effort it is to live with the pressure created by persistent anxiety. It is like trying to keep the lid on a pressure cooker all the time. It tires us physically, emotionally and mentally. However, once that anxiety is relieved, we feel benefits all through and our physical symptoms soon respond.

Perhaps Dr. Meares' greatest contribution has been to show that meditation reliably treats stress and anxiety regardless of cause, and, more important, it works even if what caused it is unidentified. Meditation is so effective because it short-circuits the stress cycle. It provides a reliable means of moving quickly and easily from those changes in body chemistry that are an integral part of the physical effects of stress. Releasing stress in this natural way heralds a return to normal function and health.

This rationale explains further why we benefit from starting the meditation technique with relaxing the physical body and why the "release," or the relaxation of body and mind, promotes a return to normal health. Once we trigger that state of release, the body chemistry returns to normal and the normal state means health. What we really need to do quite simply is to let go!

Spiritual Benefits

Spiritually, many people find meditation leads to a peace of mind they had not imagined possible. A member of our group, Cathy, recently told me that her body had never been worse but she had never felt so good! Her face was shining, full of enthusiasm and she said she was experiencing a quality of life she had never known before.

This peace of mind comes at a level so fundamental that it becomes in reality a true, direct experience. Many people who have firm religious beliefs to begin with are surprised by the depth of this experience. While some are apprehensive that meditation may conflict with their beliefs, the usual experience is that it leads to a heightened appreciation of their particular religious tradition and a greater level of personal joy.

This experience is often even more noticeable in people with no fixed religious views. I am sure that we all would like confirmation that there is more to life than just this mortal coil. In the past, most people seem to have relied on the word of others that this was or was not so. By contrast, in modern times there has been a common disenchantment with formal religion and an urge to seek direct experience. Frequently, however, as the immediate material world is explored more fully, it is found to be exciting, but lacking. There has to be something more. Meditation often leads to a direct experience of that something more. You only have to see the smiles on the faces of many of the people I have known who have learned to meditate to realize that this is a fact.

Does Meditation Lead to Survival?

How long am I going to live? That question can lurk in the recesses of our minds to catch our breath whenever we are unaware. If we are a cancer patient, that question can be a constant nagging fear unless we reach acceptance, unless we regain our peace of mind. This does happen.

There is plenty of evidence from recent research that lifestyle factors do extend how long we live, as well as how well we live. Regarding meditation specifically, there are many studies confirming the quality-of-life benefits. Remarkably, while meditation has been shown to be therapeutic for many illnesses and enhance or lead to recovery from them, to date there have been no good outcome trials with meditation and cancer. What we can say is that many long-term survivors greatly valued their meditation and believe it to be a major factor in their recovery. My own case attests to this and so do the stories of many of the people in the book *Surviving Cancer*.[8]

There is no doubt in my mind that these techniques work. I am consistently surprised by the large number of people who tell me their lives are the better for having had cancer and responding to it in the way they have. Speaking personally, I now feel my whole quality of life to be vastly better than before I had my leg amputated. I meditate because I want to. Meditation is a regular part of my day. As Judy, another person with cancer, said recently, "Cancer changed my life for the better. It has taught me so much and I have gained so much through it. I cannot imagine myself having done it all without the prompting cancer gave me."

A SUMMARY

Meditation is so important because it leads to

1. A clear mind
This enables us to think clearly and to make good decisions.

2. A calm mind
This frees us from stress and reestablishes balance in body, emotions, mind and spirit. Inner peace and contentment follow, along with a quiet confidence in all we do.

3. Healing
This flows naturally from the balance we experience in deep, natural peace.

4. The truth of who we really are
As we relax deeper and deeper, our awareness opens in such a way that we experience our inner essence, the truth of who we really are. Now the confidence and the smile come from deep within, and they last throughout the ups and downs of life.

CHAPTER 5

Meditation

The Practice

HOW DO WE DO IT? HOW DO WE MEDITATE IN THIS WAY?

It is such a simple thing this meditation, and yet we are used to great complexity in our modern lives. How do we relearn simplicity? How do we learn to be still? How do we "let go"?

It helps to understand something of the process. The type of meditation that will help us most to heal is very specific. In meditation that is intended to be therapeutic and lead to recovery, the intention is for the body to be deeply relaxed and for the thinking brain to relax, to become calm and to become still. But what is this meditation really like?

We can explain a great deal of the nature of meditation, how it works and what it does. But the true essence of meditation needs to be experienced to be fully comprehended. Dr. Meares asked a venerated Yogi in Nepal what it was like to meditate. The Yogi replied by asking him how he would describe the taste of a banana. You can use words to make comparisons and descriptions, but in the end the only way someone else can really know that taste is to peel a banana and try it! It is a matter of direct experience.

I hope these words give you the impetus and the confidence to try meditation. I trust they will leave you free to enter into this experience with an open, willing mind, knowing you are embarking on a very personal, exciting venture.

I have felt meditation transforming my life for the better and I have seen it happen often in others. It is probably the most pleasant thing I can do on my own and the most beneficial. Meditation has a place in everybody's life.

As we set out the techniques, we are aiming to deeply relax our body and our mind. We are seeking to let go and regain our balance at a very deep, fundamental level.

The technique we shall use is set out in four easy steps: preparation, relaxation, mindfulness and stillness. Each of these steps is easy to learn; each has healing benefits in its own right and each flows quite naturally into the next.

STEP 1 • PREPARATION

Start with the Right Attitude

The attitude with which we begin and then continue to practice our meditation is very important. In modern society we are used to striving for achievement. If we want something, we normally expect to have to work or struggle for it. Not so in meditation. Once we actually start the procedure, we need to abandon any sense of striving, for if we sit down with the intention to "meditate or bust," we can be sure of an unhappy result! The only striving may be in making the time to do it, exerting the will to say, "This is my time for meditation and nothing else takes precedence." That can be effort enough, but once we commence, the accent is on effortlessness. It needs to be a focused but relaxed process.

Use an Affirmation

Next, to reinforce the attitude that this is a health-promoting procedure, many people find it helpful to begin with an affirmation. Nothing rigid or forced, just a gentle statement of intention. Usually, when I lead a meditation I begin with:

Let your eyes close gently.
Turn your thoughts inward.
Remember that this is a time for healing.

However, for you at home, simply repeating the last line works very well.

Some people feel comfortable following this with prayer and, of course, prayer can be highly beneficial. Something brief like "Not as I would, O Lord, but as Thou will" seems particularly appropriate, while many repeat longer prayers. Of course, prayer can have real benefits in its own right. More advice and a summary of interesting research in this field forms Appendix D.

Where to Meditate?

It makes obvious sense to be in as conducive an environment as possible. You will find it easiest when you feel secure, free from the prospect of interruptions and distractions and when you are in a quiet, comfortable space. A group of people all doing the same thing is very supportive, but meditation can easily be embarked upon in private.

Choose a room where you feel comfortable, preferably a room that is away from any bustle. If necessary, ask other people to leave you undisturbed. Be prepared to ignore the front doorbell or telephone should they ring. Initially it is good to use the same place regularly and to practice at the same time each day, if possible.

Posture

Now, what position should we use? The position you choose needs to satisfy only two criteria—it needs to be a position that is symmetrical, and a position that has an element of discomfort in it.

Discomfort—why should we be uncomfortable to begin something that is intended to be relaxing, pleasant and beneficial? Using this technique, the mild, initial discomfort soon fades from our awareness. It is essential to begin with it, however, as it makes us concentrate more. This works to make the relaxation more profound. The more uncomfortable we are when we begin, the deeper our level of relaxation has to be for us to regain a feeling of comfort and ease. Please just try this, as experience will soon show that this mild discomfort is a really useful ingredient in the process.

For most people what works well is to simply sit in a fairly upright chair, feet flat on the floor, just a little apart, hands resting comfortably on your thighs or cupped in your lap. Not much discomfort in that, but enough to be useful. Ideally, it is helpful to have your back fairly straight, although if the need is strong, you can lie down. As a beginner, closing the eyes is an effective way to start, but as you advance, they may just naturally open a little. As you meditate more, you may even like to experiment with sitting cross-legged on a cushion on the floor. However, the main thing is to take up a position you can relax into and stay in for the period you wish to meditate.

STEP 2 • RELAXATION

Now we are ready to use our body as the tool to guide us into the experience of meditation. We do this by training our body to relax, feeling what that relaxation is like, and letting it flow into our mind.

In the beginning we use a simple, formal procedure to capture the feeling of relaxation. Once we have done that and can reproduce the feeling, we can speed up the technique and simplify it, but every time we begin a session of meditation, we do take the time to consciously relax.

Remember that what we concentrate upon in this technique is a feeling— in this case, the feeling of relaxation.

Start by Becoming Familiar with Relaxing Individual Muscles

Be assured, this is a very simple technique. How it works is that we concentrate on one area of the body at a time. First we feel whatever sensations we can notice in that area. We simply notice how that particular area is feeling at this particular time. Then we contract the muscles in that area and make them tense. As we do this we notice the different feeling created by the tension. We feel the tension and then we relax the muscles. By repeating this technique through all the areas of the body we quickly learn how to relax the body very deeply indeed.

To do this as a complete exercise, first we need to go through the different areas of the body, learn how to feel them, create tension within them and then relax them.

We begin with the feet. Having taken up our chosen position, we let our eyes close gently and put all our attention on our feet. To do this exercise really effectively, we shift our center of awareness. Normally, our center of awareness is in our head, around about the space between our eyes. We feel as if that is the central point of everything for us. Now, by closing our eyes and concentrating on our feet, we feel as if they have become our center—almost as if we are "in" our feet. We then find that the feet do have a particular "feel." If you find that hard to realize at first, the second step makes it more obvious. You now contract all the muscles in the feet to impose tension on that area. In effect, you are making the feet rigid so they are tense and immovable. The feeling of tension is quite different to the feeling of relaxation. Feel that difference. Next you let the muscles relax, and you pay attention to the feeling of the muscles relaxing, the feeling of letting go.

So there is the simple process. Feel the area, contract the muscles, and let them go.

Learning to Relax the Muscle Groups in Our Body

Another necessary step in learning this technique is to familiarize yourself with how to contract the different muscle groups. Remember that this is the introductory part of the technique and that if you follow it, you will soon experience meditation proper.

When it comes to relaxing physically, the forehead and the hands are particularly important, as over 60 percent of the body's nerve endings are in these two areas. The more nerve endings we relax, the more the message goes back to the brain to relax. Therefore, the more we feel the relaxation, the more we become truly relaxed.

As the body first relaxes, often it begins to feel very heavy. It is so loose and relaxed—it feels as if it could just melt into the floor. Then, as it goes deeper into the process, it begins to enter a phase that we describe as "letting go." A new lightness comes over it. Sometimes there can be a tingling, a sensation of warmth; invariably there will be a sense of comfort, pleasure and ease. If we let our mind go along with this feeling, we soon lose all awareness of our body and surroundings. Noises seem far away and inconsequential and we are left with an expansive, floating feeling. This feeling of "letting go" can be likened to a sensation that is similar at first to floating peacefully in warm water. Then it is as if we were dissolving out into that water. We feel as if we are taking up more space than just the normal confines of our body.

The Progressive Muscle Relaxation Exercise

Having become familiar with contracting the various muscle groups and relaxing them, we are ready for our first meditative exercise—the progressive muscle relaxation (PMR). We need to go with this a little, to trust in its simplicity and allow ourselves to move into it. The body is the guide. As we feel the body relaxing, we notice our thinking processes winding down, and as the body enters the state of "letting go," we allow the mind to flow with it.

To lead ourselves through this technique based on physical relaxation, we speak quietly to ourselves. In our mind, we talk ourselves through the

Contracting and Relaxing the Muscles

Sit symmetrically, let your eyes close gently, and contract the muscles of the feet. If you find it hard to work out how to make the muscles move, pull the toes back toward the heels while at the same time resisting any movement. This locks all the muscles tightly and gives a good impression of what tension is like in that area.

Then relax the muscles.

The calves: Imagine someone was going to pull your ankle in any direction and you wanted to resist. This locks all the calf muscles as desired. You may notice some of the muscles in the thighs become involved and that they also contract. Keep this to a minimum but do not be concerned by it, while it is helpful to concentrate as much as possible on what is happening in the calves.

Next, the thighs: These are the largest muscle group in the body and it is easy to feel the tension in them. If you need help to make these muscles contract, try to lift the feet off the ground while at the same time holding the thighs down with the hands. The tension is then obvious.

The buttocks: These are contracted by squeezing the big muscles of the backside and so lifting a little off the chair. However, we want to be aware of the whole pelvic area, so feel the relaxation flowing right through that region of the body, including all around the pelvis.

The tummy: We begin with this area by contracting the tummy muscles as well as those of the lower back. If we imagine that we are lying on our back and someone is about to drop a heavy ball on our tummy, the right muscles will be working! With the tummy, the need to feel the relaxation all through the area we are focusing upon is even more evident. So when we relax, we feel the muscles relax and also feel that inside the tummy is relaxing as well as all through the lower sections of the spine. There is no need to try to imagine a relaxed liver, a relaxed spleen, etc.—just feel that same deep relaxation all through the tummy, in a general, nonspecific way.

(continued)

(continued)

The chest: The same principle applies as with the tummy. We contract all the chest muscles and make the chest tight like a rigid barrel. Then we relax the muscles and feel the relaxation all through the chest and around and through the upper spine.

The arms: We do the arms as one unit. Make them completely rigid as if resisting movement in any direction. Stiffening them produces the feeling of tension very readily; then feel the relaxation.

The shoulders: This includes the neck and the throat as well. Here we contract the muscles by lifting the shoulders and pulling the head down. Feel the relaxation then in the shoulders, neck and throat.

The jaw: Grit the teeth and feel the tension in the big muscles we use for chewing. Relaxing, feel it in the mouth, lips and cheeks as well as the big muscles at the side of the jaw.

The eyes: Closing the eyes in a squint makes the tension obvious. Relax and feel it in the eyes and across the nose.

The forehead: Some people find it easier to frown than others! Contract the muscles, feel the tension and let it go. Maybe you raise and lower the eyebrows. Feel the forehead smoothing out.

exercise using the simple, abstract phrases reproduced opposite. In the group situation, I lead people by saying these words aloud. At home you can begin by learning them, then repeating them quietly to yourself, or you could use a CD or download with the words recorded.

The words need to be repeated slowly and rhythmically. Many people find it helpful to repeat one phrase every second breath. That is, you breathe in and say a phrase as you breathe out; then breathe in again, breathe out, breathe in and say another phrase as you breathe out the second time.

You will notice in the exercise that follows, each phrase is separated by a number of dots. These are to remind you to breathe, to proceed slowly and steadily. You will find that as the relaxation progresses, your breathing is likely to slow down automatically. There is no need to emphasis the breathing at all. It will adopt its own slow and steady rhythm in a natural way.

Now we are ready to give our attention to this key exercise. So when you are ready, take up your position and begin.

The Progressive Muscle Relaxation Exercise

Let your eyes close gently . . . Turn your thoughts inward . . . And remember that this is a time for healing . . .

Turn your attention to the feet . . . really concentrate on the feet . . . perhaps move them a little . . . really feel what they are like at the moment . . . now contract the muscles of the feet . . . feel the tension . . . feel the difference . . . and let them go . . . feel the muscles relaxing . . . feel it deeply . . . completely . . . just simply letting go . . .

The calves . . . feel them . . . contract the muscles . . . and let them go . . . feel it deeply . . . it is a good feeling . . . a natural feeling . . . feel it deeply . . . feel the letting go . . .

The thighs . . . contract the muscles . . . and let them go . . . feel it all through . . . the legs feel heavy . . . as if they could merge down into the floor . . . more and more . . . deeper and deeper . . . letting go . . .

The buttocks . . . contract the muscles . . . and let them go . . . and feel it all through the hips and the pelvis . . . sometimes it helps to imagine there has been a belt or a band around the hips that has just been released a little . . . just simply letting go . . . letting go . . .

The tummy . . . contract the muscles . . . and let them go . . . feel it all though the tummy . . . it is a good feeling . . . a natural feeling . . . feel it deeply . . . feel the letting go . . .

Now the chest . . . contract the muscles . . . and let them go . . . feel it all through . . . more and more . . . deeper and deeper . . . letting go . . .

The arms . . . contract the muscles . . . and let them go . . . and feel it in the hands particularly . . . maybe you notice a warmth or a tingling flowing down into the hands . . . calm and relaxed . . . maybe a feeling of lightness . . . as if they could be just floating there . . . just going with it . . . letting go . . .

The shoulders . . . contract the muscles . . . and let them go . . . deeply . . . completely . . . and feel it up through the neck and throat . . . more and more . . . deeper and deeper . . . letting go . . .

(continued)

(continued)

Now the jaw . . . contract the muscles . . . and let them go . . . feel the jaw drop a little . . . feel it deeply . . . the tongue, soft and loose . . . feel it all through the mouth . . . it is a good feeling . . . a natural feeling . . . feel the letting go . . .

And feel it up over the nose and across the cheeks . . . now the eyes . . . contract the muscles . . . and let them go . . . deeply . . . completely . . . feeling it all through the eyes . . . almost like the eyes could be floating in their sockets . . . more and more . . . letting go . . .

And feel it around the ears . . . the back of the head . . . up over the top of the head . . . calm and relaxed . . . just going with it . . . calm and relaxed . . .

Now the forehead . . . contract the muscles . . . and let them go . . . feel it in the forehead particularly . . . feel the forehead smoothing out . . . feel it all through . . . more and more . . . deeper and deeper . . . letting go . . . letting go . . .

After a period of silence, we usually finish by saying, "That's good . . . Let your eyes gently open now."

And so what happened? Most people, on first doing the PMR are struck by the deep sense of physical relaxation it produces. They find this a new and exciting sensation they want to repeat more often. Just recently, David, a cancer patient who is fifty-eight, said he had worked hard all his life and enjoyed doing so, but on trying this exercise for the first time, realized he had never before known the joy and pleasure of being so simply, so deeply relaxed.

As a beginner, what is recommended is to start with this PMR exercise and use it as your main meditation practice for some weeks at least. Actually, for many people I helped in the early days this was all they used. However, in current times, people often find it useful to take the time to learn how to simplify and deepen the relaxation aspect of the PMR, and then proceed, giving added emphasis to the mindfulness and the stillness. The explanation for all of this follows and the main meditation practice to move on to once you have mastered the PMR is at the end of the next chapter.

STEP 3 • MINDFULNESS

As we do come to feel more relaxed, we actually become more aware. This is another key point. We relax our body, feel the relaxation in our body and feel that relaxation flowing into our mind. But this is not a sleepy thing. We keep our awareness awake and, in fact, it becomes more vivid. It is like we are awake, aware and at the same time deeply relaxed.

How we do this is expressed in the word *mindfulness*. Now *mindfulness* may be a new word for some but it is very simple, both in concept and in practice. Mindfulness describes how we concentrate in a particular way. It helps us with the next step, what to do once our body is deeply relaxed and our mind calm.

Mindfulness has been defined by Jon Kabat-Zinn[9] as paying attention, deliberately and nonjudgmentally, to our present moment experience. Another way to say this is that mindfulness is concentrating on what is going on right now, in this particular moment, in a way that is focused and non-judgmental. It is to do with observing, with being aware of what is happening right now, without judging what is happening as being good or bad, right or wrong. It is to do with simply being really interested, really curious, really attentive to what is going on right now, in this very moment.

This then is the ability to be mindful. It is as simple as being able to give your full attention to whatever you are doing. And doing this in a way that is not distracted by old thoughts, doubts or fears from the past, or anxious wondering about how things will turn out in the future.

Mindfulness cuts through stress and anxiety by focusing on what we are doing now. And think of it: If we give our full attention to what we are doing now, how can we do any more? With mindfulness, we learn to give our best, to give our full attention, to whatever we do. This is why developing mindfulness is so valuable for more than meditation and healing. Mindfulness frees the mind to engage fully in sport, business, relationships, creativity, feeling good and being well! You name it—everything goes better when you do it mindfully.

Sometimes it is helpful to have the contrast and to realize what mindlessness is. Mindlessness is the opposite of mindfulness. Mindlessness is when you are not paying attention, when you are spaced-out as if no one is home.

It is like when you do something, know you actually did it, but have no memory of it at all. Like you get home after being out, travel home, arrive at your front door and have no real memory of the trip. Or you plan to listen to something like the weather on the radio, it comes and goes and there is no memory of it. It is like you missed it altogether. That is mindlessness and we all do it pretty regularly.

Mindfulness is where we begin to change that and we learn to be present more often, more fully. Where we learn to give our full attention; where we learn to give our best to whatever we do.

Now what most people do notice when they start to become aware of mindfulness is how often they are mindless! This is why this practice, this mind training is so useful. Not only does it help us to learn to be more mindful, more often, but it teaches us how to go easy on ourselves.

There is this natural tendency to judge ourselves harshly, so now we want to change all that. What is known from experience is that many people have a history of feeling badly about what they do and do not do. Most of us when we begin these mind-training practices do tend to notice our mindlessness, and as a result we feel awkward, unhappy, sometimes embarrassed or even ashamed. Why am I like this? Why do I do this? We tend to judge ourselves as meditators, judge our capacity to be mindful.

Now of course, we do not want our meditation to become another source of stress. So what to do? Well, it is simple. Everyone has fairly frequent moments of mindlessness, unless they have trained their minds. All of us as human beings have the tendency to be lazy, to be forgetful, to be mindless, to be judgmental. This is normal. So while it may be a bit disappointing as a beginner to even notice all this, go easy on yourself.

Be inspired! Isn't it wonderful that there is a part of us that can actually become aware of all this and do something about it! Any progress is a step in the right direction and becoming more mindful helps to let go of the judgments of others and of ourselves. The thing is to persevere. Do not be put off by what is the common starting point for so many people. We can all learn these new skills. We can learn to master our minds and feel the benefits. Here then is how we add the next step and begin to practice and develop mindfulness.

Relax and Become More Aware

As we begin to experience the relaxation, quite naturally our thoughts settle a bit and we just simply start to notice what is going on around us a little more clearly. This is the beauty of this technique. It simply unfolds from one step to another. So as we relax, we become more aware, more mindful.

Perhaps it is the sounds we notice first. We notice any sounds that may be around about us. And what we aim to do is to simply notice these sounds as they come and go. We let go of any judgment, let go of commentary. So we aim to avoid thinking about the sounds. It is fine to be aware of what is making the sound; for example, an ambulance may pass by in the street. But we avoid wondering where it is going or will we be in an ambulance one day. We simply register there is an ambulance passing by and let it go. Simple as that.

Then maybe we become a little more aware of the sensations in our bodies, and again we choose to notice these things more nonjudgmentally. We aim to let go of any sense of good or bad, right or wrong, and focus our awareness on just simply noticing what it is that we are aware of. We take up the stance of being an impartial observer; a nonjudgmental observer. We are aware, we are interested, we are curious. What is happening right now? What is our body feeling like at this particular moment? We are coming into the present moment with awareness. This is mindfulness.

And so then we might take some time to focus our mindfulness more deliberately. To begin with, it can be very helpful to focus our awareness more particularly on our breath. We feel the breath coming in. Feel the breath going out, and we feel the natural release, the relaxation, the letting go that flows quite effortlessly, quite naturally with the out breath. Almost with a sigh of relief we can let go, we can relax a little deeper.

Now it can be helpful to bring the focus of our mindfulness more particularly to our body. Again with that open curiosity, we notice the sensations in our body. We scan our attention through the body, starting from the feet and moving up to the head. If any area does feel a little tight or tense, sore or painful, we simply notice that, aiming to be free of any judgment, free of reaction, free of commentary. Maybe there is the feeling of letting go a little. That natural feeling of relaxing, releasing, letting go. Quite effortlessly. Effortlessly. We feel the natural ease of it all.

We are content to relax, to be aware, to be mindful.

STEP 4 • STILLNESS

Having prepared well, relaxed deeply and become more mindful, now we begin to notice something really interesting—we begin to become aware of a deeper stillness. In time it becomes more apparent that this stillness is like an all-pervasive background. It is like when all the activity stops, the stillness is naturally revealed.

This is just like being in a room full of people, all talking, all busy. While initially it may be the noise and movement that is most obvious, we know there is a potential silence in the room all the time; it is just with all the activity it is not so easy to notice it. If we were to ask everyone to tell the others to be quiet so we could hear the silence, they might all rush around anxiously and the noise become louder! Some people attempt this with their meditation. They spend their time trying to tell their minds to shut up and just get caught up in one form of mental activity after another.

This is why the mindfulness is so useful. We let go of trying to do anything other than to be aware. This is the key to it. Do it effortlessly, in a kindly, nonjudgmental manner. Just be curious to notice whatever happens and quite naturally the activity will settle and the stillness will become more obvious.

It is like having a glass full of muddy water. If you continue to stir the water, you just get more and more muddy water! But when you put the glass down and leave it undisturbed, the nature of water is that it clears. The mud settles to the bottom and you are left with the clear water. The mind is just the same. Leave it undisturbed and it settles.

So what is this like in practice? As we relax, our body and our mind settles. As our mind settles, thoughts invariably continue to come and go. So now, we choose to observe the thoughts. No need to try to push any thoughts away or to dwell on any thoughts in particular. We just simply notice them, again free of reaction or judgment. We are curious. What thoughts are coming into my mind right now? What am I actually thinking about right now? We turn our mindfulness to being aware of our thoughts.

We can understand what this mindfulness of thoughts is like is if we consider what happens when we watch a movie. We go into the movie theater, sit down and wait for the film to start. We are conscious of being in our seat, in the theater with other people around about us. We are watching the screen and then the lights dim and the movie starts. Almost invariably, we soon forget we are in our seat and it is like we are in the movie, lost in the projection of light and sound that is the movie. Then from time to time it is like we snap out of the movie and remember we are in our seat, observing the movie. Mindlessness is when we are caught up in the movie. Mindfulness is where we have our awareness, we are the impartial observer, and we are aware we are watching a movie. When we can adopt this attitude with our thoughts, we give them no strength. If we allow them to just roll on, to come and to go like scenes in a movie we are watching, they do just that—and soon they slow down and settle.

What becomes obvious as we relax and become more mindful is that as we go with all this, we become a little calmer and importantly, our thoughts do quite naturally begin to slow down. Again, we do not need to do anything more than what we have been doing for this to happen. This is a process based on relaxation—focused relaxation, it is true, but relaxation, mindfulness and natural ease. We just focus on doing the exercises, go with the flow as they say, and by doing so we progress quite easily and reliably.

And as we do this, a remarkable thing unfolds. As we notice our thoughts more clearly, we notice how each individual thought has a starting point, a middle and an end point. Obviously each and every thought we have has to start somewhere, and to finish somewhere. And as we relax more, as we become more mindful, this fact just becomes more obvious. We notice when we first become aware of a particular thought, we notice it passing through our awareness, and we notice when it finishes.

Then another really useful observation. As our thoughts begin to slow a little and we notice them more clearly, we notice that after one thought finishes, and before another thought starts, there is often a small gap.

Now in the gap between our two thoughts, there is obviously a moment of silence, a moment of stillness. So now we turn our attention, our awareness, to noticing the gap between the thoughts. And again, when we do this mindfully, free of judgment, just with an open curiosity, not only do we notice the stillness but often enough it lasts a little longer; there is a bigger gap before the next thought comes. But again we make no effort to force this or to manipulate it. We just notice it. We are patient. We are the impartial observer. Just simply curious to notice what happens.

More stillness? Another thought? What is it? We take the attitude of a patient, curious, impartial observer and do just that, we observe. We aim to treat the stillness and the thoughts in just the same way. Nonjudgmentally. With curious awareness. So we notice the stillness. We notice if and when another thought comes. We remain aware and undistracted.

And what we do notice is that the thoughts do come, and they do go. Thoughts are just like white clouds drifting across a blue sky. They come when they are ready. They go when they are ready.

The blue sky is there all the time. Vast. Pure. Pristine. Always there. The clouds just come and go. And even on the cloudiest of days, we know the sky is still there, we just cannot quite see it because of the clouds.

Meditation is like getting into an airplane on a cloudy day. When we take off, all we can see are the clouds everywhere. We fly up through those clouds, break through, and there it is again, like a big canopy stretching above us, the vast, blue sky. It was always there, it was just that we could not see it from the ground. We needed the plane. We needed to learn how to fly.

So it is with our thoughts. Sometimes our mind is full of them. Sometimes it may even seem as if we have a raging storm going on inside. But we can always use meditation to reconnect with that other aspect of our mind, that deeper stillness.

Sure our thoughts can be really useful, but sometimes they can be too much, too problematic. Sometimes we can suffer from excessive thinking! What a relief to know that there is a way out. That there is always the possibility we can turn our attention from the active thoughts, to the stillness. It is like on a cloudy day, we choose to focus on what we can see of the blue sky rather than what we can see of the clouds.

And in our meditation, as we move our attention from the thoughts to the stillness, we come to realize that the stillness is just like the sky is to the clouds. The stillness is ever present. It is there all the time. Vast. Pure. Untouched. The thoughts come and go but the stillness, like the sky, is always there.

Now be reminded once again that while thinking can obviously be very useful, there is great benefit in letting go of the thinking for a while—of going beyond the thinking into that deep natural peace of this stillness where balance is restored and sustained for body, emotions and clarity of mind. We may even reconnect with the essence of who we really are in that stillness.

And there is another powerful truth here. You must have noticed that even after the darkest clouds, the worst storm, sooner or later it does actually clear and the blue sky reemerges. And despite the worst storm, the sky is never stained.

Sure, there is a part of us that can feel pain, we can be ill, we can have troubling thoughts. Our personal storms can take many forms. But this is one of the really wonderful discoveries that comes with meditation: No matter how difficult things have been or may be now, no matter how stormy, there is always a part of us that is unstainable, untouchable and inviolable. There is this inner essence, this core of our being that is good, pure, whole and unstainable.

Knowing this brings a deep inner satisfaction and contentment. To experience the truth of who we really are, to directly experience that in our essence we are whole, pure and good—this is the real heart of meditation. This is what brings a confidence to all we do. This is what helps to bring out the best in all we do. This is what brings a gentle smile to the face of so many meditators. This is the truth of who we really are and the truth of how we can be.

SUMMARY • HOW TO MEDITATE

To put it really simply: Having prepared well, we relax. Relaxing more deeply, we become more mindful. As our mindfulness develops, the stillness naturally reveals itself. We rest in open, undistracted awareness. Easy as that.

This is the essence of mindfulness-based stillness meditation, and this, the main meditation technique that is recommended, is set out at the end of the next chapter.

Time to Practice

Finally then, what level of commitment is required? Quality of life or quantity of life? Your aims and priorities must be very clear. Any time allocation has to be balanced by your needs, your beliefs and your other commitments.

Quality of life is vastly improved by doing ten to twenty minutes once or twice daily. To make an impact on quantity of life, to aim for recovery, three longer sessions per day from forty minutes up to one hour each are recommended.

I feel it very important to set yourself a goal in this regard. Work out your priorities and set a goal for the coming week. It is far better to set a conservative goal to begin with and succeed in meeting it than to fall short of an overambitious target.

So having set your goal, practice for a week. Then assess your results, reassess your goals and priorities, and reset your target. Remember that it is probable that you will have what seem to be good sessions and ordinary ones to begin with. The more meditation you do, the more repeatable and the more satisfying it becomes.

When I first began, my situation was critical and I did about five hours a day for three months. I then did three hourly sessions for the next year, then around an hour each day ever since. Also, for many years I have continued to regularly attend (or give) more intensive meditation retreats. This is obviously a big time commitment. I did it when I was ill because it felt good and it gave me results. I continue to do around an hour each day for the same reasons.

If quality of life is your aim, and time appears short, ten to twenty minutes twice a day will help you a lot. I remember the story from many years ago of a man who had been estimated to have three weeks to live. He went to Dr. Meares full of enthusiasm for his ideas around meditation and was keen to begin. However, on being told he would need to spend three hours a day at it, he replied, "Oh, I haven't time for that" and left!

I am sure meditation improves both quality of life and quantity of life.

Only you can do it.

CHAPTER 6

Meditation in Daily Life

Calm, Clear and Relaxed

THE BODY'S NATURAL ABILITY TO HEAL ITSELF IS REALLY QUITE PHENOM-enal. While we often take it for granted, this ability is nothing short of miraculous.

For example, take the healing of a broken leg. First there is a trauma, a solid bone is broken in two and the shattered ends displaced. There will be torn muscles, probably internal bleeding—a lot of damage. Surgery is often required to stabilize the situation, and perhaps a steel pin is inserted to fix the broken bones together and keep them stable. Yet, once the right conditions are created, that bone will automatically reunite itself, the muscles will regenerate, and normal function return. In six months' time an X-ray will show the bone to be healed, and actually often where the break was, the bone will now be even stronger. What an amazing process!

RELAXATION, BALANCE AND HEALING

Let us see this process in perspective. First, the right conditions were created and then the body healed itself. The medical intervention was necessary to provide those right conditions. However, the doctors did not actually heal anything. What they did achieve is that by realigning the bones, they created the first requirement for the healing of a fracture to proceed. The patient then had to look after the leg and make sure the healing process could continue. The patient did not have to think of the intricate process of the bones reuniting. The body's natural healing power was what returned the leg to normal. The body, given the right conditions, healed itself—automatically.

The body's normal state is health. It has a tremendously varied and complex set of mechanisms to maintain it in good health. Whenever the body is out of balance, these mechanisms swing into action to re-create health. If those mechanisms are thwarted or unsuccessful, then we have disease.

So, what is the problem in cancer? Why does the body appear unable to cope? It is just the same as with the broken leg!

If we are able to provide the right conditions, the body has the potential to heal itself.

In the acute situation of a broken bone, the medical intervention is a very obvious first step. Surgery provides the right conditions by realigning and stabilizing the bones. The patient maintains those conditions by keeping the leg still and having a diet and an environment that permit the normal healing functions to proceed.

However, cancer is a chronic, multifactorial, degenerative disease. It takes a long time to develop and has a multiplicity of contributing factors, as we shall discuss later. While surgery and other medical treatments clearly have their place in treating cancer, correcting the causes of the disease is more involved; while providing the correct environment to allow the body's potential for healing to proceed is also more involved. All of this requires consideration of far more than the body mechanics involved in surgically repairing a broken leg. It involves consideration of the whole person—body, emotions, mind and spirit.

What we are concerned with here is investigating the potential for each of us to be directly involved in re-creating our own health. What we seek is the ideal environment for healing in general and cancer in particular. What we know is that this all comes back to that simple principle of balance. Balance equates with good health, and good health does not include cancer. Balance equates with healing.

Again, a healthy body cannot have cancer. There was a man in America who had kidney failure and was given a kidney transplant. Unbeknown to anyone, the kidney he was given in the transplant was already cancerous. Naturally, he was placed on immune-suppressant drugs to prevent his body from rejecting his new kidney and this meant his body's normal defenses could not operate properly. In a very short time, not only was the new kidney engulfed by the cancer, but it had spread throughout his lungs. With his life threatened, the immune-suppressant drugs were ceased, the new kidney was removed, and he was returned to a dialysis machine. What happened? The immune-suppressant drugs wore off, his normal bodily defenses rapidly reasserted themselves, and all the cancer in his chest disappeared—automatically, with no outside intervention. His body's normal ability to heal itself did just that. His body, with its immune system working again, had the ability to recognize the cancer should not have been there and so eliminated it.

We want to create the conditions in our body so that it can do the same thing. We want to reactivate our own immune system and provide the right conditions where healing can take place. We can do it.

There is a very close link between the function of our body and the function of our psyche. That is, if we are relaxed and easy in mind and emotions, our body will be relaxed. If, on the other hand, we have anxiety or are affected by stress, our body will suffer from subtle but far-reaching changes in body chemistry and it will also show up as physical tension. I believe that this reflex is a key factor which we can use in the process of getting well.

Equate stress, anxiety and tension with immune-suppression and illness.
Equate relaxation and balance with health and healing.

If our body and psyche are relaxed, we will be in a state of balance, and that balance means health. If we are deeply relaxed, our body's natural tendency will re-create health for us—true, deep, meaningful health, including a healthy body.

The first step, the starting point that we can readily appreciate and learn, is to lead the body into deep relaxation. Relieving emotional and mental stress is hard to begin with, as causes of anxiety are difficult to isolate and often difficult to treat using conventional means. However, if we relax the body, that reflex produces relaxation of emotions and mind.

Mental anxiety, stress and physical tension are intricately connected and interdependent. They are all disease-producing factors. However, truly break that connection at any one point and relaxation spreads all through. Healing begins.

Pause to consider a cat. A lithe, graceful cat. Watch it on the move. It moves with an ease and smoothness that is a joy to watch. In slow motion it is a sight to behold. Yet, if it has to react in a hurry, it can—in an instant. It will pounce in a flash, or turn and run with amazing speed. So too, it will often stop, consider a situation at length and then go on with its business. Concentration and relaxation are mutually supportive. All so easy, so relaxed.

This, to me, shows what relaxation is all about. It is being physically relaxed and so being free to make an appropriate response.

If we are relaxed we react appropriately. We do not rush into things and overreact; neither are we sluggish and unable to take appropriate action. What we do is simply appropriate.

There is no need to avoid the problems of everyday life. Life should have challenges and a zest of endeavor. Such challenges become causes for stress only when we do not handle them appropriately.

If we do not react to challenges well, tension and anxiety cloud our normal processes. They interfere with judgment and reactions, so that responses become inappropriate. If our mind is confused or anxious, we have great difficulty thinking clearly and are highly likely to make poor decisions. However, the more relaxed our being, the more calm and clear is our mind, the more likely we are to make good choices and to do the appropriate thing.

COMMON FORMS OF RELAXATION

Where then, do we find this relaxation? Some of the common ways we relax in a healthy way are through sleep, exercise, hobbies and holidays. All have their place.

Sleep

Sleep is an excellent way of dealing with acute stress. Even sleep imposed by drugs will often provide the time and space necessary for adjusting to and dealing with a major, temporary stress. We certainly need a regular amount of natural sleep to avoid fatigue and added stress.

As an aside, here is an important tip. We can significantly improve the quality of our sleep by doing our relaxation exercises when we go to bed. When you get into bed at night, spend five minutes, perhaps ten, doing your relaxation. This is important. If you have muscular tension when you get into bed, your body is like a spring and you will spend half the night unwinding. Researchers have observed people sleeping and documented the muscles of tense people struggling to unwind. In a series of jerks and twists, the body tries to get itself relaxed. For some people this can take most of the night and so they wake up without having much profitable relaxed sleep. So do spend a few minutes before you go to sleep and practice the progressive muscle

relaxation exercise. As you get that good relaxed feeling all th
find that you can put yourself to sleep. You could well find th
sleep than you used to, as well as waking feeling the better fo

In chronic stress situations, however, while sleep may prov
it changes very little. We wake up with the same problems and responses that
accompanied us to sleep. We need to look further.

Exercise

Exercise is well worth considering. In the right amounts, it helps to relax
physical tension by tiring the muscles and so creating a natural form of relaxation. Also, it certainly invigorates and makes the body feel better, as well as
being well proven to relieve depression, promote well-being and aid the healing process generally. Exercise warrants being a feature of our healing program and more detail on the best forms of exercise for recovery comes in the
next chapter.

Hobbies and Holidays

These can be very pleasant diversions. They also provide an opportunity to
relax, to release and to let go a little. They can certainly aid our general level
of well-being. They are well worth considering, but frequently they produce
little change in our overall situation.

Meditation and Deep Relaxation

The practice of meditation has the potential to produce the most profound
and effective levels of deep relaxation. Another reason the specific meditation technique we recommend for healing works so well is that it starts with
deep physical relaxation. Then, relaxing the mind enhances the effect.

However, let us be clear about this. While meditating once or even three
times a day is clearly beneficial, if we get up from our meditation and spend
the rest of the day just as tense and uptight as ever, the benefits will be relatively small. What we need is to take the relaxation, along with the calm and
clear mind, from the meditation into our daily life.

This is most important. The relaxation we feel during our formal meditation periods needs to become a way of life for us. We need to aim to be as
relaxed as possible because except when we are faced with an immediate
threat, relaxation is our hallmark of the balance we seek.

This is not to say we will be sluggish or lethargic. On the contrary, we will react quickly and be sharp and alert but, like the cat, be relaxed at the same time. There are a number of ways to achieve this.

INTEGRATING RELAXATION INTO DAILY LIFE

The Automatic Flow-On Effect

As you begin meditating, you will notice the calm you feel during your formal sessions of practice remains with you for a short while after. Meditating regularly in this way throughout the day enhances this effect, so that one session's benefits soon begin to flow on to the next. This is why it is useful to spread a number of meditation sessions throughout the day. While initially you will seem to have good and bad sessions, soon you will notice a cumulative effect that means you get more benefit from each experience of meditation.

This effect can be increased still further by improving the quality of the meditation and by becoming more aware of relaxation throughout the day.

Speeding Up the Process of Relaxation

Initially, as we learn to relax and meditate, the progressive muscle relaxation (PMR) is a very helpful technique. Using the physical act of contracting muscles and letting them go leads to a very reliable experience of relaxation and helps us to appreciate what it feels like to be deeply relaxed. But we can then progress and learn to relax more quickly and, in fact, more deeply. Here is how we do it.

The next step is to experience the same level of relaxation we did through using the full PMR, only this time we do so without physically contracting the muscles. We simplify and speed up the process. So now, we focus our attention on the muscles in each area of the body, and using the same sequence as we did with the PMR, this time we feel those muscles relaxing without having contracted them first. Once we have mastered this step and can feel that same deeply relaxed body we felt with the first technique, we go even further.

Now we learn to relax the legs as one unit, rather than the feet, then the calves and the thighs. We learn to relax the torso as another "block," and then the head and neck. Ultimately, it is like we can sit to meditate, bring our attention to our bodies, and, almost like throwing a switch, feel the whole body relax as one unit. Now we have arrived at that ultimate point where we do not even need to spend time relaxing individual areas. We can just sit down and feel a wave of relaxation move throughout the body, producing that total, deep calm.

However, there is no hurry to speed up the procedure. We need to feel confident at each phase before advancing. The accent is on ease. No effort, no striving, just a natural progression to a faster, easier way. Again, the point to emphasize is that we arrive at the end point where the body will be deeply relaxed and so will the mind. If we do need to employ the PMR exercise to achieve this, we do so. If we can relax just as effectively but more quickly, we do so.

Using Discomfort to Deepen Relaxation

Once we begin to develop the capacity to relax at will, we are ready to use a more uncomfortable starting position. What, more discomfort? Yes, just a little at a time. Why? Well, a measured element of discomfort makes the physical relaxation a little harder to achieve and this makes us focus more on what we are doing. Undoubtedly, this in turn heightens the effect of the meditation. It is like when you go to the gym, work out, and develop your physical muscles. Here, we develop our "relaxation" muscles. You really do need to try this, the results will be obvious.

The suggestion is that if you began learning to relax and meditate in an armchair, once the technique is working well, try it in an armless chair. The change is very little, but I am sure you will notice a different effect. Once you are comfortable with that and it has become easy and effortless, go on to trying it on a stool. Harder still, but still fairly easy and, again, a greater benefit. Then you could go on to experiment with sitting cross-legged on the floor, or going outdoors. In the open air the sounds and smells increase the potential distractions while adding to the naturalness of it.

In my own situation, I generally meditate sitting cross-legged on the floor or on a chair in the morning and at lunchtime. My back can often be tired after a day on one leg, so frequently I lie on a hard surface in the evening, as this allows it to relax better. I notice that lying down produces more benefit in terms of relaxing my body, but there is no doubt sitting cross-legged produces a better overall effect, particularly when it comes to the mind.

Using Imagery to Focus Relaxation—The Radiant Light Imagery Exercise

We will be examining the benefits and techniques of imagery in chapters 8 and 9; however, when it comes to deepening our relaxation and meditation, there is a particular form of imagery that is easy to learn and can be of great benefit. This is what we call the "radiant light" imagery exercise. This is an "extra" technique worth experimenting with. If you warm to it and find it helpful, continue on with it; if not, simply move on to the next step. What you may discover is that this exercise has the added advantage of leading on to a heightened body awareness. Using this technique you will be in better touch with your body and more responsive to its messages. Similarly you will be able to control it better.

To practice this technique takes around thirty minutes. It can be done in any position, but I find this particular exercise does work best if you lie down on a hard surface. The floor is ideal. Choose a carpeted area, or place a blanket underneath yourself to begin with. Lie flat on your back, hands loosely by your sides. Legs should be out straight, just comfortably apart and the feet allowed to flop loosely outward. Some find a pillow under the knees quite helpful.

When you have taken the time to practice this a little, and you can do it well, you will have a means to relax yourself deeply and revitalize yourself amazingly. Practicing this technique regularly, once a day for a few weeks, will produce a new dimension in body awareness and relaxation.

The clarity of visualization, how clearly you "see" the different body parts, is not so important. Obviously, someone with detailed anatomical knowledge will be able to build up a more detailed image than others. The important thing is to feel that close contact and awareness of each part of your body. So, in a large complex area such as the abdomen, you feel as if your mind is moving through the whole area. You feel the deep sense of relaxation and then the glow.

When it comes to areas affected by cancer or other disease, just do the same thing. No effort or striving, just feel your mind moving through the area, relaxing it and letting the light build up to the same level as in the rest of your body. This produces a feeling of uniformity throughout the body—a vital, healthy uniformity and it promotes the healing response.

Sometimes, relaxing areas affected by disease causes some initial dis-

The Radiant Light Exercise

Begin by putting all your attention onto just one big toe. Form an image in your mind of your toe and travel through it, examining each part in your mind. It is as if in your mind, you travel around the skin, under the nails, through the joints, tendons, ligaments and muscles. As you do so, you aim to relax each part in minute detail. So this is a process to take slowly. You really do dwell on each part of the toe, feel into it and feel it relaxing deeply and completely.

You may well notice feelings of warmth flowing into the areas you relax in this deep way; maybe even a light tingling almost like mild pins and needles. This is a sign blood is flowing more freely through the area and relaxation is deepening.

Next, you build up an image of radiant white light suffusing each area of the toe. It is as if that toe was a light globe with a dimmer switch. You turn on that switch and gradually increase the light until the toe is full of vibrant white light. You will find it feels marvelous. When you do it well, you will be thinking of nothing else, just experiencing the vibrancy of it all.

So, having begun with one toe, then move to the next and so on, until the whole foot is "lit up." You may find that at the first session attending to just one toe takes all your time. That would be fine. Next session you will find that you can recapture the feeling in that toe more easily and more quickly and so you can start with the next toe. At each session work on more areas until you can capture the feeling throughout the body. It is the feeling of relaxation, lightness and vitality that is the main thing. You aim to complete the exercise feeling deeply relaxed, filled with the radiant, healing, vibrant light.

comfort. This is because we often have long-standing tension in the region around them as a defense mechanism. These exercises relax that tension and often produce sensations of temporary discomfort, occasionally tingling, even brief muscle spasms or jerks. Be assured this soon gives way to a feeling of warmth and ease. Also, this radiant light technique is very helpful for pain relief, and we will discuss this in detail soon (chapter 10).

The aim of the radiant light exercise is to lead us to a point of profound relaxation, with an accompanying sense of wholeness and vitality. So this exercise really serves to add another means of reaching the stillness of passive meditation. It is that end point which is the really important thing.

Relaxation Trigger Points

As you become more aware of your body, you will almost certainly find that some areas feel more tense than others. Common areas of tension are the muscles of the forehead, jaw, shoulders, tummy, hands and lower back. You will find that when you are placed in a stressful situation, one or more of these areas may tense up first. Just watch what happens next time you are "pushed." These areas are called trigger areas and they are very useful! Remember the reflex?

Anxiety + Stress = Muscular tension
Muscular relaxation = No anxiety, no adverse effect from stress

Having identified localized areas where tension shows up, we can concentrate on relaxing those areas, and when we succeed in doing so, we are well on the way to being relaxed. This is a very good defense mechanism to use if you feel stress is still affecting you. If you feel a situation is causing stress to build up, concentrate upon relaxing your trigger areas. You will find that if you keep your body relaxed, the whole situation will be defused.

Relaxation in Daily Life

Once you have experienced the "feel" of relaxation in your formal exercises, you will be able to recapture it at will during the day. Soon it will become your natural state. Free from tension, you will be able to react appropriately and will not be affected by stress.

Ideally, we aim to be relaxed all day and impervious to potentially stressful situations. Practicing these techniques goes a long way toward this end and we can do still more to achieve it. At every opportunity through the day, at every idle moment, take the time to check your level of relaxation. Do an internal inventory. Start with the trigger areas and make sure they are relaxed.

When you begin doing this, you may find that every time you think of your trigger areas, they need help to be more fully relaxed. That is fine. It is good to simply notice such a fact; and then to realize you can do something about it! That is why we practice. That is why we persist with these exercises. Relax. Smile. Know that the worse the tension to begin with, the more benefit you will get in the long run by relaxing!

Seek to experience the feeling of relaxation at every opportunity. After a while you will stay relaxed and you will feel a wonderful difference.

Relaxing Moments

Use your time wisely. When in the car, do not just waste those precious seconds at the red lights. Relax as much as you can and feel how good it is. Maybe take a deeper breath in; breathe out, and let go. The muscles softening and loosening. The feeling of relaxation all through.

And then remember the cat. Relaxed but alert. As we watch a cat in slow motion, the foreleg flows gracefully forward. All the muscles at the front of the leg are contracting to draw the leg forward. The muscles at the back of the leg are relaxed. There is nothing to hinder the flow of the leg or stilt the action. Look at a tense person walking—they jerk along in a most ungainly way. The relaxed cat flows. When the leg moves backward, the muscles at the back of the leg contract, and those at the front relax.

So even while driving along, be aware that your trigger areas are relaxed. Ideally, your whole body is inherently relaxed. And at the same time, you are quite alert, focused and mindful, ideally poised in body and mind for the driving.

The key to this is the principle that you use only the muscles you need for any given task of the day. To avoid stress, to maintain a relaxed state, muscles are either working at a specific function or at rest. They do not need to hold any residual tension.

I have seen many people take on a new elegance and charm merely by learning to relax properly. Perhaps this was most marked in Edna, an elderly patient. As she learned to relax, the worry and tension left her face. Coupled with the benefits of the diet, a new vitality and vigor came over her, producing a genuine, radiant glow that was obvious to all.

Very soon, using these techniques, your body will be relaxed, your mind also, and the benefits of the meditation will have entered your daily life. You will be reacting appropriately and you will be heading toward profound healing and long-term good health.

PUTTING IT ALL TOGETHER • The Main Meditation Practice:
Mindfulness-Based Stillness Meditation

This completes all the background and preliminaries we need to be aware of and to have practiced so that we are ready for the main meditation practice of mindfulness-based stillness meditation (MBSM).

Remember the simple summary: having prepared well, we relax. Relaxing more deeply, we become more mindful. As our mindfulness develops, the stillness naturally reveals itself. We rest in open, undistracted awareness.

Here is the "script" we can learn to lead us through mindfulness-based stillness meditation:

The Mindfulness-Based Stillness Meditation—Main Practice

Take a few moments to adjust your body . . . and then, when you are ready . . . relax into your posture . . .

Now, let us begin by letting go of what we have been doing recently . . . and bringing our attention more particularly to this present moment . . .

To do this, it may help to bring the focus of our attention to the breath for a few moments . . . to simply be aware that as we are breathing in, we are breathing in . . . and as we are breathing out, we are breathing out . . .

And as you do bring your attention more particularly to the breath . . . you will probably notice that as you do breathe out, there is a natural feeling of relaxing a little with the outbreath . . . of letting go a little . . .

Breathing out . . . and letting go . . . relaxing . . . releasing . . . letting go . . .

Feeling it deeply . . . completely . . . and feeling it all through the body . . . and the mind . . . it is a good feeling . . . a natural feeling . . . just going with it . . . calm and relaxed . . . calm and relaxed . . . going with it . . . quite effortlessly . . . effortlessly . . . letting go . . .

And just allowing your breath to take up whatever rhythm feels comfortable for you at the moment . . . breathing out . . . relaxing . . . releasing . . . letting go . . . breathing out, and the breath becoming longer . . . finer . . . subtler . . . then a pause . . . and simply allowing the breath to come back in of its own accord . . . quite effortlessly . . . effortlessly . . . going with it . . . relaxing . . . releasing . . . and feeling the ease of it all . . . the ease of it all . . .

And now, it might help to take your attention to that point between the eyes, a little into the forehead . . . and notice there what is like a still, quiet center . . . a point of stillness . . . and relax your eyes . . . and soften your gaze . . . and hold your attention lightly, on that point of stillness . . .

And if you do notice any sounds coming to your awareness . . . just let them come when they are ready . . . and go when they are ready . . . a bit like white clouds, drifting across a blue sky . . . they just come when they are ready . . . go when they are ready . . .

Holding your attention lightly on the stillness . . . and simply letting go . . . letting go . . .

And if any sensations in your body do come to your awareness . . . just the same . . . just simply notice them . . . free of any judgment . . . free of any reaction, or commentary . . . and feel the letting go . . . your body relaxing . . . and releasing . . . holding your attention lightly on the stillness . . . and simply noticing whatever may come to your attention . . . simply being aware . . . a gentle focus on the stillness . . . and letting things come when they are ready . . . go when they are ready . . . letting go . . . letting go . . .

And if you do notice any thoughts coming to your attention . . . just the same . . . just let them come when they are ready . . . go when they are ready . . . gently holding your attention on the stillness . . . and feeling the ease of it all . . . the ease of it all . . . just simply letting go . . . letting go . . .

And then it is almost as if you can merge into that stillness . . . relaxing . . . releasing . . . simply resting in the stillness . . . aware . . . free of any judgment . . . free of any commentary . . . and feeling the ease of it all . . . the ease of it all . . . just simply letting go . . . and

(continued)

(continued)

resting in the stillness . . . quite effortlessly . . . effortlessly . . . letting go . . . letting go . . .

LONG GAP—for your meditation

And if at any stage you do notice your mind wandering or becoming distracted . . . as soon as you become aware of that . . . gently bring your attention back to that point of stillness . . . relaxing . . . releasing . . . just going with it . . . melting . . . merging . . . simply resting in the stillness . . . quite effortlessly . . . effortlessly . . . letting go . . . letting go . . .

LONG GAP—for your meditation

That's good . . . good . . . good . . . When you are ready now . . . just let your eyes gently open once again.

MEDITATION CONCLUSION

The aim of our meditation is to relax deeply and to rest in the balance of deep natural peace. In any given session of meditation, we do the simplest things that will help us to this end. So if we need to, it may be wise to start by taking the time to go through the complete progressive muscle relaxation exercise. But if we have practiced enough and it works for us, it may be enough to simply take a deeper breath or two and feel the body relax quickly and deeply.

Once we feel the body to be relaxed, we become more mindful. We notice whatever does come to our awareness, free of any judgment or commentary. We just allow things to come when they are ready, go when they are ready, and we remain in undistracted awareness.

As time goes on a deeper stillness becomes apparent. Sounds may come and go, thoughts may come and go. They do not disturb us. We rest in deep, natural peace. And as we do so, there is the knowing that we are in a state of deep, natural balance. And the healing flows.

Happy meditating. Happy healing.

CHAPTER 7

Mind Training 1

Positive Thinking: The Conscious Mind at Work

IT WAS HENRY FORD WHO SAID, "WHETHER YOU THINK YOU CAN OR YOU think you cannot, you are right!"

What is the most important thing when it comes to any treatment you may be considering, whether it be a medical or a nonmedical treatment? Clearly, it is your mind, as your mind will decide whether you agree to that treatment or not. Your mind will decide whether you continue with the treatment or cease it. Further, your mind has the very real potential to significantly influence the outcome by reinforcing or sabotaging the treatment.

What is the most important thing when it comes to the food you eat? Clearly it is the mind, as it is your mind that will decide what you eat and how much you eat, as well as what you drink, and whether you exercise along with that.

Clearly, the mind is responsible for the choices we make, the knowledge and experiences we remember, the habits and the beliefs that shape our lives. However, everyone who has studied the mind, from the ancient mystics to the modern neuroscientists, says we use barely a fraction of our mind's potential. In these next three chapters we will learn how to train the mind and how to activate its potential for restoring health and for maintaining well-being.

To provide some structure and so that we can understand the various aspects of the mind and their potential for healing, here is an outline of what we will cover:

THE FOUR WAYS IN WHICH THE MIND INFLUENCES HEALING

1. Consciously—Via Positive Thinking

We will learn that positive thinking is about making good decisions and following them through. Positive thinking recognizes that it is the mind that shapes our world through the choices it makes. Our health and our healing, in fact all that we do, will be dramatically affected by whether we make constructive or destructive decisions, and whether we follow through on those decisions or not.

2. Unconsciously—Via Our Habits and Belief Systems

i) The beliefs we hold have the potential to significantly influence the outcome of everything we do. We will examine the powerfully positive placebo response and the incredibly destructive impact of the "pointing of the bone." Together, these two phenomena graphically reveal the mind's capacity to influence healing directly. Then we will learn what we need to do to gain the full benefit from the power of belief.

ii) The habits we live with will directly affect our potential to heal. Are you lazy in some ways? Do you have trouble exercising regularly? Are you habitually bound to eating certain things? Do you have difficulty sticking to what you know you need to do? Habits can be changed. We will learn how to identify what, if anything, does need changing, and then how to make necessary changes in a way that is empowering, sustainable and actually fun! This is a crucial element of recovery.

3. The Mind-Body Connection

Here we will examine how the mind can be mobilized to directly activate healing. We will learn more about how to apply the techniques of imagery and affirmation.

4. Meditation

Meditation establishes an ideal state of balance. From this balance healing flows free of effort, almost automatically. We have covered meditation thoroughly in the previous chapters.

Let us begin.

THE CONSCIOUS MIND, POSITIVE THINKING AND HEALING

Imagine a loving mother who is giving her all to being the best mother that she can be. Do you imagine she ever feels that she is managing 100 percent? But do you imagine she ever gives up trying? Of course she does not. That is what positive thinking is all about—always aiming to do the best we possibly can, acknowledging our strengths and weaknesses, being comfortable with what we do achieve and knowing we will become better and better at whatever we turn our attention to.

Positive thinking is all about using our mind intelligently. Specifically, positive thinking involves understanding how our mind works, and then getting the best out of its vast potential.

The crucial point in this field of mind training is to realize there is a big difference between positive thinking and wishful thinking.

Wishful thinking is where you hope for the best and do nothing about it.

Positive thinking is where you hope for the best and do a lot about it.

This is a fundamental distinction and opens up our understanding to the truth of what "positive thinking" really is. Positive thinking is way more than just that optimistic hope—"If he can do it, so can I." That hope is real enough. It is true; it has to be done only once to show that it is possible. But what did she do to achieve what she did? And what are you prepared to commit to, to achieve the results you are after?

Positive thinking begins when we use our mind to choose a specific goal. But then we must act on that goal. We need to use our mind to commit to that goal and embrace all we need to do to give ourselves the best chance of realizing that goal. This is a very active process. Wishful thinking is a passive process that involves little active effort and clearly is not likely to make a big difference to anything we do. By contrast, positive thinking regularly results in the extraordinary.

Your Mind at Work

How then does positive thinking work? Let us begin with the role of the conscious mind. In practical terms, the mind is well described as a goal-orientated, decision making tool.* Here is how it works.

---

* For a more expansive definition of the mind, see Appendix E.

Imagine you ask me to come and share a meal with you and I agree. You say you live in Australia or Canada or France. Big places. A lot of homes to look for you in. So maybe you are a little more specific and you give me the district you live in—the Yarra Valley, the Rockies, the Bordeaux region. I am getting closer, but it is still going to be a while before I find you. So you give me a full address: street name and number, town, city, country. Now I will find you. I can use a map, a GPS, ask the locals. If I persevere, there is only one address that matches your home and I will find you.

The mind is goal oriented. The more specific the goal, the more potently it functions and the more reliably it works. If I have only your local region, it will be easy for me to be confused, to become disheartened, to give up. But with a specific goal, the prospect of success becomes very realistic.

However, clearly the specific goal is just the beginning. Once I decide to pursue that goal, to come to your address, I need to decide how best to make the journey and I need to actually complete the journey. So if I decide to come by car and the battery in the car is flat, I can either give up at that point or persevere. Having managed to start the car, I am then faced with many choices. As I begin to drive forward, I need to decide which direction to take, and I base that decision on what is most likely to lead me to your address. So I choose left, right or straight ahead, over and over, at one intersection after another, until I find you.

That is how it works. It is simple. The thinking mind is a goal-oriented, decision-making tool.

We are all positive thinkers. We all use our minds in this way many times over, day after day. However, some people become overwhelmed. "You want me to come to dinner? I don't know about traveling on the roads just for a meal. What if I get lost? What about all the dangerous drivers on the road? Maybe it will be dark on the way home and I get scared in the dark." Some people manage to talk themselves out of even simple things.

Of course, the truth is some people do set out in their cars each day fully expecting to reach their journey's end and do not make it. Fatal car accidents are real. People do get lost, have flat tires, run out of gas and have minor accidents. Does this mean we stay at home and do nothing? Well, some do, but not so many when it comes to simple journeys. We accept the risks and persevere.

Consider this. Healing from a major illness like cancer can well be described as a journey. Often it is a lengthy journey, with many choices to deal with, many decisions to make, and often enough there are unexpected turns for better and worse. In my experience, some people do sense the scope of this particular journey and decide "to stay home." Some may be paralyzed by fear. Others are deeply concerned by the fear of failure. What if I make all this effort and it does not work? Will I feel like a failure? Will I have let myself down or let down those around me?

Face the Fear and Do It Anyway!

The fear of failure is related to the notion of false hope. In many of the early media interviews that focused upon my work, presenters would ask if I was concerned about giving people false hope. Some doctors have also expressed a related concern—what happens to people who try hard to recover and still end up dying?

The answer to this is simple. Any major endeavor carries some risk. Recovering from a difficult diagnosis is not easy. If it was easy, everyone would be doing it and it would be commonplace. We know it is possible, but we do need to be realistic; it requires a good deal of effort. And the truth is I have seen people who have tried hard and still died of their disease. Long-term recovery is not easy, but it is possible.

When I had widespread secondary bone cancer in 1976 and was expected to live for a few months, I could have just accepted the disease as my fate and sat by hoping for the best, waiting to see what happened. My guess is that if I had done so, I could have died quite easily. But I dared to believe recovery was possible and, being realistic, knew that if I was to recover, I would need to do something dramatic. I knew I needed to do the best I possibly could with everything I took on.

When I became sicker before I began to recover, I simply became even more determined, more thorough. I knew I did not want to die with regret. I did not want to be near my last breath wondering if things would have been better if I had an extra carrot juice, or meditated a bit longer. Now, obviously there is a limit to how much carrot juice one should or could drink, and a balance in how much meditation to do. What all of us need to do is to decide for themselves how much carrot juice we drink, how much meditation we do, and then do it. That is the essence of positive thinking.

Commitment and Outcome

What can be said after many years helping people to face difficult situations is that these people fall into three broad categories. A number find that all this positive thinking and the lifestyle-based approach is simply not for them and they drop out. By contrast, most people recognize the truth in what is on offer, and the possibilities. However, even among these people, there are two types. We call them the 100 percenters and the 70 percenters.

The 100 percenters set clear goals and do them, 100 percent! Maybe they miss a little here or there, but essentially they do what they turn their mind to. By contrast, the 70 percenters consistently fall short of their goals. Maybe they set unrealistic goals, maybe for a multitude of reasons they just cannot persevere. But the gap between what they plan to do, what they set as their own personal goals, and what they actually do creates an inner tension. This tension commonly leads to unhelpful emotions like anger, blame, shame or guilt.

Now this latter situation is where help is urgently needed. I often suggest to people that if there is a big gap between what they believe is best for them to be doing and what they are actually doing, they need to treat that situation as if it is a medical emergency. It requires urgent attention. Either the expectations need to be brought into line or the questions of commitment and discipline addressed. To remain with a significant gap or disparity between your beliefs and your actions, between what you believe you need to be doing and what you actually are doing, for any length of time is an invitation to misery and poor outcomes. One way or the other, it needs to be resolved. More on how to do this is coming soon.

Once beliefs and actions are in sync, people invariably do well. Giving 100 percent to what they do has resulted in many people making a full recovery. But perhaps not too surprisingly, even those who give 100 percent and still go on to die of their disease, they do well too. They invariably have a good death. Maybe there is a natural disappointment and a sense of regret about dying itself. But there is no regret about having not done all that was reasonable. There is no guilt or shame. No anger or resentment. They do not die wondering. We will discuss this more in the chapter on death and dying (chapter 18), and no, it is not being "negative" to discuss dying. We will all die one day, so let us plan for a good death. That certainly is possible and perhaps a good death is a testament to a good life, a life lived well.

However, we are focused here on getting well, then living well and dying a long time later! So for those who are keen, we need to observe that positive thinking can be an innate trait or a learned skill. This is more good news. I have seen really pessimistic, "negative" people learn the three simple principles of positive thinking and transform their health. However, before we learn these three principles and clarify how to apply them, there are some really useful preliminaries.

Positive Thinking 101—Choose to Be Positive

We begin our move toward becoming more positive by giving attention to our basic state of mind. The first question is, just how positive are you? Are you content with your current attitudes, or do you need to work at being more positive?

If you already have a positive state of mind, count your blessings. You have the starting point in place to develop the power of your mind more fully.

If you doubt your own level of positivity, or know it to be lacking, the first step is actually one of clear-cut choice. You are either positive or you are not. This may seem somewhat simplistic, but it is a fact: you can choose to be positive, hold that intention, and then follow through with the steps that develop it. This act of choice is a crucial one.

We literally can choose to be positive. It is that simple. This is one of those basic choices in life that can be made consciously. We can decide, we can have the intention to be positive, commit to what is effectively a state of mind we choose, and then carry it through. To do this, the intention needs to be one that is firm and one that we strengthen at every opportunity.

One of the best ways to reinforce this intention to be positive is with the aid of contemplation. Contemplation is a reliable way to think something through in a way that brings clarity of mind, understanding and confidence. To do this, we begin by taking up our usual meditation position and consciously relax the body as normal. Then, instead of aiming for a still mind, we actively think about what positivity means to us. We consider it from every viewpoint. We think of how we would define what it is to be positive, we compare it with negativity, think of positive people we know, think of positive aspects of our own character. Think of why we want to be more positive, why we need to be positive.

A hint here to assist your contemplation. Positive thinking may be as simple as being clear about what you are aiming for and being confident you can achieve it.

As we reflect and contemplate more, we will generate a very comprehensive understanding regarding positivity and what it means. This may take one or more sessions and so we repeat the contemplation until we have thought it through and gained real insight into what being positive means to us, why it is helpful and why we choose to adopt the positive approach.

What If I Do Not Feel So Positive? Use an Affirmation

Be reassured. Many people start this program knowing they are not very positive. Others have been rocked by their diagnosis, had their confidence undermined by all that can be a part of cancer. More than thirty years of experience tells us many people have turned all this around. That is why we learn how to train our mind. That is the joy of using positive-thinking techniques.

So to consolidate and to reinforce our intention to be positive, we use an affirmation. An affirmation is a short statement that accurately reflects our goal, our intention. We will discuss them more in the next chapter, but it will be very useful to begin to build your positivity straight away. The affirmation in this case is: "I am a positive person now." What we do is to repeat this short statement, this affirmation, over and over until it has been imprinted onto our mind and carries conviction.

Affirmations are wonderful things. They work! By using such simple, positive statements and repeating them regularly, we can condition our thoughts so that they lead on to the actions we intend.

So, when you first get up in the morning, repeat to yourself, "I am a positive person now," for a couple of minutes. Make time to do it again at least twice more during the day. Especially when driving in the car, say it out loud—even sing it if you like! Adding a sense of fun can be helpful, so put it to different tunes; be theatrical and keep doing it.

What will start to happen quite quickly is that when a new decision needs to be made, you will now have a little voice in the back of your mind saying, "I am a positive person now." And bingo! To satisfy that inner voice you will make a positive decision! As you become more positive, you see the system work and it becomes that much easier to be positive the next time. As the intended actions are put into practice, the cycle of positivity is completed and all of this will steadily help to build healing and a better life.

You will soon find that you have a new feeling, a feeling of being responsible for your own situation. You will be doing everything because you feel positive about it. You will want to do it; it is your choice. You will feel in control of your situation and you will find that your inner resources will be strengthening and developing rapidly.

You will come to recognize that if you were not positive before, you almost certainly suffered from "victim consciousness." This is the "Why me?" syndrome, the attitude that leaves people feeling a powerless pawn of random fate that has slated them for doom! It is the most negative and destructive attitude in which you could have become stuck. If you recognize it from your new vantage point of positivity, be gentle with yourself. You are a positive person now. Quietly remind yourself that is not the way you are now. Seek out how you can change those negative aspects and not repeat them again.

You can reasonably expect to have ups and downs, so you need to be prepared to persevere. When you do act positively, congratulate yourself. Quietly, of course! But happily. Reaffirm your new attitude and seek the next opportunity to practice it.

Armed with our positive attitude we are now ready to sort out all the challenges cancer presents and set ourselves clear goals. The next step provides us with a major key with which we can unlock the power of the mind.

THE THREE PRINCIPLES OF POSITIVE THINKING

Before the details, a short summary of the three principles:

Principle 1. Set a clear goal. Remember, the mind is a goal-oriented, decision-making tool, so the starting point is a clear goal. When it comes to healing, there are many choices. We will explore reliable methods for good decision making and for setting clear goals.

Principle 2. Do whatever it takes. Once we have a clear goal, we need to accomplish it. Sometimes the commitment required will flow easily, other times we will need to work at it. We will investigate how best to take a good idea and put it into action, how to do whatever it takes.

Principle 3. Choose to enjoy doing it. Those things we enjoy doing we tend to persevere with; we keep doing them. Things we do not enjoy doing we tend to avoid, forget, become disenchanted with, find excuses to let go of. The value in enjoying what we are doing is obvious enough and we will discover how simply and effectively we can achieve this final key to positive thinking.

But we begin with the first principle, goal setting.

THE FIRST PRINCIPLE OF POSITIVE THINKING: SET A CLEAR GOAL

Step 1. Who Decides?

When it comes to setting your goals, when it comes to deciding what to do, who tells you what to do? Is it some external authority figure like a doctor, a counselor, a natural therapist, a parent, a child or a partner? The lady over the back fence? Or is it you?

Who decides?

Authority figures can be really useful; genuine experts are invaluable. It is always sensible to consider seeking help from people who are knowledgeable, passionate and confident in what they recommend and what they do. But who takes the ultimate responsibility for what is done to you, or what you do for yourself?

Here we need to talk of fear again. Fear has this uncanny knack of disempowering people. Often when fear is strong, we feel so anxious, so uncertain of what to do, we want someone else to fix it, to tell us what to do. This is perfectly understandable and maybe in times of crisis it is wise to defer decisions to the people we trust the most.

However, if you value your own integrity and prefer to take more responsibility for your own choices, this tells you that making big decisions when fear is strong is fraught with danger. Fear commonly causes us to overreact and become frenetic, or to underreact and become too passive, too inactive. Again that reminder, it is wise to give yourself time for major decisions. Particularly allow time for any shock to settle so that you will be more relaxed and be in a better place with fear. Then with a calmer, clearer mind you will be able to gather all the information you need, make your choices and set your goals.

Step 2. Use Both Sides of Your Brain to Make Good Choices in the Decision-Making Process

The human mind has intelligence and wisdom. We think logically and also we can think more abstractly, more intuitively, more wisely. Clearly, both logic and wisdom are useful; in fact, logic without wisdom can be dangerous.

However, in the world we live in, where science has such a high value, it makes sense to begin by assessing things logically. Then we need to add the wisdom. Wisdom in its most ordinary form may be as simple as "common sense," but we will investigate developing wisdom more fully soon.

START WITH GOOD INFORMATION AND LOGIC

Ideally, it is wise to obtain the best opinions, the best advice from the most experienced experts in whatever field you are considering. It is wise to ask them for an opinion. What would they do in your position? What would they recommend or where would they send you if you were their child, their parent or their partner? Then, informed by this expert opinion, do whatever additional research you consider warranted or within your capabilities.

But consider this, and a warning, if you do not want your head messed with a little, perhaps it will be wise to skip the next paragraph!

There was a major study carried out some years ago in the United Kingdom with the aim of developing best practice recommendations for women with breast cancer. Two hypothetical case histories were formulated: one for a typical woman with primary breast cancer, the other for a typical woman with a recurrence. These were circulated to all the major cancer hospitals and treatment centers around the UK seeking consensus as to the best treatment to recommend. The results were somewhat disconcerting. While the recommended treatments had some similarities from all the centers, there were enough variations for the study to report that a number of different recommendations were received. For the women with primary breast cancer, the number of treatments regarded to be different was put at thirty-five! For the typical case of secondary breast cancer, the woman with a recurrence, the number was forty-five! So if the woman with primary breast cancer had been a real woman rather than an hypothetical case and if she had gone to one major cancer hospital, then decided she wanted a second opinion, she could have gone to thirty-five other centers before finding a match. What do you do with that if you only use your logic?

In real life, a woman with a breast lump is likely to start with her family doctor. If breast cancer is suspected or confirmed, she is likely to be referred to a specialist. She may have known the local doctor for years or not, she will almost certainly have no prior experience with the specialist.

The logic of what the specialist has to say regarding her condition and treatment options will be really useful information. It is likely to form the basis of the decision-making process. But logic also says there may be other ways to consider treating her condition. Is it worth seeking thirty-five other opinions? Of course not. These days, many major cancer centers aim to resolve this potential problem by using a team approach. There is a trend toward gathering together surgeons, oncologists, radiologists and other health professionals to discuss the individual needs of individual people.

But what of the person him- or herself? I strongly suggest there is more to decision making than pure logic. If we talk of a broken leg with major damage, the logic is compelling to have surgery and a cast. In that situation one does not need to dwell on the choices too much. But in cancer medicine, the choices are not always so clear. The reality is that many cancer treatments are tough on the patient. Often the risk of side effects is considerable and the potential gains debatable. Unfortunately, in this and many other situations, logic does not always provide an obvious answer.

However, with almost all decisions, it will make obvious sense to gather the best information you can, based on the best evidence available. An example of how to achieve this was given in chapter 3, where we discussed how to decide what treatment to commit to.

ADD CONTEMPLATION—DEVELOP CLARITY, CONFIDENCE AND WISDOM

Contemplation is a methodical way to think something through and to gain a deeper understanding of it. Also, contemplation provides a way of directly tapping into our intuition. All this helps to dispel doubts and reliably builds clarity and confidence. As a consequence, commitment develops more strongly and it becomes easier to follow through with our decisions.

Contemplation is easy to do and comes highly recommended for all our major decisions, and for setting all our positive-thinking goals.

So we can investigate and learn how this technique works. We will use the example of reviewing our eating habits and deciding on what sort of diet to follow. Here are the steps.

Goal Setting Using Contemplation

1. Decide what the issue is (e.g., in our example, to set dietary goals) and determine to reach a conclusion.

2. Express the issue as a question (e.g., What will be best for me to eat?).

3. Do the research. Use your intellect and your logic. Read the books, get on the net, speak to the experts, discuss it with friends, listen to CDs. Ideally, make notes. This person said that, this book the other, etc. With food it is usually easiest to write lists of the different recommendations.

4. Set a time for the decision to be made. There are two ways to do this. If you were to buy a new washing machine, probably you would wait until you gathered all the relevant information. Presuming you have determined your price range, you could find out the makes and models available and collect all their details within a reasonable period of time. However, with food you could collect information indefinitely. So you probably need to say to yourself something like, "I will collect all the information I can in the next two weeks [this two weeks is just an arbitrary figure I have used—there is no need to take me literally on this one—choose your own time frame] and then I will make the best decision I can."

5. On the day when the decision is to be made, give yourself some time—half an hour to an hour is ideal—and some space—either where you meditate regularly or in any quiet area. Make sure you can be free from the telephone and other possible distractions. Take with you any notes you have made and any other material you have gathered. Also, take a pen and some paper in case you want to write on it.

(continued)

(continued)

6. When you sit down, begin by reviewing your research material and in this way refresh all the knowledge you have of your subject. If you do not have written material go straight to the next step.

7. Consciously relax your body and calm your mind. This will be a familiar process if you have some experience of meditation. The aim is to relax your body and to calm your mind so you are in a better state of mind to progress into contemplation.

8. Once relaxed in this manner, focus your attention on consciously reviewing the facts as you remember them.

9. So, in our example, you might recall the style of food you have been eating, the broad issues relating to why you are considering changing your diet, what different people have recommended to you, what you have read in different books and so on.

10. If at any stage you become distracted or your mind wanders off onto other thoughts, as soon as you recognize this, be gentle with yourself and simply come back to concentrating on issues relating to food and diet.

11. This first part of the process then is clearly a rational, "left brain" exercise. You actively think about the topic and all issues relating to it. You are actively focusing on the topic and thinking it through.

12. What happens next, as you continue to concentrate on the topic, is that at some point your mind will automatically shift into more abstract, intuitive, "right brain" contemplation. It will be as if all the facts you have been reflecting upon and analyzing, all the pieces of the jigsaw puzzle as it were, come together and now you can clearly see the bigger picture. This will give you a new sense of comprehension and understanding and usually leaves you with a clear sense of what to do. This can all come with a moment of clear insight, almost like an "Aha! I've got it," moment of revelation.

13. The more you practice this technique, the more reliable it becomes. It is a wonderful and dependable way to solve problems, develop creativity and instigate lateral thinking. (As another aside, this is an excellent way to prepare for and complete creative writing.)

14. Once the sense of clarity dawns, usually it is best to write the ensuing insight down. Perhaps you can remember having the experience of a moment of insight like this before. Perhaps you were in the shower, or was it when you were half asleep, and suddenly like a bolt out of the blue, it seemed as if you had the perfect solution to a problem you had been wrestling with. Yet by the time you got dressed and ate breakfast, it had flown from your memory! Insight during contemplation sometimes comes like that too, so it is best to write it down. I always do this exercise with pen and paper close by and as soon as the answer begins to form write it down.

This contemplation technique can be used to solve any problem. It leads to a clarity that is backed by a deep sense of your own inner wisdom. As a result, the directions that come with it, the goals that emerge from this exercise, will feel very "right" for you.

So when it comes to contemplating food, we may think through specific issues like whether we will eat tomatoes or not, and whether we will cook them or not. Or we may arrive at a more comprehensive overview and, for example clearly understand why eating organic food makes sense and come away deeply committed to doing just that.

People often ask me, "How can I trust the result of an exercise like this?" Well, if you come out of this exercise with no clarity and are still clouded by doubt, all that has happened is you have spent time simply thinking about the issue. No harm done, but no profound insight, either! The insight we are talking of has as one of its features the confidence of certainty. It comes with a deep inner knowing and no doubt. You really know what to do with the tomatoes! No one else will need to confirm such an insight for you; it will be easy to feel confident about, easy to commit to, and it is highly likely to work well.

But what if you do all this and you still have doubts?

Step 3. When in Doubt, Do Something!

It would be nice to think we will arrive at a point of certainty before making all the decisions in front of us. Maybe we will. But doubt remains a real possibility—and does that mean you are unable to set a goal effectively?

One of the benefits of contemplation is that it does clarify the choices. When you reflect on this, with most things you either do them or you do not, or you put them off. Now, while there is the old Irish saying, "If you put something off long enough it will take care of itself," maybe we need to be a bit more proactive when it comes to cancer.

Faced with lingering doubts, what many people find works well is to accept the doubts and make a decision anyway. With a decision made in this way, it is still useful to decide to commit to whatever it is you are planning, make the commitment, and to embrace it. But then it is always healthy to review your progress from time to time and adjust accordingly.

Here it is helpful to appreciate another facet of how the mind works. As we have established, the mind is a goal-oriented, decision-making tool. In this regard, however, it is more like a heat-seeking missile than an arrow. Pardon the warlike images but they serve as useful metaphors here. When an archer takes aim and lets fly an arrow, the arrow is at the whim of the archer's aim and the elements. If a wind begins to blow the arrow off course, it has no self-righting mechanism. A heat-seeking missile is quite the opposite. A heat-seeking missile locks on to its target, and then receives feedback. If the target moves, the heat-seeking missile adjusts its course.

Step 4. Make Friends with "Mistakes"

Our mind functions like a heat-seeking missile. The mind is designed to manage the complexity and changing nature of our lives. It is designed to receive feedback, to compare our progress to what we are aiming for, to adjust, to change course regularly and to persist until the goal is reached.

Some people feel badly about mistakes. Some mistakes are regrettable, and we will consider later how to transform common feelings of guilt, shame, embarrassment and blame that often accompany mistakes (see healthy emotions, chapters 16 and 17).

However, here is another possibility. Mistakes are feedback. Mistakes can be really useful feedback. It is reported that Thomas Edison made ten thousand experiments before discovering how to produce a lightbulb that worked. When asked what it felt like to make 9,999 mistakes, Edison replied that he had not made 9,999 mistakes. He had completed 9,999 attempts to achieve his goal and with each experiment he learned something. In the end, courtesy of all he learned from what appeared to be his "mistakes," he revolutionized the world with his 10,000th attempt.

Be brave. Make a start. Stick to your goal. And be flexible with how you achieve that goal. Respond to feedback. Be prepared to hold to the big goal and be prepared to be flexible when it comes to how to get there.

Step 5. Rambo or the Martial Arts?

Pardon me again but we need to discuss the state of mind that goes with our positive thinking. While what we do is of great importance, the state of mind we do it in can be even more significant.

Most people are familiar with the Rambo image. Isolated, tough, uncompromising, resolute. Very driven, a fair bit on edge, high energy. Not much inner peace or calm. Contrast this with a martial artist. There is the same resolve, the same willingness to do whatever it takes, but there is a deep calm, a palpable inner peace. Meditation leads directly to this inner peace. Meditation can provide the background, the milieu, the atmosphere for our positive thinking, so that we will find it easier to make good decisions, easier to follow them through, easier to enjoy doing what we need to do to achieve them.

Step 6. Your Primary Goal—How Healthy Can You Imagine Yourself?

When it comes to cancer, what are you aiming for? What can you imagine as the best possible outcome? Whatever that is, that becomes your primary goal.

Can you imagine yourself fully recovered? Free of cancer, with a normal life expectancy again, fit and well? Is that easy to imagine, or a struggle? Is it easier for you to imagine yourself living well with cancer? Is it just a good quality of life you are after and you do not want to focus on the disease itself? Can you imagine your illness becoming stable? Or is there a deep sense of fear, or maybe an acceptance that dying of the disease is a likely outcome?

Challenging questions. Doubts are OK. Most people have doubts. Positive thinking is not about denying doubts. Or denying fears. Positive thinking is about recognizing the doubts and the fears, and using our minds intelligently to move through them, past them, and to accomplish our goals anyway.

The limit in positive thinking is what you personally believe is possible. Not what someone else believes. What *you* believe. Some people do accept they will probably die of their cancer; we spoke of this earlier. But maybe at the moment the limit of your belief is that you can genuinely only imagine the cancer becoming stable. If you consider that prospect for a moment, we know cancer tends to multiply, to increase in size exponentially. That is why once it is large enough to be detected, it commonly grows quite rapidly. (Please note, this is a broad generalization. Some cancers do grow very slowly indeed.) Therefore, when a cancer becomes stable, it is a sign of real progress. Maybe once stable, you can imagine the cancer receding a little.

Positive thinking works well with progressive goals. While some people go for an all-out, big goal like total recovery right from the start, others find it more manageable, more realistic and effective to advance in stages.

Step 7. Write Down Your Goals

With any significant goals you have, write them down in a journal, in a special notebook or simply on paper you can easily refer to. The writing will lead to even greater clarity, and you have a good chance of remembering what is written!

Step 8. Finally, Decide How Important Each Goal Is

Once you have clarified your goals, the next question is simple. How important is each goal to you? Is it a casual thing? If it works out, would it be nice but no big deal? Or is it a matter of life and death? Something you choose to give your all to?

When my secondary cancers appeared, I became totally uncompromising. For the next few years, until it was clear that I was well again, everything I considered, everything I did, needed to get past the first big filter.

Will this help me to recover?

If it did not pass that test in the affirmative, I was not interested. Of course, having fun passed that test. Some people seem to be of the impression getting well is tough work, which it can be, and unpleasant, which it has no need to be at all. In fact, I had a wonderful time during my recovery. There was this fabulous excuse to do all the things that were good for me, all the things that caused me joy and happiness. I had cancer. I could change whatever I liked, do whatever was needed. I had a great reason, a great excuse, and when I did it all in this uncompromising fashion, I was fortunate indeed: I fully recovered.

Positive thinking is a measure of what you are committed to and how committed to it you are. The first principle, having a clear goal, leads naturally to the second principle.

THE SECOND PRINCIPLE OF POSITIVE THINKING: DO WHATEVER IT TAKES

The three principles of positive thinking tend to flow on, one to the other, fairly naturally. When we have a clear goal, it often seems easy to commit to doing whatever it takes to achieve that goal. If so, it is as easy as that. If not, if it seems hard to do whatever it takes, then planning and concerted effort makes sense—all in the right state of mind!

Step 1. Embrace All That You Do

When it comes to positive thinking, the key recommendation is to embrace all that you do. To think through your options, decide upon your goals and embrace them. So to not just passively accept a treatment, or put up with dietary changes. Not just go along with things because someone else wants you to do it. Take ownership. Take control. Embrace everything you do. Welcome it. Commit. Believe in what you are doing. Then your mind will be activated and the placebo response will be working courtesy of your conscious mind, your conscious commitment.

Jill was a lady who came to our groups in a heightened state of anxiety. She was having chemotherapy for secondary cancer and was deeply concerned for her own future and the fate of her two young children. Amid the emotionally safe environment the group created, for the first time she shared her fears and cried openly. Quiet understanding supported Jill as she released her deeply held pain. She reported feeling as if a weight had lifted from her shoulders.

Up to this point Jill had been experiencing major anticipatory nausea even before she went into the hospital for her regular chemotherapy treatments. It transpired she was quite undecided in her own mind regarding this treatment. There was the hope of some benefit and another deep fear for the potential side effects. Once the emotion had cleared, Jill subsequently talked through her choices regarding the chemotherapy.

Now, with her mind somewhat clearer, she could think more logically and she decided she was doing the right thing for her. She embraced her treatment and went to the hospital looking forward to doing something she considered to be in her own best interests. She embraced the lifestyle program, ate well, meditated regularly, exercised and so on. When Jill arrived at the group, she had not been responding to her treatment. Two months later her tests had improved dramatically. Her main doctor remarked on this and encouraged her, saying whatever she was doing, she should stick to it!

Step 2. Check Your Clarity

This is a major point. In my experience, the most common factor behind a lack of commitment is a lack of clarity. The answer? Revisit the first principle! Set a clear goal.

Step 3. Use Ideals Wisely

A great deal of what is presented in this book is made up of ideal ways to use our lifestyle, our own inner potential along with our actions to generate healing. Remember, however, ideals are just that, ideals. As such they may be unattainable in their entirety. However, ideals do give us a goal, they do give us a sense of direction, and they do give us a strong sense of what to aim for. Obviously, we will be the better for any step we make toward an ideal.

So as we lay out these lists of things to do, these ideas, be comfortable with where you are, start where you can, do what you can. It is obvious. If you are really tense and anxious to begin with and you relax 10 percent of what is ideally possible, you are 10 percent better off. That is quite a good start! It will serve you well to be pleased that you are 10 percent more relaxed, rather than to worry about being 90 percent short of being fully relaxed. Positive thinking is acknowledging the 10 percent gain, focusing on that as progress, and being committed to making even more progress as time goes on.

Step 4. Seek Inspiration

Emphasis has been given to the pivotal role of hope. Many people find it useful to collect a "bank" of inspirational material to read, view or listen to when they need inspiration. Perhaps at the place where you meditate, you keep photos of inspiring people or landscapes, whatever inspires you the most. Even simply bringing inspiring people to mind can powerfully lift your spirits and these people may be family, friends, community leaders, spiritual or religious figures.

Step 5. Develop Constructive Discipline

The discipline we are talking of here is best described as a "personal kindness." This type of discipline is not a discipline imposed by someone else, it is a self-discipline. This self-discipline is based upon having the clarity of mind to understand what is in our own best interests, what is needed for our own welfare and well-being. This self-discipline is about having the resolve to actually do whatever is good for us. It is the capacity to do what is appropriate. That is what it is to be kind to ourselves. Simple as that. It may not always be easy, but it is always kind.

So when we wander off track we need to notice, to be vigilant and to gently and firmly bring ourselves back to what we know is good for us.

There is a very useful and practical recommendation here. Do something each day purely as an exercise in discipline. Perhaps go without a piece of food you would have had for pleasure's sake; do exercise as an act of discipline; even do as I do—finish your daily shower by turning the hot tap off and the cold full-on. This for me takes great discipline! Although it is extremely invigorating and I have been doing it for years, it still takes effort for me to do it. Practicing discipline by choice makes it a little easier to use self-discipline when it is more important—such as persevering through the ups and downs of the healing process.

Another way to develop personal discipline is to develop the capacity "to go without." Perhaps simply to go without that piece of cake. Perhaps to fast through one meal or one day. Build your discipline muscles!

Step 6. Develop Your Communication Skills

As a group, people affected by cancer tend to keep their thoughts and especially their emotions to themselves. Reversing this can help to change the dynamics of the illness.

- Start with a diary. Research has actually shown this is good for your immune system. When you write, aim to be brief on fact, long on personal detail. It is helpful to record what happens day by day, but the real benefit from writing a diary comes when you elaborate and recount how you felt, how you were affected by what happened. This helps "get it out," to express your feelings in a safe, private environment. And writing it down makes everything clearer and that little bit easier. I made diary entries virtually every day of my recovery and found doing so to be very helpful.

- Letter or e-mail writing can flow on from keeping a diary. What many people find useful these days is to set up a personal blog or Facebook page where news can be shared. This can help to reduce time spent by the patient or the family retelling the same details of what has happened recently. Also, it means that phone calls or face-to-face meetings can be used for more personal exchanges.

- Decide who your "listening post" will be. Seek a safe environment. Maybe a group, maybe an experienced counselor, maybe a trusted friend can become your listening post. This is someone or some group who is stable enough to listen to you. They do not need "an answer" for your problems. They do not need to fix anything. Their job is to listen in an open, nonjudgmental way and by doing so, allow you to express thoughts, feelings and emotions that otherwise may remain bottled up inside. To be able to provide this service of being a compassionate, nonjudgmental listener is a great gift if you are supporting someone with cancer.

Be increasingly open with family and friends. Brian had a brain tumor with a poor prognosis. He wanted to protect his eleven-year-old daughter and thirteen-year-old son and so only told them he had migraines. He reported that the son became increasingly hostile toward him and the daughter withdrew. Brian's wife, Kath, was deeply concerned and felt great pressure attempting to secretively manage phone calls to doctors, the friends who called in, the discussions she wanted to have with Brian and the children. The whole family was suffering. Brian became increasingly anxious and, as time went on, it was increasingly clear he had been withholding from the children. On discussing the dilemma, he finally decided to tell the children. They took it well, his son later confiding to Kath that he had known for quite a while. Kath reported both children soon appeared much more at ease and welcomed being able to discuss what Dad was doing.

Step 7. Laugh and Be Selective

Laughter is good for just about everything. There is a good deal of research to prove it, even if your common sense does not know it already! The trick is, how do we manage to laugh when things are grim?

First, avoid the grumps in your life. Avoid the people who feel compelled to tell you about Uncle Ted who had the same cancer as you, tried everything, and died anyway. Tell those people to take a holiday. Do not call us, we will call you.

Then hang out with the people that make you feel good. Use a simple test. If a guest leaves you feeling worse when they leave than when they got there, strike them off the invite list. You want to be with the people who can be serious when needed, but lift your spirits and ideally make you laugh.

Lighten up. It is bad enough being sick, there is no benefit in feeling miserable as well. So develop a store of funny DVDs and books. Read humor. Watch the comedy channel. Maybe even join in with a laughter club from time to time. People are different. Find out what gets you laughing.

Step 8. Recognize Your Sexuality May Change, and Adjust

Cancer has the potential to impact upon every facet of life and our sexuality is no exception. Treatments may directly affect sexual function and some people find the worry and concern they feel affects their interest in sex or their capacity to engage with it.

The important thing to be aware of is that sexuality and sexual function is another area that needs to be discussed and sorted out. While meditation is very effective in alleviating worry and helping people to be more open and loving, many find that they do need to adjust their sexual life. Of course with couples this may well necessitate both people adjusting, so communication is vital. Many couples do work this out in their own way, but it may be helpful to seek couples counseling if needed. Like everything else, satisfying solutions are found when we communicate and plan accordingly.

Step 9. Monitor the TV

Looking back, one of the best things I did at the start of my illness was to give the TV away. In those days I would watch anything. I was used to working an eighty-hour week as a veterinarian, training for the decathlon a couple of hours each day and then collapsing in front of the TV. I used it as an anesthetic. It was a second-rate way of relaxing and attempting to clear my mind. However, by giving it away, I freed up hours of my time. Without the TV I read two to three books each week, I meditated, I even talked to some people!

If you can manage the TV and regulate what you watch and how often, then of course there are some good things on it. But if the TV becomes a distraction, or at worst a barrier to communication between you and those you are close to, reconsider your options.

Step 10. Exercise Regularly and Within Your Limits

Exercise is profoundly therapeutic as demonstrated by research with several major cancers. Also, exercise is a powerful antidote against depression and leads to a generally more positive state of mind. Aim to exercise for about half an hour each day and then if you miss one session occasionally you will still receive the benefits.

Exercise that is helpful therapeutically is best if it is on the moderate to gentle side. There are two criteria that help you to monitor how hard to go at your exercise, taking into account your own level of fitness and health.

First, when you finish your exercise, you need to feel better than when you began. This means you come back feeling refreshed and invigorated. If you were training for a marathon, it would make sense to extend yourself and to need time to recover, but if healing is your motivation, you have overdone it if you need to lie down for half an hour after exercising.

Second, while exercising you need to be able to keep up a conversation. If you are walking up a hill and puffing so much you cannot string a sentence together, you are overdoing it. Slow down, take a rest, get your breath back.

Step 11. Get Creative

Creativity is another proven method for improving your state of mind and prospects of healing. Maybe you already paint, knit, play music, or build things. Keep doing it and know it is doing you good. Maybe you had a hobby in the past you felt passionate about. Anything that becomes a vehicle for creative passion is highly beneficial and is to be engaged with enthusiastically.

Step 12. Immerse Yourself in Nature

Nature is healing. Fresh air, tall trees, open spaces, the seaside—nature inspires us, comforts us, shares her natural healing gifts freely with us. For those living in cities, find the best parks nearby. Make the effort to travel into the countryside or to have a day by the water. Relax into nature. Sit with your eyes open. Contemplate. Meditate. Feel the deep natural peace and the healing qualities so ever present in nature.

Step 13. Develop Patience

Many people I have met approached an initial diagnosis of cancer with gusto. As if preparing for a sprint, they used a lot of energy to do all they could to overcome the challenges and gain the benefits. For some, recovery actually turned out to be relatively easy and quick, but for many others, more like a marathon.

So be patient, use the chapters on healthy emotions and overcome any tendencies to lapse into destructive, negative states of mind, while building the ability to be resilient, to endure, to persevere and to prevail.

Step 14. Practice Gratitude

Before bed each night, reflect on your day and find three things to be grateful for. They may be simple things like the sun was shining or the rain was falling. They may be acts of kindness you experienced or lessons you learned through the circumstances of the day. This simple practice of gratitude is a proven antidote to depression, but more significantly, it can really warm your heart and result in a positive attitude to all you do.

Step 15. Meditate

Out of the balance of meditation, a positive state of mind naturally arises. Maybe this is to do with the clarity that comes with meditation, the inner confidence, the natural optimism. Maybe the fact is that our natural state is to be positive and the balance of meditation simply reasserts that state.

Step 16. Consider Using Affirmations and Imagery

These will be explained in the next chapter.

Step 17. Celebrate What Is Good

Aim to find joy in what is healthy, positive and wholesome! This is a crucial point. If you do all the so-called right things in a grumpy, resentful and miserable state of mind, you will undermine the benefits and you run the risk of becoming quite miserable!

Find joy in doing what is good for you. How? This recommendation links directly with our third principle of positive thinking—choose to enjoy doing it. Remember, when you are aware you can decide your state of mind. Become informed regarding your choices. Decide what is in your own best interests and choose to be diligent; choose to enjoy doing it! Celebrate life.

DO WHATEVER IT TAKES • Where to Start

Quite a list! Obviously it is not possible or recommended to aim to be doing them all tomorrow. Besides, some you are bound to be doing already and others will just leap out and you will recognize their immediate value. Start with them. This whole art of positive thinking is something we can continue to develop and continue to gain more benefit from.

THE THIRD PRINCIPLE OF POSITIVE THINKING: CHOOSE TO ENJOY DOING IT

We have delved into the first two principles of positive thinking in some detail, learning how to set a clear goal and do whatever it takes. The third principle concerns the attitude with which we do the things we do, given that what we enjoy we tend to persist with, and what we do not enjoy, we tend to let go of.

Now another key principle, one that has transformed the lives of many people. The operative word in the third principle is "choose." We "choose" to enjoy doing whatever it is that we do. This is one of the great lessons the mind can teach us. We can choose how we respond to our circumstances.

Many people are literally slaves to what is happening in their lives. "Of course I am angry, look at what he did to me." "Of course I am sad, she left me, didn't she?" "Of course I am laughing, listen to this!" "Of course I am miserable, don't you know how sick I am?" There is no freedom in being a slave to your circumstances. You can rise above your situation and decide how you will respond to it.

Viktor Frankl was a world-renowned psychiatrist who was confined in the Nazis' concentration camps in the Second World War. He survived and wrote *Man's Search for Meaning*,[10] which highlighted two powerful observations. What Frankl realized first was the power of the will to live. In this toughest of environments, it was easy to die. Frankl observed that those who had a reason to live seemed to do so more often than those who lost it. Whenever anyone gave up hope, they seemed to die quickly.

So consider this, what inspires you to live? Why do you want to recover? What will you do when you regain your good health? The more heartfelt that motivation, the more Frankl would say you are likely to survive.

The second observation is more directly relevant to our discussion. Frankl was in a concentration camp where every effort was made to deprive the captives of their freedom. This was carried through ruthlessly and thoroughly. Most human freedoms can in fact be stripped away. Yet Frankl observed that there was one freedom that no one could take away if the individual had the state of mind to recognize it and to preserve it. That ultimate human freedom is the freedom to decide how we respond to our circumstances. So in the camps, that may have been the freedom to decide how to go into a gas oven. Would one go in kicking and screaming, or walking with their head held high? Either would be understandable. No one could decide which it would be other than the person involved and no one could take away the freedom to choose how to do it, if that person was clear-minded.

Marjory had experienced a blessed life. In her early seventies, still married to her teenage sweetheart, her three children all doing well, she developed an aggressive, painful cancer. Marjory had a strong Christian faith. A regular member of her local church, she was active across her community. She had led a charmed life free of any real suffering. So why this tough illness? What sense did it make? It really challenged Marjory's Christian view and caused her deep introspection. "Why me?" seemed a profound mystery to her.

Marjory's response was extraordinary. She decided that her faith in God, which she had believed to be strong, had never been tested. Having had such an easy life, for Marjory it had been easy to have faith. Now it was not so easy. Marjory decided the test was to find out if she could suffer well, if her faith could withstand a real test.

What anyone else might think of this response is to miss the point. Marjory's illness progressed steadily, attended by bouts of serious discomfort and pain. But a strange thing happened. She grew in strength. Her faith shone through and she only had one problem. As her illness advanced and her physical condition deteriorated, more and more of her friends wanted to spend time with her. Her family told me they felt Marjory was demonstrating how to suffer well and how to die well.

Maybe you do not think this is such a positive story, but I suggest that again, this would be to miss the point. As Marjory approached her death, her body became increasingly frail, yet her spirit shone through. It was there for all to see. In my experience of this, Marjory found her own way to conquer cancer. She died with a deep satisfaction, a deep peace. Marjory died knowing she had chosen how to respond to her situation and she had seen it through without wavering. She died with her faith stronger, her confidence assured.

And her family? They felt the loss deeply. But they told me how meaningful the experience was for them also. They had the mixed emotions of grief and elation, and the knowing they had been a part of something extraordinary.

So choose to enjoy doing it! Sure, if things are tough you may need to work at it and revisit all the items we listed for reinforcing your good intentions. But it can be done. It is an act of choice. You can choose to be positive. You can choose to enjoy doing whatever you turn your mind toward and remarkable things can be accomplished.

FINALLY, A SUMMARY

Positive Thinking Requires:
- A sound understanding of how the mind functions, particularly the three principles of positive thinking.
- A commitment to be positive.
- Good information on which to base our decisions.
- A calm clear mind that is free to make the best choices possible. To have a calm and clear mind we need:
  - freedom from stress and confusion;
  - freedom from conflicting emotions;
  - freedom from unhelpful habits and prejudices;

- the ability to draw on the rational, logical mind, as well as our intuition and inner wisdom.
- The most reliable technique that delivers a calm and clear mind is meditation.
- Diligence—the capacity to commit to our goals, to embrace them, to persevere and to accomplish them.
- Good support.

Put all this together and extraordinary things are possible; in fact, what seems extraordinary can become commonplace!

However, some of us will be familiar with the New Year's resolution syndrome. This is when we have a good intention that makes really good logical sense, and yet we struggle to do it, or even worse, just forget all about it. So in our next chapter on mind training we need to investigate and understand the power that beliefs and habits can have in our life, and put them to good use, as well.

CHAPTER 8

Mind Training 2

Habits and Beliefs, Affirmations and Imagery: The Unconscious Mind at Work

THE UNCONSCIOUS MIND IS THE STOREHOUSE FOR OUR BELIEFS AND OUR habits. Our beliefs and our habits powerfully shape our lives. We know that what we often describe as "negative" beliefs and habits can be powerfully destructive, while when we use them effectively, strong beliefs and healthy habits can set us free and catalyze profound healing.

For example, if our belief is that cancer always proves fatal and there is nothing we can do about it, we are in deep trouble once diagnosed. If we believe we can overcome cancer, then that outcome becomes a real possibility. If we conclude we need to change our way of eating to give ourselves the best chance of recovery, and yet we are stuck in our old habits and cannot change, again we are in real trouble. If changing unhelpful habits or adopting new ones comes naturally, or we learn how to do it, then the whole process of change can be enjoyable and a source of pride, as well as being highly beneficial to ourselves and to those around us.

Our beliefs and our habits can bind us, or set us free.

The potential that the unconscious mind holds is another crucial factor in recovery and so in this chapter we aim to understand its role and how we can use it to best effect. The focus will be on developing beliefs and habits that actively support the process of recovery, along with the use of affirmations and imagery. To begin with, we will investigate how beliefs have the remarkable power to both destroy life and to restore it. Please note that my own book *The Mind That Changes Everything*[11] is recommended as a companion piece for these chapters on the healing power of the mind.

THE DESTRUCTIVE POWER OF BELIEF • The Pointing of the Bone Effect

One of the most extreme examples of the destructive power of the mind comes from the ancient peoples of Australia. As we discussed in chapter 2, the pointing of the bone is a potent ritual that involves no direct physical force, yet it routinely results in death. The only known cases of a traditional Australian Aborigine successfully surviving being pointed is when an antidote in the form of another ritual has been applied and, in doing so, convinced the victim that the second ritual had more power than the first.

When we examine it closely, the key element in the first ritual, the bone pointing is that it creates hopelessness, a powerful belief that there is no other hope, no other expectation, than to die. What the antidote provides is a satisfactory rationale, congruent with the belief system of the victim that validates the real possibility of recovery. The antidote replaces hopelessness with hope.

Knowing about all this provides two more keys to recovery—the power of hope, and the power of the placebo.

THE HEALING POWER OF BELIEF • The Placebo Response, Hope and Recovery

If the pointing of the bone demonstrates the negative impact of beliefs, placebos clearly reveal their positive effects.

When new drugs are tested, people believe they may be useful. It is well-known in the medical world that this belief on its own can produce very positive results, so a sugar-coated pill with no active ingredients is used to measure how much benefit that belief will produce. Then, the results gained with the new drug are compared to those of the placebo to measure the new drug's real value. The sugar-coated pill is called a placebo. In many conditions, "treatment" with a placebo manages to produce a 30 percent improvement. With pain, placebos given with enthusiastic conviction, "this will really help reduce the pain," have regularly produced pain relief comparable to heavy-duty narcotics. Just what the mind is capable of when beliefs are activated effectively is literally extraordinary.

Take the incredible story of an American "hillbilly" with a difficult throat cancer that had little prospect of a medical cure. This story is as extreme as the pointing of the bone, only in this case the outcome was extremely positive. Diagnosed by his local doctor, the patient was told that he was being referred to a large city hospital to have a new form of ray treatment that would cure him. Arriving in awe at the hospital, he was given a basic checkup. When a thermometer was put in the naive man's mouth, his clinician was astute enough to realize that the patient thought this was the new wonder treatment. After several sessions of this "treatment," the cancer disappeared completely! While we might smile at the mental picture of a simple "hillbilly" being cured by a thermometer, let us not lose sight of the importance of the principle he demonstrated so well.

The message is that the placebo works. Maybe in cancer medicine we could call the role the mind has through the power of belief "placebo medicine." For while it is clear that we can explain a good deal of how the mind has such positive effects in very practical ways, such as how it leads to good choices and commitment, it is also clear the mind on its own can dramatically affect our chances of recovery. What we are seeking through studying and using the power of belief is to avoid any downside comparable to the pointing of the bone effect, while we access the positive benefits demonstrated by the placebo response. However, rather than being "tricked" by a placebo, we seek to use our intelligence to harness that same potential.

How do we do it? The answer is simple. The more we believe in whatever we do, the more we will get the best out of any treatment we have, the more we are likely to reduce any potential side effects, and the more we will gain from all the self-help techniques we utilize.

Jim's story provides a glimpse of what is possible. Jim was diagnosed with widespread cancer of the prostate and given months to live. He plunged into feelings of despair and hopelessness. A self-made man, Jim stopped work and spent his days at home behind drawn curtains. He did this so no one would glimpse how he spent those days—crying! When it came time in the evening for his wife and children to return home, he did his best to pull himself together, attempted a brave face and struggled on. Jim said what he was really doing was simply waiting to die; he felt hopeless and he felt miserable.

One day, not long after this book was first released in 1984, Jim's gaze fell on the title at his local newspaper shop. *You Can Conquer Cancer*. Maybe there was something he could do for himself after all. He bought the book and then he asked his wife to take a look. This was all happening in Melbourne, and Jim's wife, Angela, knew of the groups I was running not far from where they lived. He came, but remained confused for the first few weeks. Jim could not comprehend at first how attending to his diet, becoming positive, using the power of his mind and meditating could achieve what the doctors could not. But hope was kindled.

Soon the curtains were open, the tears gone. Jim began talking to his wife and three boys. They enthusiastically embraced the dietary changes and supported him fully as he began to meditate regularly. The first sign of real progress was when the pain subsided. Jim said later that when the meditation brought him pain relief, it helped him to believe in what he was doing. It gave him the confidence to persevere and then to intensify what he had begun somewhat tentatively. Jim went on to have a complete, long-term remission.

The important conclusion we must take from all this is that if we do feel hopeless, if we do have doubts or fears, at the very least they have the capacity to undermine whatever we do, or worse as in Jim's case, render us passive, depressed and miserable. In extreme situations, they could have the same impact as the pointing of the bone.

WHAT IF MY BELIEFS ARE FRAGILE? • Building Hope

Doubts and fears are normal to begin with. Reread Jim's story above. Nearly everyone who ever came to one of the cancer groups came with some degree of fear, doubt, confusion, and uncertainty. That is normal. That is where most people begin. It is because we know this to be true that we need to address all these issues. This is not something of itself to be fearful, but it is something to act upon. The good news is that we can do something about it; the bad news is that those who do not know about all this, or do not act on it, severely limit their possibilities and often have a miserable time.

Here is what will help.

Step 1. Hope

To restate it, the starting point is hope. Hope is real. It only has to be done once to show that it is possible, but in fact we do know recovery happens quite regularly. Maybe this is a good time to revisit our discussions in earlier chapters around hope, statistics and individuals (see chapter 2), and not only dare to believe in what is possible, actually reconfirm the logic in the possibility of recovery.

However, what we hope for and believe to be possible is a combination of the knowledge we hold and the emotional overlay that affects that knowledge. We are all bound to know some people whose emotional life overrides their logic and whose hopes are more about emotion than reason. This is not always a problem, but if for example, fear overrides your sensibility, then that may well be a big problem.

Step 2. Clarity

To build hope, clarity is vital. Clarity begins with clearing our emotions and we will discuss how to manage this in the chapters on healthy emotions (see chapters 16 and 17). What we also need to appreciate is that clarity comes with knowledge and so we do need the best information possible. This is challenging amid the information-saturated age in which we live. We need to revisit the earlier sections on decision making that addressed how to sort out our choices, how to decide who and what to trust, who and what to believe (see chapter 3). The crucial point is to make the time to set clear goals and to commit to them.

Step 3. Action

Once we have hope, we need to do something with it. Do be reminded, however, that hoping for the best and doing nothing about it is what we call wishful thinking and we know that particular state of mind is a far cry from the potency of positive thinking. To convert hope into reality we need to act.

So next we need to apply the positive-thinking skills of the previous chapter. The eight steps that support the first principle of positive thinking—to set a clear goal—are where we begin. Following these guidelines helps us to make good choices and to develop confidence in those choices. Then we use the second principle, to do whatever it takes to follow through.

So do be reassured. The doubts and fears are normal to begin with; hope can be rekindled, the confidence and certainty we call belief is something that can be developed—reliably!

BELIEFS AFFECT ALL THAT WE DO

The next key point is that the benefit of whatever we do is a product of the actual thing itself, and the overarching and additional impact of our beliefs. Will you add the pointing of the bone effect or the placebo effect?

If we sit in front of a fantastic, really healthy organic salad, and the only thought going through our head is "Oh no, not another salad. I must be crazy to be eating this stuff!" then it is easy to imagine the physical benefit of the good food is significantly undermined by our state of mind. If on the other hand, we sit in front of the same salad and we think, "Wow! This is terrific! This is really going to do me good. I can feel myself healing," then not only do we gain the benefit from the good food, we gain the benefit that our mind has to offer.

So the message is to think through all that you do. Decide what is the best you can do. Accept that. Believe it to be true—it is the best you can do. Commit to it. Do all you can to reinforce it. Hang out with those that support what you are doing. Read books that reinforce what you are doing. Use all the positive-thinking techniques. This is how we utilize the power of belief and how we can be assured of getting the best out of whatever we do.

Next, we need to address the role habits play on the road to recovery.

THE HEALING POWER OF HABITS • Getting the Job Done

Habits are really useful. Imagine if we were not in the habit of cooking. Then, at each meal we would need to start from scratch. We would need to think about everything we planned to do and there would be a huge amount of information and technique to sort out. It would take forever. By contrast, most of us do cook pretty much on automatic—we do a lot of it by habit and it is quick, easy and satisfying. So a habit provides us with a fairly automatic way of doing something that often is learned by repeating that thing over and over.

The main point is that on the healing journey, habits can really free us up and support us to do the things we enjoy and that are good for us, or they can severely restrict us. We need to break free of any limitations and to ensure our habits do work for us. Good habits make for good health.

BREAKING FREE OF OLD HABITS AND REALIZING YOUR GOALS

I imagine most of us at some time in the past have suffered from what we can call the New Year's resolution syndrome. You know the one: this year I am going to give up smoking; or this year I will exercise every day; or this year I will transform my anger. These good intentions always make so much sense. They are logical choices, obviously in our best interests. Everyone around us it seems would welcome and support the changes. It should be so easy! Yet how often is it that only a week into January, rather than enjoying having made the changes, there is that nagging, recurrent guilt born of not only not having made the change, but often enough, not even being able to remember exactly what the resolution was.

One of the major challenges in using your own efforts to heal is that you are the one who has to do most of the work. You need to make the time to meditate. You are the one who needs to eat a healing diet, to exercise and so on. It is clear that on the healing journey what we need to do is develop and maintain healthy habits. Often this will require us to change our habits, and often to do this effectively, we will need to overcome the New Year's resolution syndrome.

It must be easy for each of us to reflect on times when goals seemed easy to achieve, when we decided to do something and just simply did it. But almost certainly we will have had other times when we seemed content (in a funny sort of way) to give up on a good idea all too easily and all too soon. We need to be aware of how the mind has the potential to restrict us, to bind us to old patterns, and notice too those magical times when the mind sets us free.

The question is, does all this happen at random or can we have some control? What we need now is to investigate the workings of our mind a little more deeply, to understand how our habits develop and how when we need to, we can change them in a way that is easy, sustainable and even enjoyable!

HABITS AND BELIEFS HAVE A LOT IN COMMON

Just as habits are a fairly automatic, somewhat unconscious way of doing things, beliefs could be said to be fairly automatic, somewhat unconscious ways of thinking about things. We can consciously remember, identify and discuss our habits and our beliefs, but both are held in the domain of the unconscious mind.

So that we can use both habits and beliefs to better advantage we need to establish how they develop and then learn the techniques of affirmations and imagery. What is to come is really empowering as it holds the potential to set us free from binding, limiting beliefs and habits, while enabling us to do what we need to do!

HOW HABITS AND BELIEFS DEVELOP • The Five Steps

Step 1. Habits and Beliefs Are a Product of Our Experiences

Our habits and beliefs begin to develop early in life. We have a range of life experiences that we take in, learn from, and use to form our habits and our beliefs. We become aware of these experiences, these life lessons via our five senses. So we see things, we hear them, we touch, smell and taste them.

What is important for us to realize is that what we do perceive with our five senses we generally take as being real. However, we often see something, hear something, feel something which we take to be real, only to find out later that we were wrong. If our perception is inaccurate and it concerns a major life issue, we could develop an inaccurate belief that affects our life in a major way. Further, our perception is not only affected by the physical senses.

Step 2. Our Perception Is Colored by Our Emotions and Our State of Mind

The perception of our experiences, the meaning and the relevance we place on them, is affected by our emotional and mental state. For example, it is claimed that when angry, our capacity to perceive and take in the truth of events happening around us is diminished by up to 90 percent. Furthermore, we will all know of people with befuddled minds. Minds that lack clarity for one reason or another. Maybe drugs, old age, limited knowledge or intelligence—all these things can dramatically affect perception and the capacity to develop really useful belief systems.

So sometimes we only see something once, or have something happen to us once, and because it is so emotionally charged it makes a deep impression. Other times things happen of little moment in our lives and we forget them almost as soon as they happen. Some things happen over and over so that we cannot help but remember them. Some things stick, others do not.

Step 3. Our Experiences Are Stored in Our Memory

The things that do stick, those experiences are stored in the unconscious realm of the brain as memories. The emotions that accompany memories have a big bearing on how important they are to us. Generally speaking, the more dramatic, the stronger the emotions, the more prominent the memories.

Step 4. Memories Are Stored as Images

When we analyze them, we find that memories are actually made up of images—primarily pictures, sounds (words) and feelings. Taste and smell can be involved to a lesser degree.

Step 5. Memories Accumulate to Produce Habits and Beliefs

As we accumulate memories, they steadily build up to produce our habits and our beliefs. The beliefs we have developed will be the reflection of the full range of our life experiences and these beliefs will lead to both positive and negative expectations. If you notice yourself saying, "This is too good to be true," or "That always happens to me," or "It is not like me to have done . . ." then you are voicing an expectation, a direct expression of your belief system.

Our beliefs and our habits can limit us or set us free.

THE IMPACT OF UNHELPFUL HABITS AND BELIEFS

Julia was a very likable lady. Her outgoing personality had led her into a successful designing career but her personal life was dogged by emotional distress, and she had cancer. Amid the safety of a residential cancer program, Julia spoke with frustration of the many relationships she had been in with what appeared to her to be highly suitable men. Yet time after time these relationships had turned sour.

Julia quickly came to realize she had a huge problem with not allowing intimacy into her life and that she had put barriers up against deepening relationships. She realized her relationship breakdowns had not "just happened." In fact more often than not she had actively destroyed them by the way she had acted.

Then Julia made the mind connection. As a young girl she had grown up in the country amid a large family. Here, there seemed to have been much of the best of country life—close contact with nature, an easy lifestyle, lots of friends and time with her parents and extended family. Then at the age of seven, Julia had been diagnosed with measles. In the family's large farmhouse, the only place Julia could be isolated was in the rather large pantry. Julia went from living in the midst of a very large, open, loving family to being confined by her parents in an internal room with no windows, poor ventilation and quite a few rats! Julia wondered what she had done wrong. Her seven-year-old brain concluded she must have been very bad, that no one really loved her, that she was not even worthy of love!

Looking back as an adult, Julia could reason that her family really did love her, but she also realized that this one powerful childhood experience had been anchored deep inside her unconscious mind and that it had shaped her behavior dramatically. Julia came to realize her deeply held belief of being unworthy of love had sabotaged all her relationships.

Then Julia made another crucial observation. All her life she had been driven to succeed. Now she realized that her burning ambition was motivated by repeated attempts to prove her self-worth to herself, and to others. While she had become quite successful, Julia was beginning to realize the cost she had paid for that success. It was time to find another way. Julia knew that what she needed was to change the inner beliefs she held about herself.

HOW HABITS AND BELIEFS CAN BIND US • Or Set Us Free

As human beings we have a fundamental commitment to act in accordance with our beliefs. The reality is that when we are doing what we believe in, we feel comfortable and satisfied—we have peace of mind. When our actions do not match our beliefs, we feel uncomfortable, we have a deep sense something is wrong, and we become highly motivated to do something about it.

What this means, what makes our beliefs so important, is that what we believe in becomes a yardstick for our actions. This is because we are constantly striving to fulfill our beliefs, to live true to our beliefs.

So if we happen to believe eating fast food or junk food is OK, and if we are in the habit of eating it and we like eating it, we are really stuck with it. Perhaps you think this is an extreme example, but I suggest we may all have things we believe in and are in the habit of doing, things we feel comfortable with, that are not all that healthy and that could well make it more difficult for us to get well and stay well. When we do not manage to change our unhealthy old habits and beliefs and to adopt and sustain healthy ones, recovery is given a major boost!

HOW TO CHANGE HABITS AND BELIEFS

Remember, habits and beliefs are stored in our unconscious mind and are the accumulated balance of our life experiences. Happily, we can learn how to replace unhelpful habits and beliefs with helpful ones.

What makes it possible to achieve this—in fact, what makes it easy—is that the unconscious mind cannot distinguish between a real-life experience (and the set of images that go with it) and artificial, positive experiences we can choose to generate (through the use of affirmation and imagery).

To establish, change or reinforce habits and beliefs in such a way that they will be effectively anchored in our unconscious mind and responded to, we need to learn how to use the techniques of affirmation and imagery.

HOW DO THESE TECHNIQUES WORK IN REAL LIFE?

Betty was a senior lady whose life had been lived helping others. She had supported her husband in his work, raised a fine family and contributed to her community. But now she had cancer with secondary spread, and in medical terms, a hopeless prognosis. There was no medical treatment offered or given to her. But Betty loved life and felt she had more to do. She came to our groups with her rather reluctant, but duty-bound husband. Phillip took all the sessions in, while he remained somewhat distant and aloof.

Betty's condition appeared to deteriorate at first, her pain became worse, and despondency set in. Sitting in her armchair one evening, tears began to well up in her eyes. Phillip, sensing Betty's mood, asked her what was wrong. She spoke gently of how perhaps it was all too much, perhaps she should face reality, accept her fate and give up on getting well.

As it turned out, up until now, Betty had always been a rather negative person. She explained later that a string of events early in life had not worked out as she hoped. She had taken those experiences in and developed a pessimistic view. At a deep level, Betty had come to believe that things always went wrong for her.

Fortunately for Betty, her husband had been paying attention during the group sessions. He had taken in the discussion on beliefs, affirmations and imagery, and he knew Betty was working on becoming more positive with the affirmation "I am a positive person now!" So Phillip, seeing his wife sitting there with gloom hanging over her head and pervading her very being, said to her, "That's strange. What are you now?"

"What do you mean?" responded Betty rather gloomily.

"Oh, I thought you were a positive person now."

Betty told me later this was a magical moment in her amazing recovery. With her husband's words, it was as if some inner switch was thrown.

"Yes," she said. "You are right. I am a positive person now!"

From that moment on, Betty's focus was on the positive side of life. Instead of the old half-empty glass she had been dealing with, now she truly saw the glass half full. She looked for the positive aspect in every situation, found it and, in the process, discovered a wonderful inner peace. Her physical recovery was quite remarkable and over twenty years later her calm and joyful manner was a delight to all who knew her.

The strong suggestion is to spend time reflecting on these principles that have the power to transform old unhelpful beliefs and establish new, healthy, healing belief systems and habits. The more you understand all this, the more you contemplate and take to heart how it all works, the easier it will be to use the techniques and the better they will work.

Once you have this solid framework of understanding, move on to put it all into practice. It is the use of affirmations and imagery that provides us with the technology of the mind to change our mind. One of the delightful things about affirmations and imagery is that they are rather simple to use. And they work! By following a fairly easy number of steps, we can develop a practice that has the potential to bring major benefits into our lives. First affirmations, then imagery.

How to Develop Affirmations

Affirmations are short, precise statements that summarize a specific goal. By repeating the affirmation over and over, it replaces any old, contradictory habits or beliefs and imprints the new one onto our unconscious mind.

Then, when we are faced with a new situation that requires us to respond, we check our unconscious and the affirmation guides us with what to do. Betty's story from above is a great example of an affirmation at work.

For affirmations to be effective they must satisfy three essential points, and then there is some fine-tuning to do.

STEP 1. THE THREE ESSENTIAL POINTS

Affirmations need to be expressed in the first person, present tense, and they need to be goal-oriented.

First person, present tense means we start our affirmations with words like "I am . . . ," "I do . . . ," "I have . . . ," etc.

Present time is the only time the unconscious responds to. What this means is that when we check with our memory to retrieve a habit or a belief, we are looking for what to do. If what comes out is "I am hoping to be a little more positive some time off in the future and I hope I will be, but probably I won't because I tried that before and it did not work so well, but I guess I better give it a go anyway," our mind is going to recognize our confusion for what it is and not act upon it. We will remain befuddled. If, on the other hand, our unconscious tells us, "I am a positive person now," then everything we do will need to satisfy that criteria for us to feel happy to commit to it. We will inevitably become more and more positive. Therefore affirmations need to indicate the goal is already achieved or reached. The aim is to give the mind a target to lock on to—the target is the end goal, hence, "I am a positive person now."

STEP 2. THE FINE-TUNING

Be Positive

Indicate what is needed, not what is not. The mind is goal-oriented, it locks on to targets. It needs a positive direction to aim for, not something to avoid. So, rather than saying, "I am not a negative person now," for an affirmation we use "I am a positive person now."

Avoid Comparisons

There is no need to say, "I am as good as . . . ," or "I am better than . . ." Your capacity, your potential, may be to be better, or it may be to be worse.

Aim to develop affirmations that encourage the development of your own full potential.

Unless Essential, Do Not Specify a Time for Completion

As with comparisons, specifying time may slow you down or frustrate you. Part of the joy in using affirmations is that they release the power of our creativity and inner wisdom. The fact is that this aspect of our being has a wonderful talent for getting us into the right place at the right time, and if we go with it, we will be content and at ease.

Do Be Specific, Accurate and Accountable

The mind needs a specific target. The more precise the goal, the greater its clarity, and the more confident you can be of success.

Be Realistic—*Expect a Discussion!*

You will be limited by what you believe is possible. However, it is normal to expect some reaction to using affirmations.

"I am a positive person now," you say. "No, you're not," comes that little doubting echo. That is normal. The echo is the old belief having its say. If it were not there, you would have very little need to use the affirmation in the first place.

Remember, this process directs or redirects the mind's attention and mobilizes all its power and creativity. This is a process for making change, for replacing one belief with another, as well as simply establishing a new belief or goal. So do not be surprised by the echo. As long as the affirmation has more energy, more expectation, more hope, more determination, more *oomph* than the echo, and it is repeated, it will gradually replace it and soon become the guiding force for your mind.

Consider Setting Ongoing Goals

You will need to stay within the bounds of what you can believe is reasonably possible. Some people, for example, can imagine themselves fully recovered and can set that as their goal. Others may be more confident of their condition becoming stable and recognize this is a big step in itself. Set goals you can commit to and then as you observe yourself nearing completion of one goal, look for what comes next. Extend your planning and make new resolutions.

Use Action Words and Add a Sense of Excitement

The feeling, the emotion that goes with an affirmation has a lot to do with how quickly it will imprint and be accepted by the unconscious. Affirmations, therefore, work better when said with zest and excitement. One way to do this is to add "Wow!" on the end of them: "I am a positive person now—Wow!" Saying "Wow!" encapsulates that positive, expectant feeling. If "Wow!" does not suit you, use another word or phrase from your own vocabulary to enliven your affirmation.

Similarly, look for ways of expressing confidence, ease, naturalness and joy in all you aim for.

Be Precise with the Use of Your Words

Words used in affirmations are definitely words of power. Pay great attention to how they might be interpreted. You can cover your bets by adding words like "in a harmonious way." Be as clear and precise as possible, consider all angles and choose your words wisely. Meditating and contemplating on your choice of affirmations before you use them is an excellent way to check their meaning and their validity—for you.

Keep a Balance

Affirmations can have a profound effect upon your direction in life. Consider again the range of goals you are setting. Take heed of your physical, emotional, mental and spiritual needs and those of your family, friends and community. Affirmations are exciting tools to use. Aim to maintain that sense of balance.

Some Sample Affirmations for Personal Development

These are some favorite, well-tested affirmations that can act as a guide for your own needs:

FOR HEALTH

"Every day in every way I am getting better and better."

This is one of the oldest and most famous affirmations. It was first used over a century ago by a Frenchman, Emile Coué, and recorded in his book *Self-Mastery Through Conscious Autosuggestion*.[12]

It remains an extremely powerful and effective tool for mobilizing our inner drive toward better health.

"Actively engaged with healing, I experience life fully and give myself every chance of recovery."

FOR RELATIONSHIPS
"I greet this person with love."

FOR SELF-ESTEEM
"I am worthy of being here."
"I am worthy of being happy."
"I am worthy of being loved."

OVERCOMING FEAR, FACING DYING
"Prepared for death, I transform fear."
"Prepared for death, I live well, and when my time comes, die well."

Before discussing the finer practical details of how to combine the practical use of affirmations, imagery and feelings, let us examine how to develop imagery.

HOW TO DEVELOP IMAGERY

While affirmations focus on the use of words, imagery involves using inner pictures to imprint a new goal on our subconscious mind and so stimulate our motivation and creativity to achieve that goal.

Choose the Type of Imagery That Suits Your Needs
There are three classifications for the types of images we can use—literal, symbolic and abstract.

Literal Images

With this type of imagery, we aim to see an image of the behavior, event or goal literally. This means you visualize your goal the way you are intending it to happen and you repeat it over and over in your mind's eye, a bit like rerunning a video or DVD. This literal imagery is very practical and can be applied in any situation where there is a clear understanding of the goal. This literal style is widely used in sport and has well-established benefits for changing habits and beliefs.

So if you have a very tangible goal like becoming less anxious and more positive, the use of literal imagery can be a great asset. Imagine yourself in situations where you used to be negative, only now you see yourself calm and relaxed, making positive choices, acting in a way that you consider to be positive, and feeling a sense of pride and achievement. Combining this with an affirmation such as "I am a positive person now" and persisting with the repetition of both virtually assures a change in the behavior.

While literal images are highly effective in sport and for making personal changes, when the goal is clear but the mechanism for achieving it is uncertain, highly complex or to do with healing, symbolic or abstract imagery is often far more appropriate.

Symbolic and Abstract Imagery

Symbols can be used as a vehicle to convey our conscious intention into the subconscious in a way that the intention can be recognized and acted upon. Take healing, for example. The complexity and timing of the healing process is beyond most, if not all, conscious minds. However, one does not need sophisticated instruments to learn how to influence the body's healing functions directly. Imagery in either the symbolic or abstract form is probably the most powerful tool for this purpose and we will investigate and learn these specific techniques in the next chapter.

HOW TO PRACTICE AFFIRMATIONS AND IMAGERY

Affirmations are best repeated with positive expectation, with power, confidence and good feeling. If you have a fair degree of confidence when you first begin to use a particular affirmation, you will only need to repeat it for a minute or two a few times a day and that mind-set will soon become established. When you have a more challenging belief to establish, or if your mind is cluttered, you will need to practice more often and for longer periods.

The imagery that accompanies affirmations is used similarly and the time you will need to practice it will depend on the ease and clarity that accompanies the image. While an individual session of symbolic imagery usually takes about ten minutes, abstract imagery can be used for longer times. For instance, a session of the white light healing imagery (which will be described in the next chapter) can easily occupy thirty to sixty minutes. Also, abstract imagery can be an excellent prelude to letting go into the simple silence of deeper meditation.

Affirmations and imagery can be used together. This is the most direct and effective way. However, sometimes you may feel it more appropriate to use an affirmation or imagery on its own.

For example, an affirmation on its own may work well to begin the process of changing an undesired long-standing state of mind such as low self-esteem. You may find it more effective to begin by repeating, "I am worthy of love now" as an affirmation. Then, once some confidence in the accuracy and reality of that statement is established you may enhance the affirmation by adding related and supportive images. In the case of building self-esteem, you could remember situations where previously you had felt awkward, underconfident, and vulnerable, and now you re-create those same situations in your mind and imagine yourself to be calm, at ease, confident and feeling good about yourself. Similarly, many healing situations appear to respond well to the direct use of imagery.

With the repetition of affirmations and imagery, our aim is to imprint a consciously chosen goal onto our unconscious mind so that it becomes anchored as a habit and/or a belief. This belief will then act as a target that our mind will do all possible to direct us toward.

The process of imprinting occurs most easily and most effectively when there is a close connection between the conscious mind and the unconscious. A good example of this is when we are in that reverie state just before going to sleep. It is when our mind is relaxed, not dwelling on anything in particular, and at peace. That state of reverie before you get out of bed in the morning, or as you go to bed at night, can serve as an excellent time to practice affirmations and imagery.

Also, singing or joking with affirmations loosens the power of the conscious mind and its conditioned responses, and so facilitates the imprinting process. Making up jingles for your affirmations and singing them out loud can be useful and fun!

Looking directly into your eyes via a mirror and saying your affirmations out loud with power and conviction is extremely effective if you can do it.

Best of all is to combine imagery with your meditation. The meditation provides a poise and balance and has a stabilizing effect on the whole process.

HOW TO COMBINE RELAXATION, IMAGERY AND MEDITATION

(a) Sit in a slightly uncomfortable, symmetrical position.
(b) Relax physically, inducing the relaxation response wherever possible.
(c) Then begin the imprinting—using affirmations and imagery in combination or separately.
(d) Let go of the imagery and rest in the natural peace and stillness of meditation before finishing the session.

SUPPORT YOUR GOOD INTENTIONS, RESPOND TO FEEDBACK

Reinforce your good intentions, your affirmations and imagery with these powerful supports:

- Develop a support network. Discuss your goals with family and friends. Get them on your side. Consider enlisting the new technologies and activating your social media contacts.
- Seek out allies who can support you wholeheartedly. Avoid those who challenge you too directly or too strongly.
- Read books, listen to CDs and DVDs and attend workshops that support your goals.
- Attend a support group or meditation group that is relevant to your needs.
- Tell others of your goal—be accountable.
- Be prepared for setbacks. Changing habits can take time. Be prepared to persevere.
- Be gentle on yourself. Determine to be patient and reward yourself as you notice progress.

- Do seek feedback. Be prepared to reassess your situation, make adjustments and move on.
- Smile regularly! All of this needs to be fun to be sustained. Enjoy being alive. Change is a feature of life. If you were not changing you would be dead. Enjoy the changes by celebrating your successes.

DEALING WITH SETBACKS

While you may move steadily and uneventfully toward your goals, it may also be that life goes up and down a little along the way. Setbacks can cause you to reassess your whole situation, strengthen your resolve and lead to useful modifications and changes.

The best insurance against disappointment is to give whatever you do your best, to do everything to 100 percent of your ability. Then if you have a setback, there will be no regrets, no guilt, no wondering "What if . . . ," or "If only I had . . ." At least you will have the comfort of knowing you have been giving it your all. Then there will be a level of acceptance and acknowledgment that leaves you free from looking backward. You will be free to look forward for fresh solutions.

With this approach, answers to questions and solutions for setbacks seem to come very reliably. When I was ill, often the answers to setbacks came via books. Often when faced with another setback (there were many in my own road to recovery), it would seem as if I was drawn almost intuitively, almost magnetically, to a particular book. I would open it and there would be the answer on the page in front of me! Often too, old friends would appear unannounced and have the answers. The more I trusted in the process, whenever a question or problem presented itself, the more I expected an answer, the more rapidly it appeared. Synchronicity at work! Or is it manifestation?

ESTABLISH YOUR GOAL • Move Toward the Moment

While your new goal and the changes that go with it are bound to require your conscious effort to begin with, it is to be hoped that after a while it becomes effortless, a natural part of your life. As a part of this natural flow, be prepared to move on from using active creative imagery techniques into the quieter stillness of meditation.

Be prepared for new qualities in your imagery and meditation.

As time goes on, your practice of imagery will develop and your quality of meditation will improve. You may discover that this leads to feeling more in tune with your life and the world around you. You will move steadily into a better experience of current time. You may well find there is then less need to practice imagery and that the process of goal setting and achievement begins to flow naturally, easily and powerfully with your passage through life.

A FINAL STORY, AND A GIFT

A high-powered corporate accountant involved in management takeovers and restructuring, Robert admitted to being a tough number cruncher. He hardly knew his children, fought regularly with his wife and, despite material success, was deeply unhappy. His cancer diagnosis was devastating. He had the sense of impending doom and feared the happiness he hoped he would always get to later in life was going to elude him. He rapidly plunged into the depths of despair and strong suicidal thoughts filled his mind.

Amidst this depression Robert came to our groups and realized there was hope. He leaped at the possibilities and with his usual flair, vigor and commitment proceeded to turn his life around. He changed his attitude, he changed his lifestyle, and he changed his job. His health changed and he became another person to experience a medically unexplained and quite remarkable recovery.

Many years later, Robert thanks the cancer for what it has done for him. Like so many others, he says it was as if before his diagnosis he was living his life on automatic. He was putting up with so many compromises in his life and hoping that some time off in the future he might find happiness and might have time to be happy. The cancer changed all that. With the diagnosis, his future became uncertain.

Realizing he may not have long to live, Robert felt he had to address what was happening now. The old compromises became unacceptable; he realized the value of relationships. He set about healing the relationship with his wife and began getting to know his children better. He sought work where he could live his real ethics and sense of values. So much changed for the better as a result of the cancer, that Robert thanks it for helping him to reassess his priorities and values and for putting them in order.

It is an unhappy observation that for many of us it takes a major trauma before we deeply question our habits and our beliefs. So often it seems we take life for granted, put up with the compromises and hope to find happiness later. Perhaps this is one of the great gifts on offer from the many people I have worked with who have been diagnosed with cancer. Why wait? Why put it off? Life is so precious. And so uncertain. Why not take time now to reconsider what you really value and what your true priorities are?

There is a wonderful exercise (below) that is a real gift, as it provides the mechanism for working with these ideas.

The beauty of this exercise, which has been popularized more recently as "the bucket list," is that it can provide clarity and direction for everyone. For those who are well, it can provide the benefit of a life-threatening illness, without having to get sick!

The "What If?" Exercise

Give yourself time and space and sit down with pen and paper. Fantasize. Imagine that for the next three months, everything in your life will stay the same. You will have all the same possibilities, all the same limitations. At the end of this time, your life (your life alone) will end. There is no bargaining, no extensions. This is a fantasy exercise and the first question is:

If you had three months to live, what would be the ten most important things that you would do?

Take time to contemplate this question. Then write your answers down. Review them, perhaps you can rank them in order of priority.

The second part to the exercise is to consider how much of your time currently is being given to these priorities? If you are like many people, you may well find that the top priorities are getting very little time. Commonly, they are being put off. So, the second question is:

"What would it take to fulfill the priorities you have set?"

Contemplate that question.

CHAPTER 9

Mind Training 3

The Mind-Body Connection: Using the Power of the Mind for Healing

SANDY WAS IN HER LATE THIRTIES AND HAD TWO YOUNG CHILDREN AND A husband who was very successful in business. Her diagnosis of breast cancer devastated the family, particularly as the cancer had already spread into her bones. After breast surgery, her ovaries were removed in the hope this might slow down the progress of the disease.

When Sandy came to our cancer support group many years ago, she changed her diet, learned to meditate and began to use imagery. Sandy had difficulty seeing pictures to use in imagery. She was one of those people who found "visualization" difficult. However, with a little experimentation and discussion, we soon found Sandy was strongly kinesthetic—she *felt* her images. She also had a strong Christian faith. So Sandy imagined the presence of God in the sky above her. She then prayed in a way that led to her feeling connected to her God. Then, immersed in this feeling, she felt a stream of healing energy flowing down through her head and into her body.

Sandy had seen her bone scan. She had two secondary cancers in her bones—one located in the left hip, the other in one of her ribs. When she saw the scan, her attention had focused on the lesion in her hip; she had not really taken in the one in her ribs.

About eight weeks after diagnosis, Sandy and her family were required to make a major move to follow her husband's work. Sandy was keen to find out how her cancer was progressing, as this information may have affected their choices. Her doctors felt at best her condition may be the same, they strongly implied it was likely to be worse. They were quite unprepared for what they found! The lesion in the ribs had remained unchanged—no worse, no better. Yet the lesion in the hip was not only better, the cancer was gone and the bone had regenerated completely. It was fully healed!

Sandy was delighted to share her good news with the group. But then came her realization that she had formed a clear mental picture of the hip lesion, based upon what she had seen of her scan. With the imagery, she was able to feel this flow of energy, coming from its divine source, and as it came into her body, she felt a flow of warmth come with it. She said that for her, she knew the healing was flowing whenever she felt the warmth. Sandy realized, however, that while she had done this clearly and powerfully for the hip, she had neglected the ribs almost completely.

Obviously, the next step was for Sandy to direct the healing energy to her ribs. She went home to put this into practice but rang me a few days later very concerned. In attempting to focus on her rib, she found strong feelings rising up that in doing this she was neglecting the hip and that the cancer would recur.

Reflecting on this for a moment, I asked Sandy how big her God was. She said her God was infinite. So I asked her to consider that she was drawing healing energy from this infinite source and then feeling there was not enough to go around! She laughed at the limitation she was imposing, and recognized the logical flaw in her feeling of inadequacy. Interestingly enough, however, it still took her about two weeks of practice before she felt fully comfortable with the notion of healing the second lesion while she adequately covered the rest of her body.

Given what was essentially good news, with one lesion completely healed, Sandy and her family decided to go ahead with their move. This involved the usual pressures of packing and unpacking, major change, readjustment, saying good-bye to friends, renewing old relationships and making new beginnings. Shortly afterward and, conscious of the potential effects of stress, Sandy had more tests to reassess her situation. No change—the hip all clear, the ribs still affected. Three months later, a well-settled Sandy had her next tests. All clear—healed hip, healed ribs—a remarkable recovery.

Sandy's story is a dramatic example of many cases where the use of specific forms of imagery brought specific results. Coincidence? Well, maybe, but there does seem to be a lot more to it.

Sarah had a similar background and problem to Sandy—except that Sarah had eleven bony secondaries that were diagnosed three years after her treatment for primary breast cancer. Sarah had seen her bone scans, fixed that image in her mind, was very visual in her imagery and imagined each lesion healing. She received excellent support from her family and her local doctor who was actively involved with mind-body techniques and integrative medicine. Three months later, all the cancer was gone—except for one lesion in her hip. Sarah and her GP were puzzled by this until they checked with the original scan. Sarah had missed seeing that particular lesion in her hip! She had retained a clear picture of all the other spots but had missed this one. Sarah adjusted her imagery. Three months later, at her next scan, the hip was clear too.

Steven's diagnosis of lung cancer led to major chest surgery with removal of the lower section of one lung in an unsuccessful attempt to rid him of the cancer. At the point where the windpipe (bronchus) was severed to remove the lung, staples were used to seal it shut. Not long after the surgery, these staples popped open creating a bronchopleural fistula—a large cavity filled with air in the chest. A CAT scan demonstrated that a large triangular area was affected.

Steven sought several opinions, hoping the lung might heal itself or that further surgery would fix it. His doctors were convinced the breakdown had resulted from the activity of cancer that had been left after the surgery. They told Steven that the area remaining was like a buttery mass in his chest, that it could not heal itself and further surgery was dangerous and unwarranted. They offered to wait and see, and that if it did unexpectedly improve, then perhaps they could staple it again later. Steven pressed the doctors, asking if they were sure it could not heal on its own. "Absolutely. There is no way!" they stated emphatically.

Now Steven had some previous experience of meditation with Dr. Ainslie Meares. This had helped him through a period of stress some twenty years earlier. Although he had let the practice slip, there was an experience, a foundation to build upon—and a sense of the possible. After coming to our residential program, Steven returned to intensive meditation and also began a new practice—imagery. Every day, he began his meditation sessions with ten to fifteen minutes of imagery. As a bonus, Steven found that the imagery flowed easily and naturally into the stillness of meditation. The imagery enhanced his meditation.

For his imagery, Steven brought the CAT scan to mind. In a very visual way, he saw the lesion fairly literally. Then on a microscopic level, Steven imagined filling in the hole, using symbolic bricks of a wobbly, rectangular shape that for him represented new lung cells. In his mind he envisaged these bricks slowly building up, one on top of the other, re-forming healthy lung tissue and closing the gap. Three months later, a rather incredulous doctor showed Steven a healthy CAT scan, with the report that the bronchopleural fistula has spontaneously healed! Spontaneously! Steven is in no doubt that the meditation and the specific imagery work was what did it.

So how can we explain these cases, these anecdotes? Are they just coincidences? Is it just mind over matter—or is there more to it? I believe that there is a simple theoretical basis behind these remarkable true stories. While it will be wonderful when these observations and hypotheses are followed up by serious research, this theory is based upon good science and when converted into practice through the use of imagery there is the potential to help many people overcome a wide range of illnesses.

THE RATIONALE OF HEALING IMAGERY

To put healing imagery in its full context, we need to go back to basics. The body has an extraordinary ability to heal itself. It is exquisitely well designed to cope with both trauma and disease. The body's basic urge is to maintain itself in the dynamic state of balance we call health.

To understand this a little more we need to appreciate how these healing mechanisms are controlled. In the late sixties and seventies, when I went through my veterinary training, not much was known about all this. We did know, for example, that the immune system played a major role in the body's defenses. As well as the immunity made active by our white blood cells, we knew there was cellular immunity too—that the cells of the body themselves had some capacity to resist infection and even cancer.

However, these healing mechanisms were thought to operate largely independently, and in a way that was removed from any central nervous system or mind control.

Current knowledge has come a long way! It is now well-known that the brain regulates healing in two major ways—the first by the wide variety of chemicals it produces, the other via direct nerve pathways.

What we now know is that different states of mind, different feelings and different emotions produce different and quite specific chemicals in the brain. These chemicals—called neurotransmitters, neuropeptides or, more simply, messenger molecules—are then released into the bloodstream. Traveling in the blood they then flow to cells of the immune system. There they attach onto specific receptor sites on the outer membranes of those cells. By doing so, they then trigger changes within the cells that dramatically affect their function.

This, then, is another key point. It is not only a matter of how many immune cells you have, it is a matter of how actively and effectively these cells are functioning. For a long time it has been known that white blood cells are the front line for the immune system. Also, for a long time it has been known that having too many of these cells is a problem, just as it is to have too few. More recent research, however, has revealed you could have the right number, but they could still range in function from inactive and so ineffective to highly active and highly effective. Clearly an active, vibrant immune system made up of the appropriate number of cells is a strong prerequisite for both good health and active healing.

One of the key principles in mind-body medicine is that what we commonly characterize as negative thoughts readily depress immune function, while so-called positive thoughts enhance it. What this means is that if you are depressed, suffer unresolved grief or bottle up your emotions, you are highly likely to release specific chemicals from your brain that will directly suppress immune function.

Happily, on the other hand, when you are inspired, feel a surge of hope or love, or when you have a good laugh, other different but similarly specific messenger molecules are released from the brain, travel via the bloodstream, attach to immune cells, and activate them markedly.

Furthermore, quite remarkably, it is now known that cells of the immune system, the white blood cells, produce their own messenger molecules that they too release into the bloodstream. These molecules return to the brain, giving feedback and completing the loop of communication between the mind and the healing functions of the body. This is another key principle that helps us to understand how mind-body medicine works.

THE HEALING CENTER IN THE BRAIN

What all these recent discoveries point to is that there is a healing center in the brain that has a great capacity to control and regulate healing throughout the body.

This notion of a healing center is very similar to the fact we have a running center in the brain. By this I mean when you decide to go for a run, the idea starts as a conscious thought in your mind. However, when it comes to the actual process of the running, that is a very complex process. Fortunately, when you go for a run you do not need to consciously think how to move this leg and that, how to combine the movement of your legs in rhythm with your arms, and how to regulate your heart rate and your breathing. That complexity is controlled by the automatic part of the brain.

The process of going for a run begins with the conscious thought "I will go for a run." Then that conscious thought goes down into the unconscious, automatic part of the brain where "the running center" picks up the message, recognizes it, and says, "Sure, I know how to do that. How fast do you want to go?" Again, using conscious intention, we may give the message to speed up or slow down, while the actual process of running remains under automatic direction.

Now, everyone it seems has needed to go to the trouble of learning how to connect the conscious desire to run, with the automatic center that actually does it for us. I love watching young children learning to walk and run. You see them struggle up onto their feet, usually hanging on to a chair or table leg. And you see the thought form: "I'm going to walk across the room." And off they go, full of hope, full of expectations. A few tottery steps and crash! Down they go. Now I have yet to see a toddler just lie there, give up, and say, "Well, I guess I am going to be one of those kids who never learns to walk!" No, it seems so natural. They get up, try again, and again, and finally master it.

So it seems most of us have taken the time to learn how to connect the conscious mind with the brain's running center. What I suggest is that the same potential is there to control the healing center. It is just that most of us have not yet learned how to consciously connect with it.

What we need, then, is a reliable mechanism that will connect the conscious intention "I want to heal" with that automatic, unconscious part of the brain that regulates healing. We need a link between the conscious mind and the unconscious. Sound familiar?! Obviously, what provides such a link is the creative use of imagery.

In healing, as elsewhere, imagery provides a link between the conscious intention and the automatic function.

We can use imagery as a vehicle to carry a specific message concerning a need to heal in a specific way from the conscious mind, through the healing center and on directly to the body's wonderful array of healing mechanisms.

IMAGERY OR MEDITATION?

Before we move into the techniques that make all this possible, here is another important reminder of the value of meditation and balance. Do remember that in the simple silence of mindfulness-based stillness meditation (MBSM) we return to a profound sense of balance and in that state, healing is free to flow naturally.

So the question often arises when it comes to healing, is meditation enough or should I do imagery only? Or a bit of both?

I encourage everyone who is engaged actively in healing to practice simple, stillness meditation. It provides that deep sense of balance, a stable foundation from which to work and within which to heal.

About three-quarters of the people affected by cancer that I help take up the practice of imagery. What I have found through this experience is that imagery is particularly helpful for people when recently diagnosed, particularly if they have their own fears and anxieties for the future, or have been given bad news poorly and had their hope taken away. Also, imagery is usually easy for people who have active minds. As an added bonus, it combines particularly well with any form of treatment, providing a direct means to support that treatment with the active and creative power of the mind. Imagery is a reliable, intelligent way to harness the potential that the placebo response establishes.

The principles to have strongly in mind with the use of healing imagery are that as for other imagery exercises, the images need to be accurate, complete and feel good to use. This latter point is of particular importance. Often when you begin imagery you know it could be better, you have the sense that as a beginner you are learning, but it feels good. You feel confident with where you are with it, against the background of knowing with time and more practice the actual technique will improve. This sense of feeling content and basically confident with your imagery is a vital ingredient in its successful application.

WHAT TYPE OF IMAGERY TO USE FOR HEALING

Remember, too, that when it comes to technique, we can use three types of imagery—literal, symbolic or abstract. Obviously, as has been explained earlier, healing is an area where the actual physical reality is that it involves a complex interaction of many processes that really are far better suited to being regulated by the automatic, unconscious healing center of the brain rather than by direct conscious act of will. So literal images have very limited use, although, as the examples we have already used demonstrate, semiliteral images (such as CAT scans, X-rays, photographs of immune cells, etc.) can provide a useful starting point for healing imagery.

The fact is that while healing imagery is a technique that has helped many and offers great promise, it needs to be well thought through and thoroughly planned. Let us move on then to consider how we can put all this into practice.

First, here is a summary of the necessary steps for the use of symbolic imagery.

HOW TO USE SYMBOLIC IMAGERY FOR HEALING • The Principles

Step 1. Develop symbolic images that represent:
   (a) the illness
   (b) any treatment
   (c) the immune system and other aspects of the body's healing mechanisms
Step 2. Combine these images into a sequence of action in a way that removes the image of the illness and replaces it with a symbol of fully restored health.
Step 3. Check that these symbols are accurate and complete and that you can feel good using them.
Step 4. Support your practice with meditation, other imagery exercises where necessary, and the general principles of positive thinking.
Step 5. Assess your progress, and modify or adapt your imagery as required. You may well find that over the longer term the urge to practice imagery declines and you feel more fully satisfied with the ongoing practice of meditation.

SYMBOLIC IMAGERY FOR HEALING • The Practice

Step 1. Develop the Images

When using your own symbolic images for healing they need to represent the illness for you in a way that is acceptable intellectually and, even more important, intuitively. Symbolic imagery is very personal, so the best images are the ones that you can identify with directly. The best measure for assessing that you have good, useful images is that they feel good.

There are four main ways to derive images for healing:

BY BEING INSPIRED BY OTHER PEOPLE'S IMAGES

Sometimes as you read of other people's imagery or listen to others discuss it, you are inspired and your own image springs to mind, based upon what you have read or heard. Having said that, in my experience it rarely works if you try to take on someone else's images just because they worked for them.

An excellent example of what we are discussing here involved an elderly lady who came to me having read the Simontons' excellent book *Getting Well Again*[13] (a highly recommended read if you are using healing imagery). Margaret was a small woman. Petite, well dressed, conservative and polite to a fault, she had a warm, gentle and kindly quality that was very endearing. Margaret had taken in the Simontons' recommendation to use aggressive images. She latched onto their suggestion to imagine the cancer as being like lumps of meat in the body and the immune system as being a pack of savage, hungry dogs that were let loose to race around the body and greedily gobble up the meat (alias the cancer). As Margaret described these dogs in detail, I recoiled at the terrifying picture she presented. Asking her what she felt about these dogs, Margaret replied, "Well, actually, they scare me to death!" When I asked her how she felt about being scared to death by an image that represented her own immune system, she realized she needed to change the picture.

Talking on, it became apparent Margaret's passion in life was her garden. So, together we worked out she could imagine her body to be a beautiful garden, the cancer would be a particular form of weed and her immune system was a very wise and diligent old gardener. Margaret's chemotherapy would be a weed killer that had a very selective action. It would kill the weeds (cancer) very effectively, but the rest of the garden (her body) would be unaffected by it. Then the gardener would add compost to the garden, representing the good food that made up Margaret's new diet. With all this, the garden would thrive.

We now had an accurate image Margaret could feel good about and that was consistent with her nature and life. However, to me there was a sense what she was proposing to do may still be incomplete. Being a gardener myself, my experience is that once a new weed comes into the garden, you may well get rid of it, but often it comes back. Questioning Margaret on this, I found her experience matched mine. So to offset the subtle implication in the image, and the real possibility of natural recurrence, we added to the imagery sequence. After spraying the weeds, Margaret's gardener was then sent on regular patrol, to seek out any new signs of weed growth and to eliminate them before they developed into any serious problem. He also was to constantly tend and support the garden, making it healthier and stronger—so healthy that illness had no part in it.

THE USE OF SEMILITERAL IMAGES

All the examples at the start of this chapter featured the use of semiliteral images based upon scans or X-rays. For Sandy, Sarah and Steven, what they had literally seen as a representation of their cancers (the scans and X-rays) formed the starting point for very effective imagery. However, each one of them was encouraged to regard their CAT scan or X-ray as a representation or symbol of their cancer, which of course it really is. Therefore, they were using what we call semiliteral images.

It is hard to predict who will be best suited to which type of imagery, but it is easy to imagine that more literal, left-brained people may be drawn to this type of semiliteral imagery; whereas the more creative types prefer the symbols like the ones Margaret used. While there have been plenty of exceptions to these rules, people with a medical background often find the semiliteral approach appealing and easy to work with.

Tom was a specialist surgeon who had a rather rare and particularly nasty cancer intertwined around his spine. He was well aware of his poor medical prognosis and the fact his treatment was regarded to be purely palliative. However, Tom had a very detailed anatomical knowledge of the area affected by the cancer. He studied his X-rays and scans to form a clear picture of the extent of the cancer and the damage it had done to his spine.

He then formed a very clear picture in his mind of what the area would look like when healed again. Tom proceeded to imagine the cancer shriveling and the healthy tissue regenerating. He had a remarkable response to his "palliative" treatment: the cancer disappeared and normal function of his spine returned. Tom is alive and well many years later.

We have found it often helps people with their imagery and healing when they develop a strong image of what healthy, healed tissue looks like. For example, it may sound a little weird at first, but many people with liver disease have been helped by going to the butcher and actually asking to see a healthy liver. This image can then be held in mind as the end goal.

OUT OF THE STILLNESS OF MEDITATION

Very often once people have learned the background to imagery, it works well to contemplate the principles, reflect on them deeply, and then wait for the images to arise spontaneously. This is a reliable process that has worked for many people.

Henri had prostate cancer with multiple bony secondaries. He found great comfort in using imagery as a lead-in to meditation. He would imagine he was on a large flat rock, beside a river near his childhood home, then relax and let go into the feeling, the ease and the comfort of that place. As he learned about healing imagery and was considering applying it in his own situation, a spontaneous image came to mind.

While he was meditating one day, Henri imagined sitting on his rock as he often did to relax his mind and transition into meditation. However, this time a spontaneous sequence of healing imagery arose in his mind as if he were actually doing it. He felt himself taking one of the affected bones out of his arm and in his mind he had no trouble imagining washing it in the river! Next, he took a large bottlebrush from beside the rock, pushed it up through the marrow of the bone, washed out all the cancer and then rinsed the bone in the river. He saw the cancer as a dark red stain that the river washed away, and he enjoyed seeing the color trailing away downstream. Once the first bone was sparkling white and clear of cancer, he put it back and moved on to take out and clean the next. Henri went on to have a remarkable long-term recovery.

HAVE THE BODY PRODUCE THE IMAGE

Charles was an accountant who had led a highly stressed, if fairly successful, business life. When bowel cancer was diagnosed with inoperable liver secondaries, Charles attended our residential programs more out of desperation than conviction. During meditation sessions, we sometimes apply light touch in the way of Dr. Ainslie Meares. This helps people to relax more directly and often helps focus their attention on particular areas. Sometimes it helps people to form an image of their illness.

Charles had been having little success with his meditation or imagery. His busy mind seemed to be ever active, that is, until he felt the gentle hands on his shoulders while he was meditating. At first he knew they belonged to one of our therapeutic team. He felt deeply reassured by the touch, deeply calmed. His thoughts settled, he could feel his state of mind changing. Then these initial hands felt as if they lifted from him, only to be replaced by two more hands. Two hands that had an even stronger quality. Charles, a long-time agnostic, swears they were the hands of Christ! They filled him with a sense of unconditional love. They brought heat and energy to his liver. He began to sweat, he began to smile. He was deeply moved. He felt that healing had begun.

The feeling of the hands stayed with Charles as part of a powerful image. The whole experience transformed his attitude; he began on a healing path, he began the spiritual journey. Many years later, Charles had survived liver secondaries longer than anyone his experienced specialists knew of.

For others, putting their own attention into the area of their cancer, or touching the area lightly themselves, is effective in drawing forth an image from the cancer itself.

Images derived in this way are invariably very relevant, very powerful and, when used in this way, very effective.

Step 2. Practice the Sequence of Healing

This is where all the principles of imagery come into action. Most people are able to see their imagery sequence as you might watch a DVD or a cartoon sequence. Some talk their way through the healing sequence too, either just describing to themselves what is happening or repeating affirmations as the pictures run. Whenever possible, it is ideal to add a physical sensation to the imagery. For some, this means having a sensation of a flow of energy; for others, feelings of warmth attend the healing.

Ideally, it is best to imagine the healing sequence taking place in the location of the illness itself. This means rather than imagining the healing pictures are running (literally) through your head, or on an imaginary screen in front of you, aim to focus your attention where the lesions are and super-impose the images on that place within the body. Many people find it help-ful to put their hands on or over the affected areas, so the sense of the imagery taking place at that point is strengthened.

To reiterate, the aim of the healing sequence is to start with an image of the illness, for the treatment and immune system to combine to remove the illness, and for the healthy tissue to regenerate. Steven's sequence was an excellent example of an image that powerfully symbolized the healthy tissue regenerating and completing the healing.

Step 3. Check That the Images Are Accurate, Complete and Feel Good

A risk with these practices is that they may be inaccurate or incomplete, reflecting poor technique or deeper issues of doubt or self-sabotage. Very commonly the people I work with find their first attempt at healing imagery produces useful images that remain at the core of their practice. However, it is very common that these initial images have limitations and that they can be improved upon.

One of the best ways to check healing imagery is to draw your imagery sequence. All you need are a few sheets of paper and either colored pencils or crayons. The aim is to draw a series of pictures, like a storyboard or cartoon sequence. These pictures need to start with the symbol of the disease and then demonstrate the way any treatment interacts with that disease, as well as the way your body's defenses and healing capacities are both imagined and inter-act. You then finish with an image that represents you in total good health.

Ideally, you do this drawing exercise with a therapist who is experienced in the field, although a smart friend may well suffice. You explain your intention with the imagery, what the symbols mean and how they interact. Against the need for accuracy and completeness, most outsiders will pick any deficiencies.

Nancy had stomach cancer with liver secondaries. The stomach had been cleared with surgery, but the liver remained a major problem. Nancy asked me to check her imagery, as she was committed to getting well and keen to pursue every possible avenue. She had seen a scan of her liver and had a clear picture of the extent of the three lesions in it. In her imagery, Nancy repre-sented her immune system and other healing qualities with the symbol of

Pac-Man. Her Pac-Man characters had two legs and big teeth! She knew she needed the right number of them and for her this meant she needed a team of twelve. With this very personal imagery, Nancy imagined her twelve Pac-Man characters lived behind her liver. Three times a day she did her practice, bringing up the images in her mind and seeing them eat up the three cancer lesions before she put them back to rest behind her liver.

This imagery was accurate enough but clearly incomplete. Nancy was directing her healing to be active three times a day for about five minutes each time—the time she was actually doing the imagery. For the rest of the day, she was instructing her immune system to rest! Clearly, Nancy needed to have her healing operating twenty-four hours a day. This is how it normally operates, anyway. However, faced with this suggestion, Nancy was deeply concerned that her Pac-Man characters, the symbols for her immune system, would become tired and ineffective if they worked all day! After discussing this apparent dilemma, what Nancy decided she could imagine were two more teams of twelve. She set up a rotating roster, with each team working a shift while the other two rested! For Nancy, this satisfactorily represented her immune system working fully and effectively. Nancy lived for many years, longer than her doctors had ever thought possible.

Step 4. Support Your Healing Imagery Practice

Imagery becomes a vehicle for positive expectations. It puts those hopes and beliefs into practice. Therefore your imagery practice will be supported by anything that builds your confidence, develops your belief in the possibility of healing, and anything that generates faith. So far in this book we have discussed many helpful things that have the potential to help in this regard—the benefits of simple meditation and specific positive-thinking exercises with the use of affirmations and other forms of imagery. Do recognize the value of an integrated approach and be reminded of the impact the company you keep can have on your state of mind.

The attitudes, hopes and beliefs of those around you can influence your own situation strongly. We have witnessed this repeatedly with young children battling cancer. Jane had an eighteen-month-old child, Nathan, who was not responding to his cancer treatment. His doctors told Jane and her husband, Roger, that they were sorry, but nothing seemed to be working and they did not expect Nathan to live long. Jane changed Nathan's diet to simple wholesome food, while she and Roger learned to meditate and practice imagery. At least twice a day when Nathan was asleep, one or both of his parents would cradle him in their arms, enter their own state of meditation, and imagine their meditative state was also encompassing Nathan. They imagined him wrapped in a warm blanket of loving, healing light that was all around, and all through him. As his treatment continued, they did specific healing imagery for him, imagining the imagery projected onto his tiny body. Remarkably, his condition began to improve. To his doctor's amazement, Nathan went on to make a full recovery and is now a healthy young adult.

A Caution and Some Advice for Partners and Health Professionals

Partners can share meditation and imagery with the one they love, with the patient. This needs to be done as free of ego as possible—as free of desire and longing as possible. It is a big ask to let go of the selfish motives, and to move into a space of unconditional lovingkindness, but here is an important and necessary caution. If you attempt to do this type of exercise for someone you love or care for, and find you are doing it with a sense of desperation or urgency, you may be better to leave it. You need to have a perspective that understands that in doing this exercise you are not taking on exclusive responsibility for the outcome. In other words, this exercise can help but it is only one factor. Whether your partner gets well or not will depend on many issues. What is being said here is to do your best, but do not set yourself up for mental anguish or guilt. Do the best you can, that is all you can do.

Be aware, too, that the beliefs or images held by other key people around you could also have an effect. Larry Dossey's excellent book *Healing Words*,[14] discusses the power of prayer and the impact of thought on healing. It is quite conceivable that if your doctor has a strong belief as to the outcome of your disease, then those thoughts will have some impact. It is highly recommended for people with cancer who are aiming for recovery to seek out key medical people who can imagine them as long-term survivors. I regularly suggest patients discuss this sensitive issue with their doctors and persist until they find practitioners who can support them in this very important way.

Step 5. Assess Your Progress, Adapt as Necessary

When you set yourself specific goals, it is important to assess your progress. With healing, assessments can range from easy to difficult, depending on what types of tests may be needed for useful feedback. How often to seek this feedback therefore will depend upon how quickly it seems the condition can change and how invasive any tests may be. I am a strong advocate of backing up your feelings and intuition with a reality check in the physical world. While mind, heart and spirit have a major and profound impact on our lives, it is still a physical body we live in, so I value physical assessments and reassessment.

Quite often imagery does change with time and with healing progress. Tessa had secondary spread of breast cancer in the lymph nodes under her arm. She had a Pac-Man image (no legs, big teeth!) that represented her healing. Three times a day she reinforced the sequence of healing characters by imagining the characters gobbling up her cancer. Then one day, as she prepared to begin the imagery, the characters went on strike! They literally refused to do anything and stayed motionless.

Tessa was deeply concerned, so I recommended she go for a checkup immediately. All her cancer had disappeared. She was in remission and it appeared her Pac-Man characters were not prepared to waste their time! They were quite happy, however, when Tessa responded to our discussion and sent them off on patrol, roaming Tessa's body to target any loose cancer cells and to make sure no relapse could become established.

Another major issue with healing, and the repeated practice of imagery, is the question of whether or not the image needs to change with each session. For example, Judy had breast cancer that had been treated by surgery and radiotherapy. Now she had secondaries in her liver and was using imagery to assist her healing. She had an excellent healing sequence that finished with an image of her liver being clear of cancer, returned to full health. What bothered her deeply was when she went to do her imagery at the next session (she was doing it twice each day), there was the cancer again. Sure, she could imagine getting rid of it, but by going back to the beginning each time she did her imagery practice, was she re-creating it? Should it get smaller each time she imagined it, or should it disappear altogether after just one effective imagery exercise? Judy was confused.

This is a common problem for many people beginning healing imagery. The practical answer is that you are using the imagery to convey the conscious intention "I want to heal" directly to the healing center, that automatic part of the brain that controls the healing process. To achieve this goal, you are rehearsing the complete sequence of healing. What the healing imagery sequence represents therefore is the complete process of healing, from what is known of the disease at the start, to the end point of complete health.

This is similar to the way we rehearse in our mind a physical journey from one place to another. We start at the beginning, imagine all the steps along the way and finish at the destination. In the case of healing, we are using the healing sequence to instruct the automatic healing center in the brain what to do. We want it to take us from disease to health. We entrust the details of how to complete this healing journey to the healing center. What we are aiming to do is to give it a very clear message of what we want—healing—so each time we do rehearse the whole sequence.

As feedback is not as easy to obtain on the healing journey as it is when compared to a literal journey, usually we need to wait for reassessment via medical tests that we only take from time to time. Then, based on this new evidence we may modify or adapt the imagery. Sometimes, as Tessa's story indicates, the images will change spontaneously and predict or point to a change in the physical reality of the illness.

A FINAL NOTE ON SYMBOLIC IMAGERY IN HEALING

Many people have found imagery to be a vital part of their healing journey. It seems fair to me to say that for many people it has played a pivotal role in catalyzing remarkable healing. I have seen it happen often.

I always recommend people who use active imagery in this way, to reinforce it, to balance it with the practice of simple meditation. What I then notice is that very commonly, over time—perhaps six to twelve months—people come to feel they have done enough imagery, that the meditation seems complete in itself and it is the meditation which forms the basis of their ongoing daily practice. Often as time progresses, people find imagery is something they value, enjoy to use, but that they only do it from time to time when the need feels ripe. Often too, the imagery they do persevere with tends to be of the more abstract type. So let us conclude this section by considering abstract imagery.

Abstract Imagery for Healing

With abstract imagery we move from personally significant symbols to more abstract and archetypal symbols. Archetypal images are those that are interpreted with the same meaning by the majority of people. When asked for their major images of healing, nearly all cultures respond with water and light. Therefore, the abstract healing images that are recommended involve the use of water and light. The two techniques I have found to be most effective are the white light healing imagery exercise using the breath, and the white light healing imagery exercise using energy flow. These exercises will be detailed soon.

It needs to be emphasized that these are excellent exercises for people who are healthy, as well as being powerful tools for healing. For well people, becoming familiar with white light healing imagery provides ready access to a major energy boost. When tired, you can do the exercise, draw on an infinite source of energy and rapidly revitalize your system. For example, I have used this technique often on long car trips and find it works very well for me.

For healing, the white light healing imagery exercises are the most common ones people use after coming to our programs. They are simple in their technique, combine the best of imagery principles, are relatively free of complication, work well for many, and always offer the added bonus of the very real prospect of a direct and profound spiritual experience.

When used for healing there are a few details to be aware of. An image for the illness is still required. Using a CAT scan image or X-ray for this often does link naturally with the image of water and/or light. Many people prefer to imagine the body in outline with the illness as a colored lump.

This technique is highly applicable for use with cancer, multiple sclerosis and many other diseases. Once an image is formed for the disease, the light is drawn into the body with the breath, or flows in via the top of the head, and then proceeds to wash away the symbol of the illness.

WHITE LIGHT HEALING IMAGERY USING THE BREATH—THE THEORY

Using the breathing-based technique, you imagine the breath as a white vapor, seeing and feeling it (perhaps with a sensation of warmth or tingling) flowing toward the illness. Usually in this context when you imagine and feel into the illness, the area associated with the illness will feel harder and denser to you than the rest of the body. A common sensation is that it has some pain associated with it. It may also feel warmer than the rest of the body (occasionally some people feel it cooler). Usually the illness will have a color associated with it.

White Light Healing Imagery Using the Breath—The Exercise

Once you are comfortably seated, let your eyes close gently . . . turn your thoughts inward . . . and remember that this is a time for healing . . .

Feel your body relaxing . . . feel the muscles becoming soft and loose . . . feel your weight begin to settle down into your chair, your muscles relaxing . . . feel any tension releasing . . . feel yourself relaxing deeply . . . completely . . . more and more . . . deeper and deeper . . . letting go . . . feel it all through the body . . . feel it deeply . . . feel the letting go . . . completely . . . it is a good feeling . . . a natural feeling . . . feel the letting go . . . letting go . . .

And as you feel yourself relaxing more deeply, imagine as if it is in the sky above you, whatever embodies or symbolizes the highest source of power that you know.

So this may be the image of Christ, or Mother Mary; a particular saint; the Buddha; or a figure from another tradition. Or you may have a more abstract view and imagine a ball of light like the sun which represents an infinite source of energy and healing power, as well as love, compassion, all that is life affirming and that has your own best interests at heart.

Imagine you are in the direct presence of this embodiment of all you value most . . . feel that presence and relax into it . . .

Maybe you choose to say something, like a prayer or a request . . . speaking quietly under your breath as if you are speaking to this presence . . .

Maybe there is a response or something said for you . . . so you can listen for that.

And as you feel yourself connecting more directly with this presence, become aware of your breathing . . . simply giving your breathing your full attention . . . and allowing your breath to take up whatever rhythm feels comfortable for you at the moment . . . the breath moving in and out . . . quite effortlessly . . . effortlessly . . .

And as you continue to hold your attention on your breath, imagine that you are breathing in a pure white vapor that stems from the very heart, or the center of the image in the sky above you . . . so, with each breath in, see this pure white light moving down through your nostrils . . . down into your chest and filling it with a pure white light . . . and as you breathe out, imagine that you are releasing gray light, a gray vapor, that carries with it anything that is old, worn, or unwanted . . . anything you need to be free of . . .

As you breathe in again, imagine that you are breathing in the pure white light . . . bringing with it all that is pure, and fresh and vital . . . breathing out and releasing the old and the worn and anything unwanted in your system . . . breathing it out and releasing it . . . anything at all that you want to be free of . . .

And allow yourself to settle into a rhythm . . . breathing in the pure white light . . . seeing it streaming down into your chest . . . and breathing out all the gray . . . in with the white and pure . . . out with the gray, the old and the worn . . .

And as you continue, feel the white light coming down steadily into your chest, and the strength of the light in your chest growing stronger . . . and brighter . . . and purer . . . displacing any old and worn and gray areas . . . filling your whole chest with a pure white light . . . a symbol of wholeness . . . purity . . . vitality . . . and healing . . . you may be feeling the light as a warmth . . . perhaps it even tingles a little as it flows throughout your body . . .

With each new breath, draw in more white light . . . until your chest feels like it is aglow . . . filled with this pure white light . . . so that it feels like it is radiating pure white light . . . and, as you breathe in again, you feel the white light beginning to flow over . . . traveling down into your tummy . . . as you breathe out now, you can direct the white light, down into your tummy . . . and as you see the white light flowing down, feel it relaxing . . . feel it releasing . . . feel it healing . . . purifying . . . and feel the warm white light traveling down . . . relaxing . . . releasing . . . feel the warmth, the relaxation, the softness . . . releasing any old and worn energy . . . releasing any areas that are uncomfortable, painful . . . feel them being filled with the white light, with its comfort and ease . . . releasing . . . relaxing . . . letting go . . .

(continued)

(continued)

And as you breathe in now, draw in more pure white light from its source . . . see it traveling down into your chest . . . and, as you breathe out, radiate that white light down . . . down through your abdomen . . . down into your pelvis . . . releasing any tension . . . softening . . . bringing warmth . . . and relaxation . . . feeling it deeply . . . completely . . .

And now, breathe in more white light and see it traveling down into your legs . . . down your thighs . . . softening . . . releasing . . . filling with a new strength . . . purity . . . bringing healing . . . and wholeness . . . breathing in more white light . . . seeing it passing down now, into your calves . . . down into your feet . . . releasing any tension . . . releasing any old and worn areas . . . and bringing a new vitality . . . bringing healing . . . strength . . . so that now your legs too are filled with this pure, bright white light . . .

And as you breathe in again, direct the white light now down through your arms and feel the relaxation, the release . . . the softening, as your muscles loosen still more . . . right down . . . feel the light flowing right down into your fingers . . . feel them soft and loose . . . see them filled with the pure white light . . . symbol of purity . . . a feeling of natural vitality . . .

As you breathe in again, draw more of the pure white light from its source . . . see it filling your lungs . . . and now see it traveling up your neck . . . into your head . . . and, as it moves upward, feel the muscles relaxing . . . feel them becoming soft and loose . . . feeling the ease of it all . . . any worn areas . . . letting go . . . any diseased areas being freed, and replaced with a pure white light . . . symbolic of new strength . . . of purity . . . of healing . . . of whole vitality . . .

So, now feel your whole body filled with this pure white light . . . and, with each new breath in, draw more white light from its source . . . and see it filling your whole body with still more white light . . . so that your whole body is glowing intensely with the pure white light . . .

And, as you breathe in more, see the white light expanding out . . . beyond your body . . . to encapsulate you, like an egg . . . like a cocoon of bright, pure, white light . . . filling you with strength and vitality . . . feel it as a whole . . . feel its unity . . . feel yourself to be at one with it . . . allow yourself to merge in the purity of the white light . . . feel its energy moving through you . . . feel yourself to be at one with it . . . feel yourself at peace . . . be still . . . feel it all through . . . deeply . . . completely . . . all through . . . feel yourself at one . . . and be still . . .

As you feel its sense of wholeness through you, you may now like to direct that white light to someone you care for . . . to share that feeling with them . . . and so imagine this person as if they were in front of you . . . and imagine, that as you breathe in . . . the white light passes through you . . . and as you breathe out, it radiates like a searchlight to this person you care for . . . and see it fill them with its whiteness . . . see their body glowing white . . . and see them surrounded in a cocoon of pure white light . . . a symbol of purity . . . of wholeness . . . of healing . . . of renewed vitality . . .

And, as you breathe in . . . draw in more white light and radiate it to this person . . . feel it flowing through you . . . and see them filled with a new wholeness . . . a new sense of balance . . . purpose . . . seeing them whole and healthy . . . pure and vital . . . and share your experience with them . . . feel them filled with this same pure white light . . . and add your blessing . . .

Now bring your attention back to your own body once again . . . Allow yourself to merge again with the feeling of purity and wholeness of the light . . . breathe in . . . breathe in more white light . . . see it streaming down from the embodiment of your own truth . . . pouring into you like a funnel . . . a funnel coming down through your nose and filling your body . . . and this time, imagine that as you breathe out, the light radiates out from your own body . . . spreading out around you . . . and flowing through the place you are in . . . see this white light filling the space around you . . . everyone nearby . . . filling them with purity, wholeness, health and vitality . . . feel your love flowing with it . . . feeling that warm, happy feeling going with it . . .

As you breathe in more, draw in more of this energy . . . as you breathe out, radiate it beyond the space you are in . . . to the people

(continued)

(continued)

around you . . . to the buildings around you . . . feel it moving off, across the country . . . breathing in more white light . . . drawing it down, like a funnel . . . drawing it down from the image above you . . . then through your body, and out across the land . . . spreading out, so that you can imagine the whole country bathed in this pure white light . . .

Breathing in more white light . . . breathing it out, and feeling it traveling right around the globe . . . wrapping the whole planet in a pure white light . . . and now share your feeling of peace and unity with the whole planet . . . radiate that feeling out, and feel it traveling right around, so that the whole planet is held like a ball of pure white light . . .

As you breathe in more, feel that white light streaming down . . . feel yourself again merging with it . . . feel it entering every part of your being . . . feel yourself at one with its purity . . . at one with its peace . . . one with its healing . . . feel yourself at one with its vitality . . . and realize that this white light symbolizes love in action . . . allow yourself to merge into that feeling of love, that pure love, streaming down and filling your whole being . . . feel it all through . . . feel its peace . . . and be still . . . feel yourself merging with the stillness, to allow it to be all through you . . . deeply . . . completely . . . be still . . .

As the white vapor of the breath reaches the illness, most commonly it swirls around the outside of the mass, dissolving it or perhaps causing it to burn or smolder, releasing a gray vapor. This gray vapor, representing the residue of the illness, is then breathed out and released from the body.

White light (vapor) accompanies the in breath, representing healing and all the life-affirming qualities coming in; gray light (vapor) flows with the out breath, representing the disease breaking down and being released, along with anything else, old, worn or unwanted you need to release.

Many people find it helpful to breathe in the white vapor and to direct it into the center of the illness, imagining the illness breaking down from the inside out, rather than from the outside in (as above). As another option, it may help to focus a beam of light almost like a laser, and to imagine this concentrated shaft of light accentuating and accelerating the healing process.

WHITE LIGHT HEALING IMAGERY USING ENERGY FLOW—THE THEORY

Using the energy flow technique for white light healing imagery is similar in some respects to the exercise we have just done that focuses on the breath, except that now the light is imagined to have liquid properties as well. The liquid white light then flows down into the body and filters through it, quite slowly—a bit like water filtering down through dry sand. Again, this warm liquid white light gently but effectively washes away anything old, worn or unwanted! Often the disease can be imagined as a particular color that can be seen to be washed away by the liquid light—a bit like a stain being rinsed from dirty clothes under a water tap. Also, the liquid white light can be directed readily to any areas that may need it more. This technique also can be done in a similar way to a laser, where a beam of liquid white light either washes or burns the disease away from the outside in, or from the inside out.

With these forms of abstract imagery, sometimes the disease, especially when it is cancer, will be seen to clear completely in a particular session. Other times, and for other people, it may seem that only partial progress is made. This can be fine as long as you (yourself) feel confident with the amount of progress in any given session, and you avoid any temptation or tendency to worry. Ideally, to repeat, the aim is to do these exercises with a good feeling and plenty of confidence.

Please be aware that these healing imagery techniques and principles apply well to pain control, which will be discussed in detail in the next chapter.

A Final Note on Abstract or Archetypal Images

If you reflect on this for a moment, probably the most abstract imagery of all would be to use the simple silence of meditation. To accomplish this, you begin by reminding yourself that when you enter the stillness of meditation, your immune system will return to its natural balance and in that state it will be fully activated and empowered to heal you. Then, having affirmed

White Light Healing Imagery
Using Energy Flow—The Practice

Take up your position, relax physically (see the earlier directions when using the breath).

Imagine now, as if it were in the sky above you, the highest source of power that you know. The embodiment of your own truth. It may be an image that symbolizes God, or it may be the figure of Christ, Mother Mary or a particular saint. Or you may prefer a more abstract image such as the sun that could represent the source of universal energy. Whichever of these symbolic images you find most helpful, imagine that as well as a source of energy and healing power, this is a source of love and compassion, of lovingkindness, of a presence that has your own best interest at heart.

As this image forms in your mind, allow yourself to imagine what it would feel like to come into the presence of this infinite source of energy. What would it be like to feel yourself in the presence of God? Or Christ? Or the source of universal energy?

Sometimes as you feel yourself coming closer to that presence, you may wish to say something—a prayer, an explanation, a request . . . sometimes, something may be said to you, or for you . . . so you could listen for that.

Once you feel this presence as if it is in the sky above you . . . imagine that a beam of white light begins to flow from its very center, down toward you . . . an outpouring of energy and loving-kindness . . . if you are focused upon a figure . . . imagine this light flowing from its very heart . . . if you are using the sun, imagine the shaft of light flowing from its very center . . .

Now as this beam of warm, liquid, white light reaches your head . . . it not only flows down around your body . . . but also it flows through your body . . . warm . . . liquid . . . white light . . . slowly flowing down through your body . . . almost like water filtering down through dry sand . . .

Warm, liquid, white light . . . flowing from that infinite source . . . and flowing down through every part of your body . . . like having a wash on the inside . . . it washes away anything old or worn or unwanted . . . it brings with it a new energy . . . a vitality . . . a sense of healing and wholeness . . . you can feel it filling your body and your being . . .

You may see this quite visually or you may have it as a feeling experience . . . like feeling a flow of energy or a sensation of warmth moving down through your body . . .

When the light does flow down to the ends of your arms . . . it will flow out the end of the fingers . . . when it does reach the end of your legs . . . it will flow out through the feet, washing away with it anything old, worn or unwanted . . .

When this light comes to difficult, tense, painful or blocked areas . . . it washes through them . . . clearing them . . . relaxing them . . . letting them go . . . You may see the affected area as having a particular shape . . . maybe a particular color . . . when the light reaches such an area . . . you may see that color being washed away like a stain being washed away from clothes held under running water . . . you may see the area dissolving from the outside in . . . maybe you find it helpful to imagine the light being concentrated almost like a laser . . . this then burns away the affected blockage . . . either from the outside in or the inside out . . .

See and feel this warm liquid light filling every part of your body . . . feel the same all over . . . your body filled with the vigor . . . the vitality . . . the radiance of the warm liquid white light . . .

As this feeling becomes all-encompassing . . . it is as if you merge with it . . . almost as if you dissolve into the light . . . you feel it through your body . . . and your mind . . . it is as if you become at one with it . . . given that it stems from an infinite source, this can feel like merging or reuniting with the infinite . . . go with it . . . feel it all through . . . all through . . .

You conclude by merely resting in the presence of that light and the universal energy it represents and carries.

And when you feel it is time to conclude, move your feet a little, your hands and then, when you are ready, just let your eyes open gently.

this strong intention, once you do enter the deeper stillness of meditation you will be activating subtle but powerful imagery forces. When you do this you will in fact be using the most abstract imagery of all. It is my belief that when the two elements of abstract imagery and the stillness of silent meditation are combined in this way, remarkable and profound healing becomes a strong possibility.

CHAPTER 10

Pain Control

It Is Only Pain!

IMAGINE HAVING MORE CONTROL OVER YOUR OWN EXPERIENCE OF PAIN. What a relief that would be! How empowering. Transforming our experience of pain is another very real possibility that comes with training our minds and it leads to a whole new level of personal freedom and comfort.

We will all have experienced the distressing aspects of significant pain. While many people rely on external help for their pain management, and pain management as a medical specialty has improved dramatically over recent decades, what we are talking of here is our personal management of pain. How we can learn to experience pain in a way that does not even hurt! This radical approach to pain management has transformed the lives of many who have developed it. It has freed them from the fear of pain, from the hurtful experience of pain and it has left them with a life skill that is incredibly satisfying.

The crucial point is that to convert these good ideas around pain management into reality, we need to work at it a little. We need to train ourselves, starting with understanding the theory, and then we need to practice the techniques.

FIRST, THE THEORY

The basic premise centers around the fact that pain has two aspects. Pain involves a physical sensation that is overlaid with a psychological reaction. When we learn how to experience the physical sensation free of the psychological reaction, we take the hurt out of pain. Pure pain, free of any psychological reaction, does not hurt! Interested?

REDUCE THE FEAR, REDUCE THE PAIN

We have talked of fear being a basic hurdle to overcome in the process of getting well again. Cancer is associated with two main fears: the fear that it will cause pain and the fear that it will lead to an untimely death. These fears are the primary reason why society dreads hearing or relating to the word "cancer." In fact, we have created a culture that commonly regards pain and death with undue horror, and commonly treats them as unmanageable, negative events. As a result, they are often approached with a sense of panic as individuals feel powerless to help themselves through situations where either is involved. This often leads people to rely on external aids that often do little for their quality of life.

The influence of fear extends beyond the patients themselves, as often relatives and friends become preoccupied with whether their loved ones are "in pain" or not. This concern is natural and reasonable, but in my experience, is usually accentuated and often clouded by the relatives' own personal fears. This leads to an unnatural preoccupation and is frequently a cause for tension and anxiety that in turn prevents dealing with problems on a more satisfactory level. Pain needs to be managed, but total quality of life remains of paramount importance. There is no answer in being a society of pill-poppers rushing for the analgesics at the slightest twinge.

What is needed is a fresh approach that develops the individual's ability to manage most, if not all, of the pain that may come our way. Of course, we do not need to be a cancer patient to derive benefit from such an approach. I see this as a fundamental prerequisite in self-defense and well-being. When pain can be handled without fear or difficulty, it is a great thing.

There is such a concept. It makes the self-management of pain a very real possibility, but it involves techniques that are totally new to most people. However, first a warning.

PAIN IS A SIGNAL THAT SOMETHING IS WRONG

It is important to know what is behind any pain we experience, to heed any warnings and to take such appropriate action as is necessary. People can learn to be unaffected by pain so that headaches do not bother them, so that back pain does not inconvenience their movement. That is fine if the pain is chronic and the person can be sure that it does not indicate a need for other or more treatment.

Anne had three collapsed vertebrae in her spine. She used the methods we are about to learn to such effect that all the initially excruciating pain was gone and her mobility returned to normal. She then had to be extremely careful not to overdo her exercise, as her back was very unstable. Similarly, it is important to know before you turn a headache off that it is just a simple headache and does not have a more serious cause.

Always investigate and clarify the cause of any pain before setting about its management.

THE MEDICAL MANAGEMENT OF PAIN

It was not so long ago that unmanageable pain was a real concern for people with cancer. There is no doubt that if you do feel pain and it persists, then that pain can easily consume your interest and demand your attention. Everything else rapidly becomes secondary to it. If pain is a reality for you, its treatment requires top priority.

Therefore, it is important to know that these days the medical management of pain is a highly developed area of expertise. Cancer pain can be relieved reliably by external means if you cannot do it yourself. There is no need to feel bad or guilty in seeking such aid. If you are experiencing pain that is above a reasonable threshold for you, it is very appropriate to seek suitable relief. Once the situation is under control, you will be able to redevelop your own resources. It is comforting to know that most large hospitals now boast pain-control clinics where the full range of possibilities are explored. One such large clinic in England reported that in one year they admitted four hundred patients with a specific pain problem; only ten could not be relieved satisfactorily.

The range of medical options used to relieve pain usually begins with analgesic drugs. They certainly have their place, but can have their side effects. Some have the potential to become addictive, while some affect our normal thinking processes and lessen our quality of life. The additional help of counselors, hypnotherapists, acupuncturists and physiotherapists with mechanical aids such as transcutaneous electrical stimulators may well be warranted. Even surgeons can contribute by cutting nerves to problem areas.

Palliative care teams are often experts in pain management and can be called upon for their expertise in this field.

There are less drastic but more experimental methods that have possibilities. Some medical practitioners report consistent pain reduction following large intravenous doses of sodium ascorbate, better known as vitamin C. Iscador, a German mistletoe extract, has been used by injection, again with considerable results. The controversial Laetrile (an extract from apricot kernels) also has been associated with many cases of pain reduction.

At home, I found two great aids, the ever-faithful hot-water bottle applied over the affected area and the generalized effect of coffee enemas. (More will be said of coffee enemas in discussing the dietary principles. See Appendix F for details of their preparation.) Also, many people have found that transferring to a really healthy way of eating significantly decreased their experience of pain. Removing any toxic load in the body leads to further reductions.

PERSONAL PAIN MANAGEMENT USING THE MIND

Before we investigate the radical notion that true pain does not hurt, we need to be aware that there are two main ways in which the mind can change our perception of pain. They are dissociation and a version of mindfulness. We will begin by considering the very real usefulness of dissociation.

DISSOCIATION

Dissociation (dis-association) is where we move our attention away from the pain and onto something more pleasant, more manageable. We may do this in an almost unconscious way by simply becoming distracted, or we may dissociate quite deliberately using a technique based on imagery or hypnosis. Distraction is a reliable way of minimizing, avoiding or even forgetting the pain.

Vera attended a meditation group seeking relief from her painful scoliosis, a chronic recurrent back condition marked by persistent pain. Vera reported how important being busy was to her:

When I go to work and have to interact with people, it takes my mind off my back. The more involved I am, the quicker the time passes. The busier it is, the better. The worst part of the day is when I go to bed. I spend ages trying to find a comfortable position. That is when the pain is strongest.

This experience is a common one. Being busy, especially when we are engrossed in the busyness, or being distracted, like when we go to a good film, are both ways of dissociating. What we are giving our attention to comes into the foreground of our mind, and it is as if the pain slips into the background.

It is last thing at night, with all the activities of the day completed and with nothing else for our mind to dwell on, that pain often comes to the fore. There are no more distractions and our mind is free to fantasize. *How long will the pain go on for? Will it be better or worse tomorrow? What if it gets worse?* And so on. With no distractions, no dissociation, the psychological reactions of the mind and emotions are free to run riot. The pain seems more obvious, stronger and more distressing.

Understanding how this works, how the impact of dissociation and distraction affects our perception of pain, gives us more confidence to manage it. Clearly, it can be useful to use dissociation. When we engage in a pleasant and engaging activity we can experience genuine pain relief. Also, we can use the principle of dissociation in some very good mind-body medicine techniques that provide effective pain relief.

It is not the intention of this book to discuss techniques like hypnosis and self-hypnosis. It is enough to acknowledge that these are also useful applications and to say that, commonly, when hypnosis is used for pain, the principle that makes it work is often dissociation. The mind is distracted from the pain. It is paying attention elsewhere.

DISSOCIATION USING IMAGERY FOR PAIN RELIEF

We can apply this same principle of dissociation for ourselves through the use of imagery. One of the most reliable ways we have found to do this is to utilize a technique where we create a mental image of a place where we feel particularly peaceful and comfortable. This place becomes an inner sanctuary, a place to which we can retreat, give all our attention to and rest in the feeling of its space and comfort. In this exercise we move the focus of our attention quite deliberately from the pain to this inner sanctuary.

The whole intention of this exercise is to imagine yourself to be as fully as possible in your inner sanctuary. Aim to use all of your senses—see the place through your own eyes as if you were actually there, hear the sounds, notice whatever there is to smell, and feel the physical sensations. Perhaps there may even be something to taste (for example, when a person imagines themselves to be in the ocean). The intention is to transport yourself from your normal conscious reality to this place of inner peace and comfort.

Here, then, is the exercise (opposite). You might like to read it and learn it well enough so that you can lead yourself through it, or you might find it useful to have someone else read it to you in a slow, steady and relaxed tone of voice. The exercise is recorded on my CD *Effective Pain Management*.

Many people find this exercise gives them a reliable way to dissociate from pain and to find a comfortable inner haven. Children are particularly good at it, and as a technique it is very useful when there is a short-term need for pain relief.

Marty was a nine-year-old boy who needed repeated injections for cancer tests and treatment. The most challenging were lumbar punctures, where Marty would have to lie still while a needle was passed between the bones of his lower spine and into his spinal canal to collect fluid. Just one of these procedures would have been harrowing enough, but as more and more were required he began to react with great distress.

Two techniques transformed Marty's experience. First, Marty was taught how to "go all floppy." This is childspeak for relaxing the body. In a few moments, Marty was taught to make his body all stiff, and then to relax it, to make it go all floppy. Children are terrific at learning the essence of the progressive muscle relaxation exercise in this very quick, simple and effective way.

Second, Marty was taught to go to his own personal inner sanctuary. No real-life place for him, Marty created a Disney-like fantasy castle full of interesting and fun characters and animals. There was plenty to entertain and distract him.

Marty's medical staff cooperated by giving him time to do his preparations before each new procedure was performed. When Marty was advised that the procedure was about to begin, first he made his body go all floppy, then it was as if he left his body there on the table while the procedure was

The Inner Sanctuary

Settle into your posture and take a few moments to relax your body in your own way.

Allow an image to form in your mind of a place where you feel particularly peaceful and comfortable . . . it may be a place you have been to before, or it may be a fantasy place . . . just allow an image to form in your mind in a way that you can explore it in more detail . . .

What can you see in this place? . . . what is close by? . . . what is further off in the distance? . . . what can you see? . . . what shapes? . . . what sizes? . . . what colors? . . . what shades of color? . . . what time of day is it? . . . if you can see the sky, are there clouds, or is it clear? . . . what movement do you notice in this place . . . or is it quite still? . . . what can you see in this place?

Now notice what sounds you can hear in this place . . . are there any sounds coming from nearby? . . . are there any sounds coming from farther away? . . . what sounds can you hear in this place?

Give your attention now to noticing what you may be able to smell in this place . . . what fragrance? . . . what odor? . . . perhaps just the quality of the air itself . . . what can you smell in this place?

What sensations can you feel in this place? . . . you will probably be aware of the temperature . . . is it warm? . . . or cool? . . . or neutral? . . . can you feel a breeze on your skin? . . . or the warmth of the sun on your face? . . . notice too your position and what you are in contact with . . . is it hard or soft? . . . damp or dry? . . . what physical sensations are you aware of in this place?

Is there anything you might like to change to make this place even more peaceful and comfortable? . . . if so, you could do that now . . .

Now dwell on the feelings that come with being in this place . . . allow these feelings to build within you and rest with those feelings . . . just simply letting go . . . relaxing . . . releasing . . . letting go.

carried out. Instead of being present for the harsh realities of what was going on, Marty was happily off in his own magical space. When the procedure was completed, he quite readily and easily took leave of his inner sanctuary and brought his attention more particularly back to his body. These relatively simple steps transformed Marty's experience.

Therese was an older woman who had chronic rheumatic pain that had distressed her and restricted her movement for many years. When Therese attempted to meditate, she found the hurdle of her pain was too much to manage. She simply could not relax or find any peace. Even in the group setting she made little progress. However, with this inner sanctuary imagery exercise, Therese found instant relief. After her first experience of it, she explained:

> It was wonderful. I went to a tropical beach that I visited not long after I was married. We were so happy there. I could feel the warmth and I relaxed on the sand. I just seem to drift off in that place. It is the most relief I can remember experiencing for so long.

What Therese did next was even more useful for her. She was able to remember the feeling of her inner sanctuary and to keep that feeling with her.

While this inner sanctuary exercise can be a great way to dissociate from pain, by its nature it involves dissociating from life itself. To do it, we need to move our attention from our present moment, worldly reality to an inner fantasy, an inner reality. Many people like Marty find this really useful for short-term pain relief. Some, like Therese, use it to work out a method that brings long-term relief. Therese again:

> What I did was to find such comfort in that inner sanctuary, such peace and relief, that it really left its mark. I did not want to forget it. So in some way after I come out of the experience, the feeling stays with me. It is like I remember that feeling and it becomes a new part of what I experience during the day. Perhaps it is the comfort of knowing I can go back to that lovely beach any time I want to. It is like it is always there. And I feel it. I really feel it and it gives me a lot of comfort. My pain is much easier to manage than it used to be.

Dissociation, then, has its place and can be quite useful. But it does involve dis-associating—losing our association with what is actually happening in our current moment experience.

So what of the other possibility? How about, rather than avoiding the pain, we give it our full attention? What happens then?

This brings us back to the proposition of learning how to feel the pain as a purely physical sensation, free of any psychological reaction.

MINDFULNESS-BASED PAIN MANAGEMENT

This is a comprehensive system of pain management that does take a little while to learn, understand and practice. However, the time we spend doing this will be repaid when we have acquired a profoundly effective way of managing both acute and chronic pain. While as the name suggests, this technique does draw on mindfulness, there is more to it. We begin by understanding more about the nature of pain.

THE TWO ASPECTS OF PAIN • The Physical and the Psychological

The more radical premise we will now investigate is that true pain does not hurt! You will come to see that this apparently extravagant claim is true. To begin with, however, it may be well removed from your normal experience of pain. We all know from past experience that when we feel a pain that goes beyond a certain level, it jolly well hurts. Whether the pain is coming from a physical cause, such as a cut finger, or a psychological cause, such as a broken romance, if we feel pain we normally experience it as a hurt.

So, having said that, the normal experience is that pain hurts, and myself having gone through some very tough times with what reputedly is one of the most painful types of cancer, how can I say that true pain does not hurt? *True* pain does not hurt. Not many people have experienced true pain. Once we do understand the nature of pain and its basic components we can come to experience it ourselves and learn that pain does not have to hurt.

ANIMALS PROVIDE A CLUE

I recall a little puppy that came into my veterinary surgery some years ago. It was four months old and owned by a policeman. He rushed into the surgery with it, saying that the puppy had been hit by a car and he thought he ought to shoot it, but first he wondered if we could do anything.

When I first saw the animal, I could not imagine what the problem was because all I could see was a little puppy looking around the surgery with a smile on its face and wagging its tail. It reacted just like any exuberant puppy would, trying to give me a lick and wagging its tail. When I looked at its front legs, however, I found all the skin had been stripped right off them and both wrists were broken. The two open joints were just hanging loose. I am sure that, for a human, the shock alone would have put them in a very precarious position, but here was this puppy looking around the surgery as if nothing had happened.

When I went to examine him, I needed to move his legs. His initial response was to try and pull out of the way. When he could not get away from me he tried to nip me. Not very seriously, but he was definitely trying to tell me that he would rather I did not do what I was trying to do. So, the nurse held his head. Once he would not get out of the way and could not bite us, he immediately accepted his position and allowed us to examine him. His tail stopped wagging and he looked a bit unhappy about it all, but soon we had finished looking at his legs and put them back down on the table. His tail started wagging again and he went back to looking around the room as if nothing had happened.

Later, we gave him an anesthetic to clean him up as best we could and to keep his legs still while the plaster casts we used set hard. About two months later, the casts came off and that puppy was walking around again. Over the next month, all the hair grew back on his legs. He was a normal dog again!

To me, that experience really shows us what is involved with pain and how to deal with it. It was a remarkable demonstration of how pain in its proper context does not hurt. Pain is a stimulus. For the puppy, his pain was a warning signal. It told him that if he moved or was moved, his legs hurt more. He avoided movement. He did all he could to remain still. He made the appropriate response to the stimulus. If he had been in the wild, and could have kept still long enough, his legs may well have healed just as they did in our plaster casts.

The pain was a warning stimulus—not pleasant, presumably, but still for the puppy, only a stimulus. When he was in a position of minimal discomfort, he was quite ready to accept that stimulus and make the most of his situation.

THE PSYCHOLOGICAL COMPONENT OF PAIN AND HUMAN SUFFERING

Contrast the puppy's reaction with what might happen if we were to break a leg. We would have the initial physical pain of the event that caused the break. But in the same instant our mind would start to race. "Hell, I think I have broken my leg! Will I ever walk again? Is my insurance up to date? Who's going to do my work for me? How will I pay the bills while I'm in the hospital?" And on and on it goes. This is the *psychological* aspect of pain— the worry and the anxiety, the mind's response, the fear that goes with the physical reality.

The key principle that has the potential to free us from the distress of pain is that true physical pain does not hurt. It is merely an unpleasant stimulus. Psychological pain can be excruciatingly hurtful. Understanding the difference between the physical and psychological aspects of pain is fundamental to dealing with pain in the most appropriate manner.

Consider a day of 107 degrees Fahrenheit. Hot, uncomfortable—but painful? Very few people would consider it to be so. We know that the pure physical effect of such a temperature is not likely to be harmful and, anyway, it will probably be cooler tomorrow. We tolerate it and go on with our business as best we can.

Yet imagine what would happen if people started dying when the temperature reached 109 degrees. The psychological component of pain would swing into action. Faced with a reason to fear the temperature, people would no doubt become preoccupied with the weather and limit their activities dramatically. I am sure that as a consequence 107 degrees would suddenly become a very painful temperature indeed.

This psychological component of pain is very strong in humans. Surely it accounts for that wonderful phenomenon we discussed earlier, the placebo effect. Many trials have shown the effectiveness of placebos in controlling even the most severe pain just as there is ample scientific evidence of their dramatic benefits for many medical conditions.

We need to appreciate what the placebo is demonstrating. If a sugar pill can relieve pain for us, surely we can learn to do it for ourselves and derive the satisfaction that we otherwise laughingly bestow on the placebo. A placebo is an external agent that we can accept as a treatment for the nonphysical aspect of our condition. We can learn to harness the placebo effect and put it to work for ourselves. We can experience pain in its true, pure, nonhurtful and manageable form.

This to me is a basic technique in self-defense that everyone should know. Through it, we can become free of the fear of pain and improve our level of well-being enormously.

I used to have a very low pain threshold. In my athletic days, when I was fit I could run a reasonable four hundred meters, but my performance was poor at any farther distance. It hurt too much! To run a fast 1,500 meters or mile, or especially something like a marathon, you require a very high pain threshold indeed. I could not handle it. In the past, even just having stitches taken out was for me an acutely painful experience. I also remember that after my leg was amputated, I avoided analgesics wherever possible. I was afraid I might become conditioned to them. The bone cancer I had is normally very painful and, not knowing any better then, I was quite afraid of what the pain might be like if the cancer recurred. What would I do if the analgesics did not work? How could I handle chronic, severe pain?

I learned through experience and by training in pain. Seriously, we train in so many things to increase our ability in that area. In athletics I used to train hard to improve my performance. No one would consider it strange to go through the rigors of what on one level could be fairly described as quite painful training. So why not train ourselves to better our performance in dealing with pain?

By doing so myself, I have freed a whole area of my life. I no longer have fear of pain. Whereas before I used to be scared stiff of visits to the dentist, now I see it as an opportunity to confirm my freedom from the stranglehold that pain held me in. I have been able to suture my own cuts without anesthetic and again marvel at how pain, true pain, really does not hurt.

CHILDREN AND HOW WE LEARN THAT PAIN HURTS!

If a child falls over and cuts himself, comfort and treatment may well be required. However, there is no need to overreact. Children are conditioned by the emotions of those around them so quickly. Just watch the influence of a group of adults reacting to a small child's fall. "Oh, my goodness!" they cry, as the hands fly up in horror. "You poor thing, where does it hurt?"

I have seen society's effects on my own children. The eldest, Rosemary, initially had a remarkable pain tolerance. The normal bumps and scrapes she went through were only an annoyance to her. She was far more interested in getting back to learning, experiencing and doing other things like having fun than to worry about pain. Up she would get and carry on, as I struggled to contain my own anxieties.

Reinforced by her obvious lack of hurt, I was soon able to react in an appropriate way and the everyday minor accidents became nonevents. After turning two, however, it took only a couple of episodes with doting elders gushing over some minor falls for her to begin reacting in the stereotyped way. Soon these same falls became a cause for tears and apparently genuine hurt. Interestingly, however, the worse the accidents, the less the reaction. Now it was as if the minor incidents were an outlet for pent-up emotions. It then took several years for her to relearn how to accept pain and deal with it appropriately.

When she was four, Rosemary had a plantar wart deep in her foot. It was quite irritating for her. Finally, being used to watching me work in the veterinary surgery, she declared she was going to cut it out. Did she think that would hurt? "No, Daddy. I'll just make myself all floppy." Rosemary had learned how to relax herself and she is an expert at it. She made herself go "all floppy"—deeply relaxing herself so her muscles were loose like a rag doll—and then she proceeded to take to the wart with some surgical scissors and excised it completely. The hardest thing was for me to control my own reactions. Surely, it was a reasonable thing for Rosemary to cut out this annoyance and clearly it can be that easy. Perhaps we should not be surprised to see the theory at work!

THE UNDERLYING PSYCHOLOGICAL FACTORS IN OUR PERCEPTION OF PAIN • Transforming Fear and Self-Gain

For most of us, by the time we reach an early age our psychological reactions to pain are deeply ingrained. These psychological reactions commonly are the product of our fears or our attempts at self-gain.

The fears are easier to understand. There can be personal fears such as "Why am I hurting?" "Is it going to get worse?" "Will I recover?" "Am I going to die?" There can be financial fears: "Can I pay my medical bills?" "Will I be able to work again?" "Will I get my job back?" There can be social fears: "Will I be rejected?" "What will my family do?" "What will my friends think?" "Am I to be an outcast?" It does not take long to run up a list of horrors that are all too real in any disease and in cancer especially.

There are many ways available to us to transform fear. These techniques form part of chapters 16 and 17 on emotional health. But for now, perhaps one of the greatest needs in dealing with fears specifically related to pain is to learn how to accept our situation as it is, yet to still be able to act decisively, as and when we need to. This is what mindfulness teaches us: how to avoid worrying about what tomorrow may or may not bring, and how to have the clarity of mind and commitment to do what we need to do now. Also, regular meditation and actually putting the principles of positive thinking into practice consistently leads to a deep level of peace of mind, acceptance and commitment. Many people, therefore, have found that learning to be more mindful, learning to meditate and to be more positive has led to a significant lessening in their pain almost without thinking about the pain itself.

However, another aspect of the psychological reaction to pain is the fact that often we have an ulterior motive in feeling pain. We are getting, or at least trying to get, something through the pain. This idea of pain having secondary gains is often a hard one to look at in our own life. However, it is also most certainly adding some component to any pain we might feel.

Here is one challenging possibility. Many people feel guilty about being sick and so some accept that they "should be suffering." For these people, having cancer and being "in pain" is all part of their expectation and the punishment they accept. Our personal reaction to pain is very much a product of our attitudes, emotional state and level of well-being. There is no need to punish ourselves by accepting pain. Again, use the positive-thinking principles, giving close attention to concentrating on pleasant activities. Laughter beats aspirin any day!

However, secondary gains frequently involve the other people in our life. By being "in pain," relatives and friends rally to us and often fill an emotional need we feel. Again, there is no need to feel guilty about realizing this—unless you are doing it consciously! There has to be a better way. We will discuss how to do this more in the chapters on healthy emotions, when we explore ways to fulfill our needs without the involvement of sickness and pain.

The psychological aspect of pain is therefore rather complex. To deal with it appropriately we need to understand our nature honestly and to look openly at what our goals are in life and how we want to achieve them. Again, this makes cancer an exercise in self-discovery and self-development.

I remember a young man, John, who had a deep fear of the pain of injections. Being on chemotherapy, his fear caused great difficulties. Each time he was to be injected, he would reflexively pull his arm away with a rapid jerk. Often it took many attempts to get the needle into his vein, causing anguish all around. After learning to relax and to cope with pain appropriately, John told me that not only did he stop the jerking, he did not even feel the needle going in. This transformation in his way of experiencing his pain and his treatment gave John a whole new level of confidence in his own abilities. This in turn helped him to transform his disease and his life. How is this possible?

We need to learn how to experience pain in an entirely different way. First we will clarify how it is possible to experience pain free of hurt, then we will examine the amazing possibilities when we learn more specific techniques using imagery, mindfulness and awareness.

TRAINING TO EXPERIENCE PAIN FREE OF HURT

Step 1. Separate the Psychological Reaction from the Physical Sensation

We begin by accepting that physical pain is real, but that it is just a sensation. While the intensity of that sensation can vary, we know that of itself, it is still just a sensation. What we also know is that the psychological reaction to pain can be deeply distressing. Recognizing this, we aim to drop the reaction and to experience the pain in its pure form—free of hurt. To be able to do this we need to learn the theory and then we need to practice the techniques. What we are aiming for is to experience the reality of hurt-free pain.

We can do this in a set exercise by detaching ourselves from the psychological aspect of pain and then applying a controlled painful stimulus. To avoid any psychological loadings we need to feel secure, to be in control of the situation and divorced from the influence of our mind and emotions. We meet all these criteria admirably by doing the initial exercises while meditating. Here is how.

THE BULLDOG PAPER CLIP EXERCISE

Preparation

We begin by choosing a suitable stimulus. We do not want to cause ourselves any bodily injury and so a paper clip of the "bulldog" type works well as these can be purchased from any office-supply shop. They come in different sizes, so when selecting one, you may like to try them out. Actually, while the big ones look most impressive, the small ones tend to create a sharper sensation. Some would say they hurt more! Select the size you feel you can work with.

Remembering that everyone has a different pain threshold to begin with, find a convenient place on your arm or hand where the clip can be put to produce a tolerable stimulus. The upper part of the forearm has quite thick skin and is fairly tough. If the clip does not cause much reaction there, try the inner, softer part of the arm. If need be, try the webbing between the fingers, or use just one corner of the clip. The aim is to produce a strong but acceptable stimulus. Putting it on ourselves leaves us in control. We know that we can stop the stimulus whenever we want to.

Relax, Apply the Stimulus and Observe

Now we take up our normal position for meditation and proceed to relax our body thoroughly. We let the mind come to rest also. Once settled, we open our eyes a little if necessary, and apply the clip. What reaction does it produce?

If you feel any hurt you will probably notice an automatic reflex. Your muscles will tense up. Probably those in the hand and arm will contract first. If you react a lot, the whole body may stiffen. Now, if you can impose relaxation on the body again, a strange thing happens. The hurt gradually diminishes, leaving a pure stimulus. In the calm, you can experience true pain. The more you try this experiment and become confident with it, the easier it is to experience true, non-hurtful pain.

The significance of this reflex is so important to us, we must appreciate it fully. Not only do anxiety and stress lead to tension, but by doing so, they also lead to hurtful pain. Similarly, relaxation relieves tension, defuses anxiety and stress, and takes the hurt out of pain. Relaxation is again the key. When we learn how to keep our body relaxed, free of tension, we will find pain is well on the way to being controlled. This is why these exercises are easier and most effective if they are done while we are practicing meditation each day in the standard simple way.

Experiment in More Challenging Situations

Following these early, easy experiments, we need then to go on to bigger and better things. Increase the level of stimulus first by using more powerful clips. Alternatively, lie on your back with a rock under your shoulders or look for other ways of experimenting with pain.

Next, and importantly, advance to more real-life situations by relinquishing control of the exercises. Have someone else apply the clips when you are meditating and so add the element of the unknown. This will teach you more control over the psychological aspect. Similarly, going outside and sitting near a rotating water sprinkler provides another type of unforeseeable stimulus. Perhaps the ultimate test is meditating where flies or mosquitoes are active! Create the opportunities to experience the reality of true pain.

Step 2. Experiment in Real Life

Having gained confidence through the formal exercises, now it is time to experiment with the use of our new skills in real life.

For example, if you have injections, relax yourself during the procedure and enjoy not having them as hurtful experiences. Consider having dental work done without anesthetic!

I remember well my first trip to the dentist after having resolved to not have an anesthetic. I felt the techniques should work, but I had yet to test them—to know for sure. Needing a sore tooth attended to, I organized a light workload for the morning of the big day. I made sure that I practiced my meditation more than usual for days beforehand and practiced several times before setting off. Arriving unusually early at the dentist's office, I sat and meditated some more in his waiting room. My name called, I scampered into the chair to relax myself and get into meditation as quickly as possible. Mumbling that I wanted no anesthetic, the dentist did little to reassure me by replying in a startled voice, "Are you sure?" Unwaveringly, I said I was sure, and the drilling began.

The result amazed me. Not only did I feel no pain, I virtually felt nothing at all. In response to my questions, the dentist said that yes, it should have been a painful procedure. The decay was near the tooth's nerve. Definitely I should have felt it. I was elated. For the first time, a trip to the dentist had been a positive experience for me. I walked out without half my mouth feeling numb and lopsided. I had no pain or discomfort whatsoever and the tooth was repaired.

I then had a great deal of restorative dental work done, including the fitting of crowns. As I gained confidence, I found the "great meditation buildup" was no longer necessary. One morning I managed to cut one of my fingers with an electrical saw. I was lucky I did not cut it off! I sewed up the gaping wound myself without an anesthetic. And that same afternoon, I had six fillings replaced in an hour-and-a-half session at the dentist's office, again without anesthetics or any particular preparation. I could feel it all, but there was no pain in it, just a stimulus that for preference I would still rather not have had. And remember, it was not long before this that I was known as having a poor tolerance of pain.

Step 3. Take the Benefits into Meditation

Another happy side effect of these exercises with pain is that they deepen our meditation. Using pain in this way focuses our attention very well and makes sure we are attending to our stated aim. If we do happen to let our mind run free, the pain soon asserts itself and reminds us to get it right. This is a bonus from the exercises that makes them doubly worth practicing.

These pain management exercises are ideally done when we feel well. Then we can take our time and there is no urgency to succeed straightaway. Over time, we will learn to perceive pain differently and we will experience a whole new way of living and being.

Be reminded that if pain is distressing in current time, it makes sense to gain relief where best we can. There is a great deal that can be done through the medical system, and through our own efforts. Many people do learn how to train in pain management in the way we have just explored, but there is another equally amazing possibility that is highly recommended when pain is strong and present.

DISSOLVING PAIN WITH IMAGERY AND AWARENESS

Warwick was a commercial fisherman. Used to hardship and having a fairly stoic nature, he was embarrassed to be crying in pain. Warwick was attending a residential program and I found him between sessions distraught due to the relentless pain created by a cancerous lymph node in his groin that was causing his right leg to swell. Warwick also suffered from chronic back pain, a legacy of his life at sea.

The exercise we are about to share often continues to amaze me, despite years of witnessing its transformative effect. I have to admit that when I saw Warwick in such distress, at first I was a little tentative, but I suggested we do an imagery exercise together. He was ready to try anything but I know he had no idea that within five minutes all—yes, all—his pain would be gone, and several months later he told me that while it sometimes recurred, it was minor and manageable. His back pain had been present for around fifteen years and resisted all previous attempts to manage it—now it too was insignificant.

What did we do that produced such remarkable results?

If you are experiencing significant pain, the following exercise can be remarkably transformative.

Option 1. The Exercise for Dissolving Pain

Many people have found the exercise opposite to be truly remarkable, leading to rapid and profound pain relief.

There are several additional techniques that build upon this exercise and are worth mentioning, as some people find they bring additional benefits.

Option 2. Repeated Scanning

It may be necessary or useful to repeat the exercise above and to continue to scan the body, locating and examining the pain using the guidelines as given.

To aid this process, and particularly for someone in distress, you could

The Exercise for Dissolving Pain

1. Sit or lie in a symmetrical position and close your eyes.

2. Relax as completely as you can without giving this step too much attention. Do not try to force yourself to relax; do it as easily and as deeply as you can. If you have already established a practice of meditation, aim to recall the feeling of deep relaxation.

3. Move your attention through the body, seeking out an area that feels different—an area that is painful, tight, under pressure, etc.

4. Be aware of where the sensation is in your body, for example the tummy. Be as specific as possible (e.g., close to the skin, deep in the abdomen). In the upper or lower region, etc. Where is it?

5. Be aware of its shape. Is it shaped like a ball, a sphere, a rod? What is its shape?

6. Be aware if its size. How long is it? Is it three-quarters of an inch or 1½ inches, and how wide is it? Is it three-quarters of an inch wide? One? And how deep is it? What is its size?

7. Be aware of its density . . . is it hard like a rock? . . . or soft like a sponge? . . . and is it harder on the outside, harder on the inside or the same all the way through? . . . What density does it have?

8. What is its surface texture? Is it soft and fuzzy or hard and smooth? What does it feel like?

9. What temperature is it? Is it warm? Or cool? Or neutral?

10. What color is it? If it did have a color, what might that color be?

11. Now hold this area in your attention . . . and as you breathe in next time, imagine you are traveling with the breath . . . right to that area you are focusing your attention on . . . and then imagine the breath gently washes around the outside of it . . . and as you breathe out, the breath just gently ebbs away again . . . a bit like an ocean wave coming into the shore, washing around something in the sand and then just going out to sea again with the out breath.

12. And do that for three more breaths . . . so each time you breathe in, the breath comes in and washes around the outside of the

area . . . with the out breath, the breath just gently ebbs away again.

13. Now the next time you breathe in, imagine that your breath flows right into the very center of this area . . . and as you breathe out, the breath just gently ebbs away again. Do that for three more breaths . . . so breathe in and the breath goes right into the center of this area . . . and then, with the out breath, it just gently ebbs away again.

14. Good . . . Now as you breathe in again, imagine flowing with the breath as it goes to this area once again and washes around the outside of it . . . and then, as you breathe out, the breath gently ebbs away . . . Do this again for three more breaths, breathing in and the breath goes around the outside of the area . . . breathing out and it just gently ebbs away.

15. Good. And now just gently scan your attention through the body again. Notice if there is a particular sensation that your mind is drawn to. If there is, you can repeat the whole process again like this:

16. Notice where that sensation is localized . . . Which part of the body? . . . Is it close to the surface or deeper into the tissue?

And then be aware of what shape it has . . . round like a ball, or oval like an egg? . . . a rod? . . . What particular shape does it have?

And then notice more particularly what size it is . . . How long is it? . . . How wide? . . . How deep? . . . How many centimeters or inches? . . . What size is it?

And then be aware of its density . . . is it hard like a rock? . . . or soft like a sponge? . . . and is it harder on the outside, harder on the inside or the same all the way through? . . . What density does it have?

And then the surface . . . Notice whether the surface is rough or smooth . . . What is its surface like?

And what temperature is it? . . . Is it warm? . . . or cool? . . . or neutral? . . . What temperature is it?

And color . . . If it had a color, what color would it be?

And now, as you hold your attention on this area, the next time you breathe in, follow the breath in and around the area . . . the

(continued)

(continued)

breath washing around the outside . . . and then with the out breath, gently ebbing away . . . and do that for three more breaths.

Good . . . Next time you breathe in, follow the breath right into the very center of the area . . . then breathe out, the breath just gently ebbing away once again . . . and do that for three more breaths.

17. Good . . . and now you can simply rest with the feeling you have right now . . . or you can continue with this exercise and repeat step 16 once again . . . but you might like to just let go of the exercise and simply rest with the feeling . . . just simply letting go . . . going with it . . . just simply letting go . . . quite effortlessly . . . effortlessly . . . more and more . . . deeper and deeper . . . just simply letting go . . . letting go . . . letting go . . .

ask a relative or friend to read you the exercise. They would need to read slowly in an even tone, and you would be wise to reply out loud to the questions as they are read to you: Where is the pain located? Specifically? What size is it? And so on. This process is further enhanced if the support person breathes in time with the person in pain and talks in a quiet, slow and confident manner. They may need to relax themselves first and establish their own inner calm before beginning.

Another very helpful option is to be led by my voice on the CD I have recorded of this exercise (see the details at the back of the book). When using the CD, you could answer the questions quietly to yourself, or even better, get over any awkwardness you might feel and reply out loud.

Once pain is fully experienced in this manner, it will often simply fade away.

Option 3. Imagery Along with Internal Relaxation

Another option, a different way of releasing pain, is that once you have developed your own image for the pain as described above, put your center of attention inside that image and consciously relax it. Doing this may cause an initial increase in discomfort as you concentrate fully on the pain. There is no avoidance here. This is a process that will enable you to pass through the pain and become free of it.

Having already established a practice of meditation, a familiarity with consciously relaxing your body will make this technique easier; however, it can work very well for beginners. Usually, as you relax the pain from the inside, it feels like a bubble bursting in slow motion as the outer shell of the pain breaks down and a wave of warmth and relaxation spreads from the inside out. This wave usually feels as though it extends out into the rest of the body and feels very pleasant.

Option 4. Triggering Endorphins

Sometimes while this process of concentrating upon a pain and releasing it is being practiced there can be a natural release of endorphins, the brain's opiate-like pain relievers.

This is the same effect experienced by many long-distance runners. Commonly, after eight or nine miles, runners experience their "second wind" or "break the pain barrier," a stage that involves the body releasing its own pain-relieving chemicals which produce a powerful sense of euphoria. This is one of the body's natural mechanisms for dealing with protracted pain and it can bring profound relief. In fact, it often produces a deep sense of well-being.

Some people have learned how to trigger this response consciously and so top up their pain management.

Option 5. Talking to the Pain

Some people find that they can talk to their pain. This may sound unusual at first, but sometimes an image of the pain arises spontaneously during meditation or the imagery exercise above and communication can be established with the person, animal or object that appears.

What is happening here is that the creative unconscious is using an image to enable us to talk to our own inner wisdom. This often leads to an insight into the nature of the pain and to its resolution.

So you could ask:

"Is it all right to talk to the pain?"

If the answer is yes, you could then ask any or all of the following:

"What is causing you (the pain)?"

"What is your purpose?"

"What is needed to make you go away?"

Option 6. The Secret of the Stillness

Remember too that as our experience of meditation develops, we become more aware of what we call the stillness. As we become more familiar with the stillness, we learn to give our attention to that stillness and to simply allow the pain to be there—while we remain undistracted.

This technique has a number of elements. It begins with the preparation that gives us a positive mind-set with which to approach pain. It draws huge support from the physical relaxation that we practice. Then, in a way, the stillness can be compared to the ultimate quiet place or inner sanctuary. This stillness is an ever-present source of peace and calm. In fact, the more we experience the stillness, the more we realize there is this inner part of us that is completely free of pain. In the stillness comes the direct experience of that part of us that is more permanent, more enduring and, just like the metaphor of the blue sky, unstainable, inviolable. We realize that there is this part of us that cannot be hurt. This can come as a source of great comfort and relief.

Option 7. The Role of Partners and Caregivers

Support people can also be of great help in the control of your pain. Touch works wonders. The comfort produced by a loving hand reaches us on a psychological level and such contact can ease many situations.

Talking through the progressive muscle relaxation we use as a lead-in to meditation can have a profound effect. This is a particularly helpful technique if someone is restless or distressed. It works best if the patient's given name is used while talking through the exercise. So, it could be said: "Feel your toes, Ian. Contract the muscles, Ian—and let them go." The name need not be used with every phrase, but including it regularly does aid the process. The exercise needs to be talked through in a slow, steady, unemotional tone and the one who is in pain does need to follow the directions. The exercise then finishes with an instruction for the person being guided to rest quietly and to allow any thoughts that do come into their awareness to simply be there, just allowing them to come and go, while remaining undistracted.

In a similar manner, it can be very helpful to have a support person read through the inner sanctuary exercise, or the exercise for dissolving pain.

RECOMMENDATIONS

This mind-based approach to pain control has no element of avoidance in it. It is a means by which the pain can be experienced as it is, free of fear or false imaginings. Commonly, when this is done, particularly in conjunction with the practice of mindfulness and meditation, the pain can be experienced as a sensation which, while it may be unpleasant, is certainly free from distress.

This technique has great merit as once established it requires little energy to maintain it. The pain can be acknowledged and accepted, and life can carry on free from its effects.

Start where you are at. Maybe analgesics are necessary to make life bearable. Maybe you can use more natural self-help methods to take the edge off the pain. Of course you will benefit from working with all the tools discussed in chapters 7 to 9 on positive thinking to improve your self-image and level of well-being. Do not overlook the role of laughing and indulging yourself in purely pleasurable activity. Likewise, aim to reach acceptance of your situation, especially if it does, or is likely to include, pain. If you can accept and flow with the pain rather than resisting and struggling against it, it will cause significantly less inconvenience.

Then, maybe by simply practicing your meditation, any pain eases and becomes more manageable. Maybe you will benefit from the extra learning that can come courtesy of a bulldog paper clip. Maybe there is something else in the range of possibilities we have covered that speaks to you more directly. The imagery and awareness exercise can be extraordinary. And then there is the deep comfort to be found in the stillness.

It is important to be prepared to experiment a little and to find what does work best for you personally. Just knowing that genuine pain relief is a possibility is a starting point. For many who have worked at this, a genuine change in their experience of pain has transformed their life for the better.

Finally, maybe it is obvious, but surely the best time to learn pain management skills is when you are pain free. Why wait until the need is strong? This is a life skill from which everyone can benefit. Use the techniques, practice, and remember, the more reliably you experience the stillness and its deep calm, the more confidence you will have in the face of pain. Why not experiment and find out the truth of the matter for yourself. You might just transform your experience of pain in the process.

Perhaps the greatest comfort I have gained through my cancer is learning that true pain does not hurt. Pain is a physical response; suffering is a conscious reaction that we can choose to do without. Knowing this to be real, experiencing it in daily life has been profoundly liberating.

CHAPTER 11

Nutrition 1

The Principles: A Logical Approach

THERE HAS TO BE AN APPROPRIATE DIET THAT WILL HELP PEOPLE AFFECTED by cancer to get well again. This is something to get positively excited about!

If you were diagnosed with heart disease, at the very first consultation it would be incumbent upon your doctor to talk to you about what you eat. The doctor would also be required to discuss other lifestyle matters: what you drink, whether you smoke or not, your levels of exercise, how you manage stress and, these days, how you relax and probably whether you meditate or not.

If you were diagnosed with type 2 diabetes (T2D), even more so. The link between what you eat, your lifestyle, the diagnosis and your capacity to recover are patently obvious. Heart disease and T2D are chronic, degenerative, lifestyle-related diseases. They respond well—as in you can recover from them—when you attend to what you eat along with your lifestyle more generally. Cancer is just the same.

Virtually all the remarkable, long-term cancer survivors I know value what they ate as a major factor in their recoveries. Same as me. Virtually all the thousands of people I have assisted for well over thirty years found giving considerable attention to nutrition and food produced significant benefits.

However, we live in a technological age. Current-day robots are capable of delicate and intricate surgery, even when the human surgeons directing their movements are on line and at a distance from the actual patient. Computers have phenomenal memories and wonderful capabilities to help us function. Medicine is becoming more and more complex and often when we are seeking healing we think it has to come through some complex technology.

Yet every human being lives in a physical body. While that body in its way of functioning is incredibly complex and could well be described as a technical marvel, it is very much dependent upon the food it eats and the fluids it drinks. Now while it is true that our digestion and all that happens in our body is affected by our emotions and our mind, clearly what impacts on the function and structure of our body most directly is the physical reality of the fuel we provide it with.

WHAT FUEL GOES INTO YOUR TANK?

One recent, very hot summer's day, I pulled into a station for gasoline. Beside me, a hot, sweaty, overweight and grumpy man approached a nearby pump for his fuel. He had three choices—low, medium and high octane—and he seemed clear on which to choose.

Seeing his foul mood, the mischievous part of me thought to suggest he take out his grumpiness on his van and put the wrong fuel in it. The more logical part of me rapidly decided this was not such a good idea. Not to be outdone, the mischievous part rose up with: *"Tell him to do a really good job of it and fill up with diesel instead of gasoline."* No came the response, you will get hit for sure if you say that!

So I held my tongue and watched. Very attentively this man put the right gasoline into the simple combustion-engined van he was driving. Then he went into the shop, bought all sorts of junk and proceeded to put absolute rubbish into the highly sophisticated, super complex, combustion-engined body in which he was living. My guess is that as well as being so particular regarding the fuel he put into his van, this fellow was like the rest of us and regularly attended to his vehicle's service timelines.

Why the disconnect with the body? Surely, it is common sense that food builds our body and is the mainstay of running and repairing it. If you want a junk body, eat junk food. Want a healthy body? Eat healthy food. Want a body that just manages to function? Well, feed it whatever. Want a body that is capable of remarkable healing? Surely it makes sense to fill it up with the best fuel possible. Again, get excited!

THE HOPE THAT GOOD FOOD OFFERS

For me, food is another major piece of good news following a cancer diagnosis. Understanding the clear role nutrition plays in the causes of cancer helps to make more sense of the disease. Understanding the role changing your diet plays in recovery provides real hope—it gives inner confidence and feeds optimism. Understanding that improving the diet of your family, and who knows, maybe even having a positive influence on friends and others you care for, brings reality to the wish that others will not get cancer or any of the other chronic, degenerative diseases. Eat well and you can be really well!

The aim of the diet chapters is to provide hope, clarity and confidence. We will focus on what works nutritionally to support recovery and long-lasting good health, as well as how to make eating healthy food easy and tasty, practical and enjoyable.

How we will achieve this is by first examining the role our mind and our culture plays in our food choices. Then we will use our logic to investigate how food and nutrition can help us to heal. Experience tells me that when we understand the principles involved in good nutrition, the details follow fairly naturally. The intention is to understand what we do and why, and to enjoy eating for recovery.

Let us begin by examining the principles that connect food, cancer and survival.

WHAT DO THE DOCTORS KNOW?

You will have no trouble in finding cancer specialists who will tell you what you eat is very important. You will have no trouble finding other specialists who tell you it will make no difference whatsoever. Why such a big disparity?

My wife, Ruth, who is a GP with a master's in general practice psychiatry, studied at the highly respected University of Sydney's medical school, where there was not one specific lecture on nutrition in six years of medical training. Not one! This is the norm for medical education. No wonder so many doctors have no knowledge of or interest in nutrition and its relevance to healing.

Having trained as a veterinarian, I find this continuing error of omission in my colleagues' education staggering. One of my daughters, who is currently studying veterinary science, is required to complete four full semesters of study on nutrition. In veterinary science, they study seven main animal species. What is so special about the human species, the human body, that leaves medical educationalists believing that what it eats is of no importance?

I find this oversight in medical education deeply concerning. Also, what this knowledge clearly indicates is that unless your doctor has completed post-graduate education in nutrition, they will be grossly underqualified to comment on this vital area.

This problem is compounded by the food industry's infiltration of the psyche of the community and the health professions. Dietitians generally seem to believe nutritional requirements are solved by formulated and standard eating patterns of the day. In my view many of them represent the food industry far more directly than the real needs of the community.

What we do know for sure is that the current, average Western diet contributes significantly to six of the ten major causes of premature death in modern society: heart disease, diabetes, obesity, hypertension, diverticulitis and, of course, cancer.

World authorities, professors Sir Richard Doll and Sir Richard Peto, in their book *The Causes of Cancer*, first published way back in 1981, stated that the best current estimate was that diet is a major contributing factor in 35 percent of all cancers. August bodies such as the American Academy of Sciences put the figure at 40 percent for men and 60 percent for women. However, medical confirmation of the diet-cancer link had only come in the few years before Doll and Peto's work was first released. Prior to this, the connection had been vehemently denied in most quarters, as was the thought that diet could help a person to get well.

What is apparent, however, is that there is an emerging number of doctors actively counseling people affected by cancer on dietary principles. They get results that are plain for all to see, and the interest grows. Yet diet in the sense in which we are talking is still frequently, if incredibly, considered by some medical authorities to be an "alternative" area of treatment. Some would dismiss it altogether. So you will need to make up your own mind and set a clear path.

Having said that, I strongly recommend that any major dietary changes are best supervised by a qualified and experienced health professional with the necessary skill and knowledge of nutrition. This is particularly important if the disease is directly impacting on the digestive tract or there has been significant surgery in that area. Ideally, this supervision would be provided by a doctor who is qualified and experienced. Some naturopaths are very knowledgeable. In my own experience, people in a stable condition find getting their diet organized to be a safe, relatively easy, and certainly reward-ing experience. It is necessary, however, to be open to change and prepared to learn. For those in a less stable condition, a word of caution and a repeti-tion: seek suitable, qualified guidance and recognize that you may need to make an intense personal effort to begin with.

EVALUATE THE EVIDENCE

Naturally we want to make the best choices possible with our food and all else that we do. For this we need the best evidence, a clear mind to evaluate that evidence and the motivation to follow through on our choices. If it is helpful, revisit the major section on goal setting and contemplation in chapter 7.

As we investigate the role of nutrition in cancer medicine, it will be use-ful to digress a little and take the time to understand what evidence-based medicine (EBM) is, why it is so valued by the medical profession, and how in my view, it is commonly distorted.

EBM is a logical and very useful principle. Simply put, it says that all medical decisions need to be based on the best evidence available. No one would argue with that proposition. However, it is helpful to understand that EBM is commonly distorted in current usage. To understand the problem we need to turn to the definition. The definition of EBM that has most wide acceptance was published in the *British Medical Journal*[15] in 1996:

> EBM is the conscientious and judicious use of current best evidence
> in making decisions about the care of individual patients. The prac-
> tice of evidence based medicine means integrating individual clinical
> expertise with the best available external clinical evidence from sys-
> tematic research. By individual clinical expertise is meant the profi-
> ciency and judgment that individual clinicians acquire through
> clinical experience and clinical practice.

However, the problem is that frequently in medical circles where the emphasis is on "being scientific," the research from published journals is overemphasized and the clinical experience (what happens in the real world) is diminished.

Of course, the science is important. Of course, research is important and it would be wonderful to have more research funding used to investigate the foods that help to heal cancer. However, while clearly there is a great deal of knowledge and research concerning nutrition in general, when we do examine the current research evidence relating to food being used as a therapy for cancer, the first thing to notice is how little of it there is. There are multiple reasons for this as with most things, but significant facts are that nutritional research is very complex and expensive. Doctors who have no undergraduate training in nutrition and therefore no belief in its relevance are hardly likely to drive research in this area, and food is unpatentable, so only government, philanthropic donors or food industry people are likely to fund these inquiries. Unfortunately, the fruit and vegetable growers do not seem to place a high value on investigating the merits of their produce in cancer research.

However, in the absence of compelling, published research, EBM says we need to examine the best level of evidence that is available, and with cancer, nutrition and healing, that evidence comes from clinical experience.

Here is where this book comes in. My background is in veterinary science. I received a thorough, if basic, training in nutrition. I recovered from a very difficult cancer, very much against the odds, using food and nutrition as one of my major platforms for healing. I have over thirty years' experience working closely with people affected by cancer who took what they ate very seriously. It is fair to say that myself along with the foundation I helped to establish have a great deal of clinical evidence regarding what to eat when you have cancer, and that this volume of evidence probably compares favorably with anyone or any organization on the planet.

To be clear about all this, I do value the research highly. I continue to study nutrition and read widely. However, in my experience, what happens in practical reality is the real test of any diet that is proposed. What follows is the best and most practical information I can offer currently based on the accumulated experience of thousands of people and informed by the best of modern evidence.

GOOD NUTRITION STARTS WITH THE MIND

What is the single most important factor when it comes to what you eat? Clearly it is the mind. The mind decides what you will eat and how much of it. The mind will decide what you drink and regulate your levels of exercise. Your mind and its attendant emotions have the potential to completely disrupt or enhance your digestion. Obviously when under stress, our eating habits can suffer. Many people eat to fill an emotional hole. Many eat out of habit, false beliefs, neurosis or food addiction. Most of us are heavily influenced by advertising and by what those we hold in authority, like our doctors, have to say on the subject.

The aim we have here is to break free of destructive mind states regarding food and to eat for enjoyment and genuine good health. This is why we start with meditation. The calm and clear mind that meditation delivers will leave you confident to make good dietary choices, in the right state of mind to digest your food well, and confident to develop and sustain healthy eating habits. Happy meditating equals happy eating! However, along with meditation, it makes good sense to use our logical minds to examine the influences our society and our own unconscious exerts on us, and how we can use these energies to our advantage.

DECIDE WHO TELLS YOU WHAT TO EAT

There is a key question when it comes to what to eat, how much to meditate, what treatments to have and so on. Who tells us what to do? When it comes to diet, will it be a doctor, a dietitian, a naturopath, the lady over the back fence, a book—or will it be you?

Who to believe? My guess is that most people would prefer to work it out for themselves. Yet for many, when it comes to actually doing this, the choices appear complex and often confusing. If we are to take full responsibility for our own decisions and to work it out scientifically ourselves, there is an incredible amount of work to do—references to find, differences to sort out, so much learning. Clearly the amount of information available on food is vast and quite complex. The interactions of different foods that we might eat are complex. People's reactions to food are complex. So how do we simplify it?

My sense of it is that if we were to wait and not eat another meal until all the facts were clear, all the research completed and the debates settled, we would be old and gray indeed. And probably pretty hungry! There is an immediate imperative to make the best choices we can now, to do the best we can. This is what this book aims to help you with—a logical, step-by-step approach to eating for recovery.

GOING NUTS OVER FOOD DOES NOT ONLY MEAN EATING LOTS OF ALMONDS

We need to recognize the complex states of mind and the emotional turmoil that can exist for some people around food.

All of us are creatures of habit and we have discussed the role of conditioning and habitual thinking in chapter 8. But many of us could well be described as neurotic around food, while some are clearly afflicted by dietary-related addictions.

At the risk of laboring the point, it is obvious that our psychology can dramatically affect our food choices as well as our ability to actually do what we choose to do.

We need our mind to support our healing, not to sabotage it. Therefore we need to be honest with ourselves, talk of these issues, maybe even seek help through professional counseling if necessary, and make sure we use our food well.

UNDERSTAND THE INTERNAL FORCES GOVERNING OUR EATING HABITS AND ESTABLISH HEALTHY ONES

We receive training in the rights and wrongs and the dos and don'ts of food from many quarters. Family, friends, school, books, magazines, the media—all are sources of information. The problem is how to differentiate between false or inaccurate information and that which is correct. And how to take account of any biased information that may come your way. For example, the Dairy Board in Australia has created an excellent impression in many people's minds that the only way to get enough calcium is to consume regular and substantial quantities of dairy products. Yet, when you check the analysis of our nondairy, vegetable-based diet via the tables in Appendix M, you will find that it is more than adequate, containing over twice the recommended daily intake of calcium.

The reality is that to develop a healthy diet most people will benefit from clarifying what factual information they have learned already and from learning more.

Next, it only takes a little reflection to realize that our dietary choices are influenced by far more than pure information. There is the culture we grow up in, the social structure and the habits we develop. In a psychological sense, some people appear quite addicted to certain foods while others are dramatically affected by their emotions. Some people eat to excess to fill an "emotional hole," while others provide reward or punishment via food. Commonly, many of us feel the need to rebel and so we eat, smoke or drink something really daft to demonstrate our independence.

Advertising and peer pressure influence and condition the choices made by many people. Anorexia and bulimia are powerful extremes, but most children these days are growing up with their dietary choices heavily influenced by the food industry generally and the fast-food industry more particularly.

If you are embarking upon dietary change, it is really important to bring some awareness to these subtler, yet very powerful issues. These issues help to explain some of the difficulties you may experience. To change your diet is to change a major habit.

To ensure a future life, a healthy life, it may well be necessary to recognize any negative conditioning you have picked up and to develop a healthier way of thinking, a healthier way of eating. This is why we gave consideration to positive thinking in chapter 7—so that you could understand more of how the mind works, how conditioning has the potential to bind us into negative, unhealthy habits and yet how it is possible to transform all this, to make a new start and to rebuild your own good health and the health of those you love and care for.

WHO ARE YOU EATING FOR?

To clarify the psychology around food still further, we need to consider what external influences may be involved. Are you trying to please your partner? Your family? Your doctor? The advertising gurus? Or are you eating to meet your own particular health needs? Obviously the people around you are important and need to be taken into consideration; however, you do need to be clear on your own motivation.

If you do need to change your diet, it is bound to have an impact on your family and friends at least. How they react to your needs, how they support you and how you in turn deal with their reactions, could significantly affect what you do, how long you do it, and how well you do it.

This is why it is so important to communicate with those who you value. Once you have reached a decision as to what to do in the dietary arena, it is highly recommended that you write your dietary choices out as clearly as possible. You will find the charts in chapter 14 helpful for this. Then, using your written plan as a basis, discuss it with the important people in your life, emphasizing what you intend to do and why.

Regarding the family, it is clear that prevention is better than cure. It is well established that a healthy diet can prevent many illnesses, including cancer. So, as a minimum, the Wellness Diet is recommended for all the family. As an extra bonus, when others in the family are eating the same thing, it provides a sense of tangible support and makes meal preparation easier. Doing these things together assists in the healing process and helps to develop lifestyle patterns that will ensure long-term good health for everyone.

HOW MUCH CLARITY AND COMMITMENT DO YOU HAVE?

This really is a summation of what we have discussed so far. Food can help with healing, it can prevent disease, and it can make you feel good. There are many issues you will need to focus on—practical ones like cost and availability, factual considerations, emotional states, mental conditioning and habits. For many, their spiritual view, religious traditions, sense of ethics and responsibility to the environment play a prominent role in deciding their food choices.

So with all this, be clear on why you are eating and what you are eating. It makes good sense to take the time to resolve as many of these questions as you can. Many more questions are likely to arise as you proceed. Welcome this. Work with the questions, stay with them and seek your own answers.

DIFFERENT STAGES • Different Eating Patterns

It may be helpful to realize that for most people, and especially those dealing with cancer, the diet is best regarded as having different stages. When you first pay attention to your diet, it is highly likely that you will decide to make some, if not many, changes. So, there will be a transition—a transitional time where you are saying good-bye and letting go of past habits and adjusting to and welcoming new habits.

Often if illness is a major issue, people benefit from a stage of paying attention to their diet intensively. Then as the outlook improves there comes a stage of modification, experimentation and adaptation. Then it may be time to settle into the maintenance phase—that stage where you are eating in a normal, healthy, ongoing pattern.

My own experience is that food helped me tremendously during my recovery. While I am sure that it has been a major factor in my ongoing survival and good health, I now eat in the way I do because it helps me to feel the best that I can. I enjoy my food. I enjoy the fact that it is good for me and I enjoy the fact that I feel really good after I have eaten. I enjoy the fact that I am well.

ENJOY • The Message of the Big Mac and the Salad!

Is it better to eat a Big Mac and enjoy it, or a garden-fresh salad and loathe it? Is what you eat more important or the state of mind in which you eat it? Is it better to do what is good for you regardless of whether you enjoy it or not, or is it better to do what you enjoy whether it is good for you or not?

Have you read Yogananda's mind-blowing *Autobiography of a Yogi*?[16] It recounts his years as a young spiritual seeker searching through mystical India for his teacher, his guru. In ancient times, before the days of calling cards and websites, spiritual leaders needed to demonstrate their prowess to validate their capacities and to attract followers. There were different ways to do this, but commonly they developed siddhis, or signs of spiritual accomplishment. Yogananda describes many amazing feats he witnessed including "the poison eating saint." This fellow's demonstration was to eat poison and broken glass and remain unaffected—that is, as the story goes, until he repeated his siddhi on a day when he was in an agitated state of mind and unceremoniously died.

My experience of these matters is that there is a spectrum as in most things. Some people do have strong minds and strong constitutions and can manage on a wider range and quality of foods. However, it is a high level of accomplishment to be able to eat any old rubbish and be unaffected by it—especially long term.

For most of us mere mortals our health and our capacity to heal is dramatically affected by what we eat. Healthy eating leads to long-term good health and eating particularly well has the potential to assist us to recover from major illness.

The trick with food therefore is twofold. How can you be sure of what is good for you? And how do you enjoy eating it so you keep on eating it?

Easy. You need good information and the right state of mind.

Everything starts with the mind. It is our mind that decides what food to buy, how to store and prepare it, how much to eat and what state of mind we are in when we eat it.

How then to use the mind to good effect? We need to use our mind, our wits, to gather good information, then we need to train our mind to serve us—to follow through on our good choices and lead the way in deciding what we eat and how much we enjoy eating it.

Here is the kicker. Here is the real secret that so many people I met in the past were not aware of, but who on learning of it changed their lives dramatically for the better. Here is the secret to enjoying what the theory says is good for us:

Anything you do often enough you get used to. Nothing is difficult once you get used to it. Anything you choose to, you can put your mind to and enjoy doing it. It is not such a great accomplishment to decide upon the state of mind you will do something in. With just a modicum of willpower, most people can do it.

So use your intelligence. Choose the salad and choose to enjoy it!

This whole arena of nutrition is full of excitement, controversy and the definite prospect of being helpful. It is essential to be clear in your own mind as to the relevance it has for you. You need to feel good about your choices. It is very necessary to think about the whole area and to come to definite conclusions.

In the final analysis, food needs to be enjoyed. You need to be able to sit down before it, give thanks for what you have to eat, know that it is appropriate for your situation, and eat it with a smile on your lips and a song in your heart!

Let us move on now to consider how to put these principles into practice. What to put on the plate tonight?

CHAPTER 12

Nutrition 2

Foods That Heal: Clarifying Your Choices

IF YOU HAVE BEEN READING MORE WIDELY, YOU WILL KNOW THERE ARE different opinions offered regarding what is best to eat. Most books include a list that features what to avoid and what to eat, then they claim their list works well for those who use the list. So you check—you read another book or visit another authority and receive their list along with the assurance that this list works well too. Only problem is, the lists are different! So you go to the third book, the third authority, to find out which is correct, only to be enthusiastically provided with yet another list. What to do? How to make sense of it?

Many of the lists I read are actually correct—for some people. Where the confusion arises is that we often overlook the fact that people are different. One list can work really well for one group of people, another different list works well for another different group of people. The vital question is: Which group do you fit into? What will work best for you?

There is an answer. To clarify any confusion, we begin by identifying general food principles that apply to most people. Then we develop a process whereby it becomes possible to establish a way of eating that is best suited to your own individual situation and needs. We take two key steps. First, we establish what we call healthy boundaries. Then we establish personal food awareness.

ESTABLISH HEALTHY BOUNDARIES • The Wellness Diet

The first step in establishing a way of eating that will have therapeutic benefits against cancer, and will suit us specifically, is to establish healthy boundaries. The simple principle behind healthy food boundaries is that these boundaries aim to define what we are wise to avoid and what we are best to concentrate upon eating.

These healthy boundaries then form the basis of the Wellness Diet. The Wellness Diet is nutritionally sound, relatively easy to implement and will bring a great deal of benefit very quickly. This way of eating provides a good, general starting point for anyone with cancer and it provides sound guidelines for every member of the family. It is reasonable to say that if the community generally followed the Wellness Diet, overall health would improve dramatically and chronic, degenerative diseases reduce significantly. The details of the Wellness Diet form the next chapter.

DEVELOP PERSONAL FOOD AWARENESS • The Healing Diet

The second step is to develop our own personal food awareness so we can go from the general recommendations of the healthy boundaries, to the specific needs we have as an individual on the Healing Diet. This we will learn to do with the assistance of mindfulness and meditation, along with developing our knowledge of food, and increasing our personal sensitivity and responsiveness to what we eat.

The starting point is to develop your awareness. The deep stillness of pure and simple, uncomplicated, mindfulness-based stillness meditation (MBSM) leads naturally to clarity of mind and heightened awareness. This is another of the automatic and positive flow-on benefits that come with regular meditation. The more you meditate, the more you become aware. The more aware you are, the more you notice what is affecting you and how you are reacting. So as you meditate more, and become more aware, you become more likely to notice whether you react well or badly to any given food you eat. Also, as you meditate more you are likely to feel well within yourself. This means you are more likely to make good decisions. So not only are you more likely to notice what foods agree with you, you are more likely to respond to that observation and to actually enjoy eating what is good for you.

YOUR BODY AS YOUR GUIDE

However, there is more to this. Your body can become a major ally when it comes to making good food choices. It is quite possible that you can help your body to become more sensitive to what you are eating—in a way that it will help you to be able to discriminate between those foods that are good for you and those foods that are not.

We often think of this principle with animals. When they are sick, instinctively they seem to know what to eat, what serves them best. The suggestion is that as human beings, we too can regain this instinctive or insightful capacity. It is possible to help your body to develop to the point where it can assess how the food you are providing it with is affecting you. Even more important, your body can let you know what is helping it and what is not. In this way, it becomes possible to develop a really personalized diet.

Clearly, if you do want your body to be able to assess your food, you will be using it like an instrument. For an instrument to be useful, to be accurate and readable, it needs to be clean. So, if your body is full of junk, then it is hard to imagine how it would be sensitive enough to discriminate. This then is another reason to recommend a period of dietary cleansing or detoxification. Once the body has been purified it will be far more sensitive to what you put in it, and far more likely to give you helpful feedback.

How to cleanse or detox the body will be explored soon in chapter 14. It is enough for now to say that the approach that we recommend is quite similar to an allergy elimination diet, which is an approach used in mainstream food sensitivity and allergy testing.

THE HEALING DIET • A Summary

The Healing Diet is based on the principles of the Wellness Diet, but it involves applying those principles more diligently and then guides us as we develop our own specific program. Here is how we do it:

1. Start with the mind. Meditation leads to clarity and inner peace. This enhances what we learn intellectually, helps us to make good choices, and develops our awareness of what works personally and what is best avoided. Meditation also helps us to be unaffected by any potential stress that changing our diet may involve. We aim for clarity, confidence and enjoyment.
2. Establish healthy boundaries, using the Wellness Diet to ensure we have the basic elements of our food correct.

3. Go from the general to the specific by using:
   1. More meditation and contemplation—and the heightened awareness they bring.
   2. A mono diet or partial fasting for short periods of time to heighten our food sensitivity.
   3. A process of experimentation based upon elimination and reintroduction of sensitive foods.
4. Regularly use foods known for their anticancer properties.
5. Establish a cancer-unfriendly environment in our body by manipulating our own metabolism (through the use of appropriate foods) to make life difficult for the cancer.
6. Use fresh juices to increase the vital nutrients required for healing.
7. Consider using supplements. In my view, there is a hierarchy when it comes to using nutrition to heal cancer. Food is the number one priority, juices come second and supplements third.
8. Continue on the Healing Diet until cancer free, and then modify it toward the Wellness Diet.

The details of the Healing Diet form chapter 14.

As I am frequently asked to detail what I did regarding food and juices during my own recovery, I have summarized my own experiences with the Healing Diet and with the Gerson Therapy specifically in Appendix G.[17] But do remember, just like you, I am an individual. What I did may well be interesting and informative, but it is for each one of us to discover what will work best for us personally.

HOW THOROUGH DO WE NEED TO BE?

When we were developing as a fetus inside our mother's abdomen, both of us had very specific nutritional requirements. As a child and adolescent, we needed about 25 percent more food on a weight-for-weight basis to take account of our growth rate. Some parents would say for teenage boys it is way higher. Certainly if we are engaged in physically demanding sport or work, we need significantly more than someone who sits behind a desk all day.

When we are basically well, it is what we eat mostly that is important. The fact is that as human beings, our bodies are reasonably adaptable. If you eat well at home through the week and then go out on the weekend and play up a little, there is little likelihood of harm. If you play up every night, then the risks begin to build fairly rapidly.

So again, when we are well, what we eat mostly is important. However, when we are dealing with major illness, what we eat all the time is important.

This statement is made based on my years of clinical experience, and is reinforced by Dean Ornish's randomized, lifestyle-based prostate cancer trial.[18] Ornish first won international acclaim in the nineties for publishing research that demonstrated it is possible to reverse coronary artery disease using a basically vegan diet, exercise, meditation, yoga, emotional healing and group therapy—a program very similar to the one we developed at the Gawler Foundation. Ornish then went on to investigate the same program with men diagnosed with early prostate cancer who were in what essentially in those days was called the "watchful waiting phase."

The results were compelling. Not surprisingly, the cancer advanced for most of the men in the control group, their PSAs (a blood marker of prostate cancer activity) went up, the aggressiveness of their cancers went up and several required major medical treatments. Those men who made modest lifestyle changes stabilized their condition, a significant benefit in its own right. However, those who made major lifestyle changes and diligently maintained them were able to reduce their PSAs, reduce the aggressiveness of their cancers and, after one year, none had required medical intervention. After three years, the benefits were still highly significant, although a small number of the diligent men (significantly less than in the control group) had required more medical treatment.

In nearly all areas of life, how we apply ourselves will make a difference. Do nothing and the natural course of events is likely to follow. Do nothing in response to cancer and it is highly likely to progress. Intervene, use your own resources, and remarkable outcomes become possible.

So when faced with active cancer, the recommendation is to take what you eat seriously.

But if you think, "I will eat well long enough to get well, and then go back to junk food," you are missing the point. The first thing when faced with cancer is to recover. Then we aim for a long, happy and healthy life. What we eat provides the raw ingredients for healing and a healthy old age.

CLARIFY YOUR CHOICES • Make a Decision

Having read what has been presented so far, maybe it is time to begin to make some broad but important decisions. Regarding nutrition and our way of eating, there would seem to be four options worth considering:

1. Make no change.
2. Adopt the Wellness Diet.
3. Follow the Healing Diet.
4. Commit yourself to a specific intense diet such as Gerson's and seek professional help with it—preferably in a suitable clinic.

Dietary Choices—Make No Change

If you are happy with your diet as it is and feel it cannot be improved, that is fine. Skip the next two chapters and go on with the other things available to help you back to health.

However, I am convinced that dietary considerations are one of the basic tools for getting well. Most of the dietary factors associated with a risk of increasing the incidence of cancer are prominent in our Western diet. These factors are a high content in the diet of fat, protein, salt, sugar, refined foods and foods with a low-fiber content, as well as too many calories, and drinking excessive alcohol. It is likely, then, that most people need to consider making changes.

Dietary Choices—The Wellness Diet

This is a relatively easy step. It is how we establish healthy boundaries. It requires eliminating from the diet those things associated with a health risk and concentrating on what is known to be good for us.

The Wellness Diet can be described in simple terms as a plant-based, whole-food diet.

For many people, then, this type of diet does involve a significant change in eating habits, but it still fits readily into most daily routines.

The Wellness Diet is ideal for those with cancer who want to improve their way of eating without giving food a great deal of attention. It is a sound "bottom line." It is an excellent consideration for those in remission, being an ideal way to eat for those who are basically well, as well as for those who are interested in preventing disease and in maximizing their health. I feel confident in putting it forward as a basic, sensible and sound diet.

The Healing Diet

This is the more intense approach recommended for people with active cancer. The Healing Diet includes learning to develop a personalized and specific dietary program and requires a good deal of commitment. It is for those who intend to take what they eat seriously and are intent on using nutrition for recovery.

Specific Intensive Dietary Programs

I do not recommend these unless they are supervised by qualified personnel. My attitude is that a knowledgeable doctor needs to be involved in any such program.

MAKE A PLAN

Eating for recovery requires you to set clear goals. Here is how you can establish a good plan that will make it easy for you to eat for recovery.

1. Set a time limit for collecting information on the dietary possibilities.
2. Take what is written here, and add more information from all sources available to you.
3. Assess this body of information. Remember the value of contemplation to enhance the information and use the contemplation technique detailed in chapter 7.
4. Make a decision and plan a course of action.
5. Enlist the support of your family, friends and colleagues.
6. Commit yourself to a period of time to experiment with your diet.
7. For the given period of time, adhere as thoroughly as possible to your plan. Give it a chance to produce an effect.
8. At the end of that period, reassess and plan again.
9. Repeat steps 7 and 8 regularly.

There is a great deal that can be done, and remember: Diet is not the total answer to cancer, but without a good diet, there is no answer.

WHAT I SUGGEST

At the very least, the Wellness Diet is easy and reliable. Committing to this approach will avoid most problems and be significantly helpful. When the need is to recover from cancer and you want to do the best for yourself and those around you, the Healing Diet makes more sense to me. However, the choice needs to be yours. Consider the options. Meditate. Contemplate. Discuss the possibilities with those you value.

When you are ready, move on to the next chapters where we define the Wellness Diet and clarify the Healing Diet.

CHAPTER 13

Nutrition 3

Healthy Boundaries: The Wellness Diet

THE WELLNESS DIET IS BASED UPON A SIMPLE PREMISE. IT AIMS TO AVOID foods that are known to be unhelpful; it concentrates on using the foods that are known to be healthy and enjoyable. By doing this well, we have a diet that is highly anti-inflammatory and highly regenerative. It is a diet that will prevent the majority of chronic degenerative diseases, will be enjoyable to prepare and eat, will provide a sound basis for recovering from illness, and is easy to understand and commit to.

While we could say the Wellness Diet provides logical guidelines for anyone interested in eating well, another way of explaining it is via the concept of healthy boundaries. When you avoid the things that are unhelpful and eat the healthy foods, you are in safe territory.

For many who are basically well, this diet is ideal. For those embarking on recovering from cancer it provides a quick and reliable starting point. By following these guidelines you immediately take out of your diet the things that could aggravate your illness, and you immediately incorporate many things that will help you to regenerate and to heal. Once you have settled into this first step of the Wellness Diet, then you can go on to individualize your eating pattern and to gain the additional benefits available through the Healing Diet.

As we move into clarifying the detail of the Wellness Diet, we will begin with more principles. Remember the key point; by understanding the principles, we gain confidence in what we are doing and the details tend to follow on fairly easily.

Wellness Rule 1: Understand the principles to simplify the details.

So as we discuss the principles of fats, proteins, soy and so on, we will do so in a practical way. The rationale behind what to eat and what to avoid will be explained. As we examine each food or aspect of food, we will consider three questions:

- Quantity—how much, if any, of a given food to eat,
- Quality—what type of the food is ideal if there are choices available, and
- Preparation—including storage and cooking techniques.

FATS AND OILS

Making intelligent choices regarding the quantity, quality and preparation of the fats you consume is one of the most powerful ways to improve your nutrition, your health and your capacity to heal.

Nutritional Information

What is the difference between a fat and an oil? Essentially oils are liquid fats. Fats and oils have a similar chemical structure and from the body's perspective, they both have similar functions. We call those fats that tend to be solid at room temperature fats—such as lard or animal fat—while those fats that are liquid at room temperature, like olive oil, we tend to call oils. To simplify things, we will mostly use the word "fats" during this section.

Fats fulfill a wide range of functions in the body, being a source of energy and a major means to store energy. Fats also act as a buffer—they protect us from trauma, insulate us from temperature changes and importantly are a repository for dangerous material. When the body has an excessive load of toxic material or even unsafe bacteria coming into it, rather than allowing that material to impact on our vital organs, the body in its cleverness shunts the offending matter into our fat stores. There it remains until it can be metabolized and eliminated from our system. This is important to realize, as it means that eating fat from polluted, unhealthy or toxic sources means we accumulate their rubbish.

But also, if we are unhealthy and overweight, and then we lose weight rapidly, we can have a significant toxic overload to deal with as our fat breaks down and releases the offending material into our system.

On a happier note, fats also play a positive role in healthy skin and hair, and are essential aids for the transport and metabolism of the fat-soluble vitamins A, D, E and K. Fats also play a vital role in the integrity of our cell membranes or walls, which we will investigate further soon.

Quantity

Currently the average American acquires over 40 percent of their caloric intake via fats. In Australia it is in the low 30s and yet the ideal is around 15–18 percent. So for the average person, halving your fat intake would be about right. It is worth noting that to reverse coronary artery disease or atherosclerosis, the fat intake needs to go down to about 11–12 percent, which is quite difficult to do. This would require avoiding things like avocados which, while they are about 50 percent fat, do actually fit in nicely with the Wellness Diet.

How do we reduce our fat levels? Simply avoid hidden fats and use modest amounts yourself. Those who do have a high fat intake acquire a great deal of their fats hidden in fried foods, dressings, fast foods, pastries and the like, so we avoid all those unhealthy foods.

The quantity of fat that is ideal is one of the many principles that takes care of itself by adopting the Wellness Diet. What is meant by this is that when you follow the Wellness program and eat in the way recommended, the fat levels will automatically be close enough to ideal. This means you need not be concerned to measure, weigh or add up what actual fats you use. This is something you can trust.

Quality

Understanding the different types of fats available and choosing the best ones is crucial to our health and to our capacity for healing. There are several classifications to be aware of and respond to.

Saturated vs. Unsaturated Fats

Fats fall into these first two major categories: saturated and unsaturated. Saturated and unsaturated fats have one major difference—saturated fats have many more double bonds connecting the molecules that make up their structure. This fact makes them harder, more brittle and more angular in their shape. This in turn accounts for saturated fats being solid at room temperature—like lard (animal fat) and coconut oil (one of the few saturated vegetable fats). This chemical structure also explains why unsaturated fats are liquid at room temperature and why we use the names animal fats and vegetable oils.

To understand the principle behind using unsaturated fats and avoiding the saturated ones, we need to understand how these fats are incorporated into our own bodies. Our body is made up of many, many cells, each with a similar basic structure. Each has a cell membrane, or external wall within which are contained those more fluid, internal elements of the cell that are responsible for the cell's functions. Each cell membrane has what is called a double lipid layer much as a wall could have bricks or timber. Lipids are fats; we are talking of a double layer of fats being an integral part of the membrane of each cell in your body. Now the crucial point.

If you are eating mostly saturated fats, the lipids in your body will be mostly saturated; eat mostly unsaturated fats and the lipids will be unsaturated. Cell membranes composed of saturated fats will be hard, brittle and have what effectively are spiky edges. A direct consequence of this is that saturated fat cell membranes will be dense and not very permeable. This means it is harder for nutrients to get into the cell and harder for waste products to get out. The whole metabolism of the cell is compromised.

By contrast, when our cell membranes are made up of mostly unsaturated fats; those cells will be more pliable, more permeable, more efficient.

This issue is of great importance for your red blood cells. Red blood cells transport oxygen and other nutrients around your body. They can be visualized like balloons filled with water. If their outside membrane is made up mostly of saturated fats, they will be quite rigid and inflexible, as well as sticky because of the angular nature of saturated fats. This has two very unhelpful consequences. First, the blood cells cannot change shape so easily and they will find it harder to squeeze through the tiny capillaries that are intended to bring them into close contact with the other cells of your body. Even more problematic, they tend to stick together a bit like Velcro does, because of their angular shape. This increases the risk of blood clots and thrombosis—a real problem at any time, but an added risk during chemotherapy.

Most people will know of someone who has high blood pressure, or who had heart disease and was put on blood thinners. Sticky blood is a major health risk. Sticky blood refers to how thick your blood is and how easily it flows. Compare a tomato sauce bottle with tomato sauce in it, to one with water in it. Upend the two bottles; the water flows, the sauce sticks.

If your blood is sticky, it does not flow well. It is much harder for your heart to pump it around your body. It is much harder for the blood to get into and through the tiny pipes that are your small blood vessels. Hence sticky blood raises blood pressure and aggravates heart disease, as well as increasing the risk of developing a blood clot or an embolism (significant potential side effects of chemotherapy).

The best way to have thin blood that flows well is to avoid saturated fats; only use unsaturated fats and follow all the other principles in the Wellness Diet.

Wellness Rule 2: Avoid saturated fats; instead, use unsaturated fats or oils.

What are the saturated fats? All animal fats are saturated—whether from beef, chicken, sheep or pig. There are two vegetable-based ones—palm oil and coconut oil.

Palm oil is a disaster for the environment and human health. It is widely used in prepared foods, so read the labels. Most cookies and many candies and pastries contain vegetable oil. If the actual oil is not specified, it will almost certainly be palm oil. Palm oil is very cheap and, being a saturated fat, makes cookies crisp and crunchy. Some commercial cookies use olive oil, which is healthier, and they will always be labeled as such due to olive oil being more expensive.

Vast tracts of ecologically sensitive land, mostly in tropical areas, are cleared daily for more palm oil. Curiously, it is the environmentalists who are leading the push to reduce the world's consumption of palm oil and they are making useful inroads. One cannot help wonder where the dietitians have been when the health risks to people have been known for a long time.

Coconut oil has some advocates, as it is a shorter chain saturated fat and has a high resistance to cooking temperatures. I still recommend against its use, as there are better oils to choose. To understand which ones are recommended we move on to consider:

Omega Fatty Acids

There are three main classifications of omega fatty acids—the 3s, 6s and 9s—and your body needs some of each. However, the consequences for your immune system vary dramatically depending upon which one predominates in your diet.

The omega-3 fatty acids are the good guys—they act as a very positive tonic for your immune system and many other healing functions. The omega-6s are the baddies—they actually weaken your immune system and have other unhelpful consequences—while the omega-9s are neutral for immune function but do have other redeeming features.

Wellness Rule 3: Use omega-3 fatty acids regularly, omega-9s modestly and avoid the omega-6s.

Which is what? The two main omega-3s are fish oil and flaxseed oil. Flaxseed oil is highly recommended. When you hear of the benefits of eating fish, those benefits mostly relate to the fish oils. Of course, to obtain oil from a fish, you need an oily fish! Sardines and tuna qualify, but almost all varieties of canned tuna have the oil removed as the oil is worth more in a capsule than a can. Be extra careful, as several producers put unhealthy oils back in the can. More details of this soon. Also, see Appendix H for details on sustainable fish species that meet health standards.

The main sources of the omega-6's fatty acids are sunflower and safflower oils and they are best avoided. Also, it is best to avoid canola oil.

The omega-9s predominate in olive oil, avocado and most nuts.

To understand exactly what to do, there is one more vital issue with fats.

Preparation

Healthy fats have many benefits but they all share a common problem. Fats all have a high tendency to oxidize and become rancid. Rancid fats are seriously dangerous both in the short and long term. Short term they are highly toxic, long term they are carcinogenic—that is, they cause cancer.

Fats oxidize and become rancid when exposed to air, heat or light.

Wellness Rule 4: Protect your oils from air, heat and light.

This means buy oils in cans or dark bottles, which are protected from the light.

Use cold-pressed or virgin oils because they have not been heated during the extraction process.

Buy flaxseed oil from a refrigerator, not off the shelf, and store it at home in the refrigerator. Once opened, use all oils within two months ideally, three months at most.

Learn to cook without oils. Cooking can easily overheat oils and lead to oxidation. The best solution is to cook oil free and only add oils to your meals at the table. Oil is good to add to food, just do not cook with it. While this does take some adjustment, once established, it is a really healthy and enjoyable habit. As a positive side effect, it makes the washing up easier!

If you really must use some oil in cooking, olive oil has a high resistance to heat (flaxseed is very low). And if using a wok, adding water (before heating the oil) helps protect the oil.

Avoid roasted nuts or cooking with nuts or seeds, as this overheats the oils. Many nuts have around 50 percent oil content, so this is a real issue—more on nuts soon.

FAT RECOMMENDATIONS

On the Wellness or Healing Diet, the amount of fat to consume will be taken care of by following the general guidelines:

- Avoid all animal fats thoroughly (including dairy).
- Learn to cook oil free.
- Include two tablespoons of flaxseed oil daily in your food—best added to meals after cooking, although some do take it off a spoon (not me!).
- Use olive oil for variety. While it is neutral for your immune system, it has other useful properties in its own right.
- Read labels; avoid palm oil and coconut oil.

PROTEINS

Protein is another essential ingredient in the human diet.

Nutritional Information

Proteins are involved in virtually every process in our body, as well as being a major contributor to our structural integrity. Proteins are vital for our immune system and for healthy muscle activity. They make up significant parts of the enzymes that regulate our metabolism, as well as the messenger molecules such as the neuropeptides that transfer information internally around our bodies.

Proteins are made up of amino acids, some of which are called essential amino acids because we need to obtain them directly in our food, while others are nonessential amino acids and can be manufactured in our own body.

Quantity

Virtually everyone who specializes in nutrition, along with the broader mainstream authorities, agrees that the ideal quantity of protein to consume is less than what many in the general public understand.

Speaking personally, being an athlete before I was diagnosed with cancer in 1975, I was encouraged to eat a very high-meat diet. These days, most athletes train on a high-carbohydrate diet with only modest protein levels, as it is known this brings better results. Interestingly, Carl Lewis, perhaps the greatest athlete known, claimed that being a vegan led to his greatest performances. Murray Rose, one of Australia's greatest ever swimmers, was competing as a full vegan and winning Olympic gold medals back in the 1950s.

In the seventies, it was not unusual for people to be averaging 120gms of protein per day. Now the recommended level is around 55–60gm/day for the average-size person; so again, like with the fats, this may be around half of what many have been used to. We will clarify what 55–60gms looks like in the preparation section.

> Wellness Rule 5: Eat modest amounts of protein—around 55–60gms/day for the average-size person.

Quality

Why is it that so many authorities who are really serious about nutrition, and especially nutrition for healing, recommend a vegetable-based diet with little or no meat?

To understand, we need to divert a little and consider dogs, cows and digestive systems.

Digestion

There are three types of animal digestive systems: carnivore, herbivore and omnivore. A classic carnivore like a dog is designed to eat a high-meat diet. A classic herbivore like a cow runs on grass, and us human beings—well, we are omnivores trying to get the best of both worlds. Knowing about our own digestive system, and how it compares to the others, helps us to understand what we are wisest to eat, and what makes best sense when we are eating for recovery.

The Carnivore

A dog has a very specific anatomical setup to enable it to manage the food it eats. Here is the key point regarding meat. Digestion of virtually any food produces waste products. We eat a food like meat or a particular vegetable, we take what we can use from that food and we eliminate the leftovers, the waste products. With meat, the waste products are somewhat problematic; they are rich in nitrites and other potentially toxic by-products of their digestion. Vegetables do not produce these problematic waste products.

If the metabolic waste products from meat stay in the bowel for long, they can be directly toxic to the lining of the bowel, or they can be absorbed through the bowel and become toxic to the rest of the body.

Now, the dog is essentially a scavenging meat eater with a matching anatomy. It has sharp canine teeth for biting and ripping its potential meal into big pieces. Then it swallows quickly before anyone else can steal its share. Therefore, it has modest chewing teeth at the back of its mouth and actually does little chewing unless on a bone or equivalent. Next it has just one, relatively compact stomach that secretes almost pure hydrochloric acid to liquefy the lumps of food it has gulped down.

Then the key point: because of the potentially toxic nature of the metabolic waste products that come from the digestion of meat, the dog needs to get rid of them quickly. Therefore, every dog has a very short bowel, and as a result, what we call a rapid transit time. The transit time measures how long it takes food to go through the system, from front to back, or top to bottom. Hence, short bowel, rapid transit time.

The Herbivore

By contrast, a classic herbivore like the cow has a very different digestive challenge. It is eating vegetable matter and with grass, needs to be able to digest cellulose. The cow therefore has a very different anatomy. First, there is a need to start the digestive process by grinding the food very finely. As a result, the cow has no serious biting teeth, but very serious grinders! While the dog's back teeth are permanent and static, in the same way that adult human teeth are, the cow's back teeth constantly grow. Cows do so much chewing that they need to continually replace what has been ground down.

Next, the cow has four stomachs! Four. The first is like a huge tank that mixes the finely ground grass with water and saliva and literally ferments it. In the process, cows produce large amounts of methane. So these days, aware conservationists are joining the push to reduce meat consumption as the volumes of methane produced have a major impact on the atmosphere. Also, to grow an equivalent amount of beef protein compared to vegetable protein requires around eighteen to twenty times more land area. Given the huge problems with the clearing of forests and utilization of land, this is another major environmental rationale for less meat and more vegetable protein consumption.

Back to the cow. After the four stomachs the cow has a very long digestive tract and a much slower transit time than a dog.

The Omnivore

As humans, we are trying to manage eating just about anything, so our anatomical set up is a compromise. We have teeth that can bite and chew. We have one stomach with high acid content and an intermediate length of bowel. While the dog's transit time is around six to eight hours, the cow's two to four days, the ideal human transit time is eighteen to twenty-four hours.

For people, there is another relevant issue. Fiber in our diet does two important things that are relevant to this discussion. First, fiber adds bulk and regulates transit times; low fiber, longer transit time. Second, fiber acts as a sponge or a buffer. If we do eat something, or have some potentially toxic metabolic waste products form in our bowel, high levels of fiber act as a sponge to absorb the toxic material and usher it quickly out of our system.

Now, you probably know that the average Western diet has been high in meat and low in fiber. This means more toxic waste products, less buffering or absorption from fiber and slower transit times—a great recipe for provoking all bowel diseases and some others in the body generally.

Clearly, humans can manage eating meat, but anatomically, we are better designed for vegetable proteins.

Wellness Rule 6: On the Wellness Diet, reduce or preferably avoid meat consumption. On the Healing Diet, it is preferable to avoid meat altogether.

Let us now look at the various protein sources.

Vegetable Proteins

Many vegetables contain useful amounts of protein. The next issue to clarify relates to the quality of those proteins. Proteins are made up of amino acids and our bodies need quite a number of them. Some the body can make itself and these are called the nonessential amino acids. Others the body can only obtain directly from the foods we eat and they are called the essential amino acids. In general, most individual vegetables are described as being incomplete sources of protein because they do not contain every one of the essential amino acids. By contrast, meat is often touted as a complete protein because it does contain all the essentials. The two notable vegetarian exceptions are the soybean (whose popularity is partially based on the fact that it is a complete protein) and quinoa.

The protein quantity and quality in tofu (the cheese-like soy protein) is very comparable to that of chicken—both are nearly 30 percent protein and both contain all the amino acids we need. Common grains such as rice and wheat are incomplete proteins; however, they do have around half the amount of protein in them when compared to chicken, which is still a very useful amount. Legumes or pulses are the protein-rich vegetables like peas, beans and lentils.

Quinoa warrants a special mention as it is an old grain whose nutritional properties have recently come to the forefront and increased its popularity.

An alternative to use in place of rice or couscous, quinoa has a high-protein content (around 18 percent), importantly is a complete protein, is gluten free, easy to digest and just mildly laxative. It can be cooked like rice and is well suited to sprouting; it is highly recommended for regular use.

It is important to understand that the diets of many large cultural groups around the world are largely vegetable based and they know the secret to obtaining complete protein from vegetables. If they only ate one source of vegetable protein over an extended period of time, they would soon have a problem. However, mix any two grains together, or eat a grain with a pulse, and you almost always end up with a complete protein. This mixing is commonly done in the same meal, but is still adequate if done over a day or so. So most vegetarian-based cultures have their staples that manage this. The classic example is in India and other countries where rice and lentils (or dahl) are eaten together regularly.

Wellness Rule 7: When relying on vegetables for protein, eat cooked soybeans (ideally as tofu) and quinoa regularly, or combine two grains and/or legumes in one meal or one day.

Fish

The metabolic waste products from the digestion of fish fall between the toxicity from meat and the ease of vegetable proteins. Oily fish has the advantage of being a source of omega-3 fatty acids.

Increasingly, fish presents serious environmental and production issues. Intensive fish-farming practices (where antibiotics are being used more commonly) are only somewhat better than those for the intensive rearing of chickens, pigs and cattle (where what goes on can be quite problematic). So, wild fish are highly preferable; but then there are the questions of pollution (particularly for the fish that live close to the shore or built-up areas), environmental degradation (as from bottom dredging), overfishing and wastage (as from longline fishing).

Knowing where your fish came from is now a necessary step in selecting which fish to buy. Then there is the fact that the smaller species of fish are less likely to accumulate pollutants when compared to larger predator fish. Seafood like oysters, prawns and scallops are notorious for picking up pollutants, so where these foods come from is also well worth knowing before you eat them—if you eat them. Farmed prawns are better for the environment, as netting the wild ones can be very harsh on the seafloor.

> Wellness Rule 8: If you eat fish, avoid farmed fish in the main and eat the smaller, sustainable wild fish varieties that come from nonpolluted areas (see Appendix H for more details) and eat seafood only occasionally. On the Healing Diet, fish is preferably avoided.

Eggs

How eggs are produced commercially is a real concern. If you do eat eggs, only use genuine free-range eggs. Many people are also unsure when it comes to the cholesterol in eggs. Cholesterol is very useful in the body and we need some in our diet. The Wellness Diet generally is low in cholesterol and so a few eggs each week are fine inclusions. Be mindful of how you cook them; the frying of eggs is to be avoided altogether.

> Wellness Rule 9: Two to four genuine free-range eggs per week are OK on the Wellness Diet. Most people find eggs are better avoided on the Healing Diet (more on this later).

Dairy Products

It is obvious that before the development of agriculture, milk was not part of the human diet after weaning. Given how long it takes the body to adapt to major changes like this, some critics pose the logical question regarding how well our digestion is suited to consuming a food source that traditionally we never ate. Looking around, you would have to notice many cultures eat dairy, and many people seem to manage just fine. Dairy-based cultures like the Swiss and the French seem to do quite well in the longevity stakes; certainly they are comparable to many other less dairy-focused cultures.

However, there are serious concerns with dairy products that warrant consideration. Over the years, based on the research and clinical experience of working with people adding or subtracting dairy from their diets, I have become increasingly convinced the best approach is to minimize or avoid dairy on the Wellness Diet and leave it out altogether from the Healing Diet. Why? The first and most obvious issue is that natural dairy products contain a large amount of saturated fat. This can be minimized in low-fat milk, but many cheeses actually concentrate the fats and butter (nearly 50 percent saturated fat).

> Wellness Rule 10: If you do use dairy products, use the low-fat varieties.

Next, we need to understand that the protein in human milk is a short-chain protein. This means it is a small molecule. By contrast, cow's milk is comprised of a long-chain, large and angular molecular protein. When a young child is introduced to cow's milk early in life, the contrast with human milk is stark. The child's developing immune system will not be sure if this large molecule is a food that needs to be digested or an invader that must be attacked. As it is, it seems many mount a low-level immune reaction to milk—a reaction that results in chronic, low-level, generalized inflammation. While this reaction may not amount to much in ordinary daily life, given extra stress, through environment, unsuitable food, disease, emotional or mental stress, and the inflammation may flare. Children who suffer from recurrent ear infections or tonsillitis often find their conditions clear up when taken off all dairy products.

For adults, consuming dairy products may seem manageable with no obvious consequences. However, faced with stress or disease, or simply wanting to be at our best, it may well be better to leave dairy out of the diet.

What about goat's or sheep's milk? They have smaller chain proteins so that issue is lessened. Many children with full-blown allergies to cow's milk can manage goat's milk. However, these sources of milk are high in fat and naturally homogenized. That means that the fat is suspended in the liquid of the milk, does not naturally settle out and is not so easy to separate. Therefore, goat's and sheep's milk tend to be high in saturated fat with all the related issues. They too are best avoided or minimized.

Nuts

Nuts are a good source of protein but care needs to be taken with their oils, as they go rancid easily and quickly. Nuts like walnuts, pecans and Brazil nuts are all best bought in their shells and eaten within a few months of being picked to reduce the risk of rancidity. Some can be purchased vacuum-packed, which is a great advantage. When nuts taste bitter, that is the sign they are dangerously rancid. Almonds are best bought with their brown skins intact, as this protects their oils from the air and from the light. Also, it is best not to cook with nuts or to eat the roasted varieties.

Chestnuts and especially almonds are relatively low in protein and quite low in oil and are suitable for eating regularly. Because chestnuts are so low in oil they are one nut which is OK to cook and, besides, they really are terrible raw. Almonds make great snacks between meals and, interestingly, have been proven by research to help the overweight lose weight. There is no indication they cause people with a healthy weight to lose more, so they are highly recommended—ten to twenty per day.

> Wellness Rule 11: Eat up to ten to twenty almonds per day, chestnuts when they are in season, and eat the other nuts occasionally, when fresh and not roasted.

Preparation

The Wellness Diet derives a good deal of its protein from the grains we will discuss next in the carbohydrates section. What is needed is to add a modest amount of protein from the high-protein sources covered in the previous section on quality.

What to prepare, therefore, and what it looks like in practice depends on which of those protein sources you choose to use.

VEGETABLE PROTEINS

If these constitute a major source of protein for you, eat them regularly. With tofu, two slices the size of fish sticks are recommended three or four times weekly, and if you have a couple of rice and lentil dishes throughout the week, the protein levels are likely to be quite adequate.

COOKING LEGUMES OR PULSES

There are many different peas and beans. Some can be eaten raw, but most need to be cooked. French beans, runner beans, peas, snow peas, soya, kidney, lima and mung beans, chickpeas and lentils require cooking.

The dried seeds of plants we know as beans are easy to store and a good source of carbohydrate and protein—especially when combined with equal amounts of rice, wheat, etc. Most beans require special cooking because uncooked they contain alkaloids and glycosides that are detrimental to digestion, so never eat them raw. Ideally, beans are best soaked in water eight to sixteen hours and then simmered in boiling water until cooked—usually for two hours. Another cooking method is to pour boiling water over the beans, allow to soak two hours, then cook as above.

With legumes it is wise to throw out the soaking water if you use it, and replace it before boiling, as well as discarding the water used to boil them. This also means that you do not cook legumes (including lentils) in soup; cook them separately and then add them.

Sprouting many legumes before cooking can work well and also makes digestion easier, but this usually takes several days. If sprouted, legumes need only to be blanched before eating.

FISH, IF YOU EAT IT

Once or twice a week is OK. Cooking methods apart from burning are not significant, although steaming works very well.

EGGS

Two to four per week, if you eat them. Do not fry; any other cooking method is OK.

DAIRY

Avoid or just eat on special occasions if you really like cheese, for example. Remember, it is highly recommended not to cook or heat any food in a microwave (especially any dairy products).

NUTS

Eat ten to twenty almonds per day; chestnuts when in season, and eat the other nuts raw, occasionally and when in season.

MEAT, IF YOU EAT IT

Back in the seventies, again, meat was the feature on a dinner plate, the vegetables appearing more like condiments on the side. These days, if you do eat meat, the reverse is the aim—lots of vegetables with a small piece of meat. Cooking methods do not matter much except char grilling or burning;

burned bits contain hydrocarbons, which are highly toxic, so avoid these methods. When using a barbecue, this means it is necessary to use a hot plate and be careful to avoid burning the food.

If you do eat meat, the lean white meats are preferable. Rabbit may be best, veal could be considered, but chicken requires real caution. Commercially raised chicken has overwhelming problems related to what they are fed, how they are housed and the routine use of low-level antibiotics as growth promoters. If you do eat chicken, it is mandatory in my view to only eat genuine, free-range, organically fed birds.

When it comes to red meat, lean is best, while things like fatty sausages and salami are the very worst. Avoid meat that has been through a feedlot; seek organic meat.

Protein Recommendations

- Eat a modest amount—2 ounces/day for the average person.
- Follow the hierarchy of protein sources. The more thorough you choose to be, the more you commit to the Healing Diet, the higher up this hierarchy you stay (e.g., the vegetable proteins are the ideal).
  - Vegetable proteins, known collectively as legumes or pulses: soybeans, tofu or bean curd, quinoa, lentils, chickpeas, any of the beans or peas.
  - Fish (preferably small deep-sea ones).
  - Eggs: two to four per week if agreeable; duck eggs may be suitable if hen eggs are not.
  - Dairy products: especially low-fat yogurt, cow's milk if suitable, soft cheeses. Goat's milk may be suitable if cow's milk is not.
  - Meat, in descending order of preference again: lean white meat such as rabbit or veal, free-range chicken, lean red meat, fatty meats.
- Minimize or avoid meat and dairy products, especially on the Healing Diet.
- Two to four genuine free-range eggs can be eaten weekly; eggs may be better avoided on the Healing Diet.
- Eat almonds regularly; the other nuts need to be fresh and uncooked.
- All grains have reasonable protein levels and warrant regular inclusion.
- Avoid burning all foods, and high-protein sources particularly.

CARBOHYDRATES

This is where we discuss grains and sugars. Grains are the main source of carbohydrates and receive fairly universal acceptance as a major part of any dietary approach. Grains certainly figure prominently in the Wellness Diet and the Healing Diet. However, as they are closely allied to the sugars, which receive a good deal of bad press, a little more explanation is warranted.

Nutritional Information

Carbohydrates are divided into four groups based upon their chemical structure. These groups are called monosaccharides, disaccharides, oligosaccharides and polysaccharides. Of more practical relevance, these are further divided into two groups that we hear of quite a deal, the simple carbohydrates or sugars (monosaccharides and disaccharides) and the complex carbohydrates or starches (oligosaccharides and polysaccharides).

Keeping it simple and avoiding going into a great deal of biochemistry, the complex carbohydrates are made up of aggregates of the simple carbohydrates. The simple carbohydrates include various sugars such as glucose (cane or white sugar), fructose (fruit sugar) and lactose (milk sugar). They provide a ready source of energy and are used to build the nucleic acids that make up our DNA.

Importantly, both sucrose from sugar and fructose from fruits are polysaccharides. What this means is that they need to be converted in the body to the monosaccharide glucose before being used as a source of energy. The speed of this conversion in the body is the crucial point—as the more rapidly it occurs, the more we experience a spike in our blood sugar levels and the more insulin is activated. Insulin, as well as regulating our blood sugar levels, is now recognized as playing a role in the modulation of the immune system and other aspects of healing. Insulin becoming overactivated by glucose spikes is increasingly recognized as a serious problem. Also, the insulin connection may well explain the long clinical experience of too much white sugar being a bad thing and why it is avoided strongly in many healing diets, including ours.

The rate at which all carbohydrates are metabolized into glucose will vary depending upon the source of the carbohydrate. Generally, simple sugars break down much faster than complex starches but fruit sugars are slowly metabolized, while processed or refined starches are fast.

The glycemic index (GI) and insulin index provide ways of assessing these metabolic rates in more detail, but in my clinical experience, there is no need to concern ourselves with these. I have observed some people becoming unnecessarily obsessive, even neurotic about these indices, and we aim to avoid stress and enjoy our food.

The crucial point is that sucrose from white sugar is metabolized very quickly and causes glucose spikes. In practice, fructose from fruit sugars and the more complex carbohydrates like starches do not metabolize so quickly and therefore are much safer to use.

In both animals and plants, energy is stored by combining simple carbohydrates into complex ones. In plants, these complex carbohydrates are commonly known as starches and we find them very commonly in the grains like wheat, rice, rye and so on. At the table they are predominant in bread, pasta, potatoes, corn (or maize) and cereals.

In animals and humans, the complex carbohydrates are stored as glycogen. This stored glycogen then requires a series of metabolic conversions to get back to the usable energy form of glucose. Interestingly, the body can obtain all its energy from fats and protein and do without carbohydrates altogether, but in most cultures, carbohydrates actually are a major source of energy.

Quantity

Major health bodies recommend about 45 percent to 65 percent of dietary energy comes from carbohydrates with the great majority of this coming from complex carbohydrates. The less simple carbohydrates or sugar we consume, the better.

One way of describing the Wellness Diet is to say it is high in fruit, vegetables and grains. It is best not to fixate too much on exact quantities, but to include a significant amount of grains in most meals. Two to three pieces of fruit per day are encouraged in both the Wellness Diet and the Healing Diet. The concerns some people raise about eating fruit sugars in my view are well satisfied by knowing that the conversion of fructose (fruit sugar) to glucose is a far slower process than that of sucrose (white sugar) to glucose. Fruit has many benefits and is recommended highly.

Wellness Rule 12: Use grains and fruit regularly.

Quality

As well as fruit, we need plenty of unprocessed complex carbohydrates. This includes good quality whole-grain bread made from wheat, rye or spelt, whole-grain pasta, or whole-grain rice. Processed carbohydrates such as those made from white flour and white rice, as well as being nutritionally poor, are digested very rapidly and cause significant, unhelpful blood sugar spikes.

Preparation

The digestion of most complex carbohydrates, as with grains, is improved by cooking. For example, while eating raw cereals such as muesli is fine if your digestion and energy level generally are robust, for those who are more fragile or delicate, porridge is easier.

Good-quality breads are widely available these days, but do check the ingredients. Avoid white flour and artificial or chemical additives. Also avoid the addition of seeds like sunflower or flaxseed in breads or other cooking, as they will have been oxidized by the heat of the cooking process. Spelt is a good bread flour and sourdough an ideal method of preparation. Flat or unleavened breads are also recommended.

Potatoes are best eaten with their skins, as are all vegetables and fruits where practical.

Rice is best cooked by the absorption method. Add about 50 percent more water than rice and boil in a saucepan with a lid on. When cooked, all the water will be absorbed.

Wellness Rule 13: Avoid processed foods generally and processed carbohydrates particularly. Eat plenty of whole grains and fresh fruit, eating the skins wherever possible. Prepare meals from raw ingredients as much as possible.

CARBOHYDRATE RECOMMENDATIONS

- Complex carbohydrates in grains along with in fruits are recommended as daily staples.
- Avoid processed or refined foods; eat whole grains, leave skins on wherever possible.
- Remember that grains do provide protein, as well as carbohydrates and their associated energy.

FIBER

Fiber was discussed under the section on digestion. Fiber is important in maintaining regular bowel motions, as well as acting as a sponge to absorb toxic material, including the waste products from digestion, and usher them through to elimination.

Quantity

A high-fiber diet is strongly recommended unless there are specific contra-indications from an active disease process or as a consequence of major bowel surgery.

In America 20 to 35gms of dietary fiber is recommended per day. While the average American consumes around 12 to 18gms, or half the recommended level, this amount is readily achieved using the Wellness Diet and the Healing Diet.

Quality

There are two main types of fiber, so-called soluble fiber and insoluble fiber.

Soluble fiber is able to be fermented in the large bowel, producing useful metabolic substances and some gas. Soluble fiber has a good range of benefits. It is known to reduce the risk of heart disease, helps to stabilize variations in blood sugars, may reduce the risk of developing diabetes, and may reduce glucose and insulin levels for those with clinical diabetes. Soluble fiber is commonly found in oats, (bran, rolled oats and oat flour), barley (the bran and barley flour) and psyllium husks.

Insoluble fiber is as it sounds, inert. It does not break down but can absorb water and is useful in aiding bulk to our stools and stimulating movement through the bowel. Insoluble fiber is known to alleviate constipation and has been closely linked to protecting against colon cancer. A good source is organic wheat or corn bran, while other sources are nuts, seeds (including flaxseed), potato skins and some vegetables.

Both types of fiber contribute to an increased feeling of being full and therefore may help to reduce appetite and stabilize healthy weight levels.

One major study of people aged from fifty to seventy showed that a high-fiber intake reduced the risk of dying over a nine-year period by nearly one quarter. Those on the high levels had significantly lower risk of heart disease, infections and respiratory diseases and lower cancer rates (especially among the men).

Preparation

Wherever possible eat whole foods. The husks of seeds removed during refining or processing are rich in fiber, as is the skin of most fruits and vegetables. It is particularly important to leave potato skins on both for the fiber and as the skins help to reduce the sugar spike peeled potatoes trigger.

It may well be useful to add a teaspoon of wheat bran and barley or oat bran to the daily diet and the easiest way to do this is to add them to morning oatmeal.

There is a caution with too much fiber. If you are not used to it, if you suddenly increase the amount of soluble fiber in your diet, there can be a rapid increase in gas production, with bloating and discomfort to you and maybe those around you! Also, if not enough water is taken with a high-fiber diet, it is possible to create constipation, which links nicely to the next section on fluids. So if you have been used to a low-fiber diet, all you need to do is to adapt slowly over a week or two.

FIBER RECOMMENDATIONS
- Eat a diet high in fiber by using whole grains and eating the skins of all suitable fruits and vegetables.
- Consider supplementing with a teaspoon of both wheat bran and barley or oat bran—most easily taken when cooked with oatmeal but possible to add to breads or other foods.

FLUIDS

Quantity

Generally it is recommended that the average person drink eight glasses of fluid in total each day. Many do not and as such are only partially hydrated.

Wellness Rule 14: Drink at least eight glasses of fluid in total each day, ideally at times apart from meals.

Water

Fresh, pure water is an essential part of a healthy diet. Ideally, it is chlorine free, as chlorination is linked to a heightened risk of bladder cancer. As unchlorinated water has even greater risks (through infection) in most public water systems, this recommendation is not practical unless you have your own water supply or a water filter. The latter is highly recommended if you are on a chlorinated, public water system and most commercially available water filters do an adequate job. They have the added benefit of removing fluoride that remains contentiously linked to increased cancer rates and immunological impairment. I am not totally convinced by the antifluoride argument, but as adults we do not seem to need it and the chlorine risk seems well established; therefore, the filters make sense.

If you collect your own rainwater at home as we do, you need to be able to regulate its collection. We have a valve that we open after about an hour of heavy rain, which is how long it is said to reasonably clean the atmosphere and the roof, thereby ensuring good quality water is collected.

Juices

These are a feature of the Healing Diet and as such will be discussed in the next chapter.

Teas and Coffee

Black and green tea, along with coffee, contain caffeine. Caffeine is also found in cocoa, which is a major component in chocolate (and chocolate drinks), as well as Coca-Cola and of course the high-caffeine drinks like Red Bull. In the plants it comes from, caffeine serves as a pesticide, protecting the plants from being eaten by insects.

In humans, caffeine is mildly addictive. It is a potent stimulant of the central nervous system and it is the world's most widely consumed, legal psychoactive substance. It can help keep us awake and increase physical performance.

Some people are very sensitive to caffeine's effects, others adjust to them and notice very little. One of the best pointers to the downside of regular caffeine usage is the size and range of withdrawal effects. Within one to two days of stopping the use of caffeine, many people experience some or all of the following: headaches, irritability, lack of concentration, difficulty sleeping despite feeling sleepy, and aches and pains in the stomach, upper body and joints generally.

Most people I know who do cease drinking or eating caffeine report feeling much better for it. I certainly recommend avoiding or minimizing caffeine intake, especially on the Healing Diet.

Instead, use decaffeinated coffee along with herbal coffee substitutes and herbal teas.

Refer to Appendix I for the relative caffeine levels in teas, coffee and chocolate.

Alcohol

Alcohol consumption generally has been associated with a higher risk of several of the cancers of the digestive tract. The cancer link is a serious issue requiring consideration with beer. Chemically brewed beers have been directly linked to an increased incidence of colon cancer. Therefore, drink only naturally brewed beers if you drink any. There are very low alcohol, naturally brewed beer options that taste good. In Australia, Coopers Birell brand is excellent.

Of real concern is the fact that the metabolism of alcohol requires a good deal of liver activity. Alcoholics develop cirrhosis of the liver due to the excess strain involved. To recover from cancer, we need our livers to be functioning at their best, so we avoid alcohol on the Healing Diet.

See Appendix J for the approximate levels of alcohol in commonly used drinks.

ALCOHOL RECOMMENDATIONS
- On the Wellness Diet, social drinking a few days per week is acceptable.
- Ensure regular alcohol-free days.
- Consider using very low alcohol, naturally brewed beer.
- On the Healing Diet, alcohol is not recommended, primarily because of its effect on the liver.

OVERALL FLUID RECOMMENDATIONS
- Drink eight glasses of fluid, combined from all sources (water, tea, juices, soups) per day.

- Make healthy choices—with water, tea and coffee substitutes and alcohol.
- Add juices to the Healing Diet and consider their use on the Wellness Diet.

CONDIMENTS

Now we can consider those things we add to our food for taste and variety.

Salt

It is essential to know that the average diet more than meets the recommended daily allowance for salt. Unless one is working or exercising very hard in very hot conditions, there is no dietary need for additional salt.

Salt is a compound that consists of sodium chloride. The recommendation for sodium consumption for the average person is 1,500 to 2,300 milligrams per day.

Too much salt is linked with high blood pressure, stroke, heart disease and heart failure. Too little is associated with muscle cramps, dizziness and more general electrolyte imbalances that in extreme deficiencies can lead to neurological problems and even death.

More relevant to the cancer situation, and our health generally, is to understand that one of salt's primary roles in the body is to regulate the balance of water. A simple way to understand how this works is by knowing that salt, or more specifically sodium, is hydroscopic. That means salt draws water to it.

If we consume excess sodium via salt it does not accumulate in our blood. The levels of sodium and other ions in the blood are crucial for the healthy functioning of the body and as such, they are tightly regulated within fairly narrow boundaries. Our body will do its best to excrete the excess, but some will build up in our cells. Once in the cells, the extra sodium draws water into those cells, making them effectively "soggy." This is like having a waterlogged garden; everything suffers. So excess sodium negatively affects the healthy metabolism of a wide range of our cells, contributing to a general malaise and significantly impairing regeneration and healing.

Finally, some people tout salt from exotic locations claiming special benefits for their product. All salt is made up of sodium chloride, regardless of its origin. Salt is salt. Avoid adding it to your food.

Wellness Rule 15: Adopt a low-salt diet; avoid salty foods and do not add salt to food.

Peppers and Chilies

These foods warrant special mention as they are in such popular use. Green pepper is the natural form of pepper but it is rarely used. Black pepper has been cooked and dried, while white pepper has been "refined," having the shell taken from the same type of seed that is the raw product for all peppers. White pepper tends to have a milder taste.

The use of pepper dates back to antiquity and it has been suggested to have a wide range of mildly medicinal purposes. It does have mild antioxidant properties and maybe some mild anticancer action. Caution is required by anyone with an irritated or inflamed bowel and probably any cancer affecting the bowel, because pepper is an irritant in its own right. It makes sense not to use pepper when on chemotherapy, as that treatment frequently affects the lining of the bowel, making it even more sensitive.

Chilies come from the capsicum family, and have a similar history of use to pepper. Chili also has some positive but minor health claims made for its use. However, it is far more irritating than pepper and as such has a strong potential to aggravate the lining of the bowel and impair digestion. Chili is not recommended for use at all.

Herbs and Seasonings

Garlic has been shown to be a natural antibiotic and antifungal agent, to decrease blood pressure, to have anticancer properties and is a chelating agent.

Ginger, like garlic, also makes an excellent seasoning while having special properties. Ginger stimulates stomach acid production, so aiding digestion. Ginger is particularly useful for people changing from a heavy meat-based diet to a more vegetarian way of eating.

Turmeric has many good anticancer properties, such as targeting cancer stem cells. It is best taken with black pepper to increase absorption.

Other acceptable seasonings are allspice, anise, bay leaves, celery seeds, coriander, dill, fennel, mace, marjoram, rosemary, sage, saffron, tarragon, thyme and summer savory.

Most herbs that are made into teas have medicinal properties and need to be used wisely. Any of the mints make a good refreshing drink and can be used cold in summer. They have a tannin content, so do not overdo them. However, peppermint is particularly useful to aid digestion, soothe the bowel and decrease flatulence. Chamomile, a mild sedative, aids sleep, soothes upset stomach and bowel, and decreases flatulence. Chamomile can be useful before bed.

Coltsfoot is excellent for chest complaints, particularly if mucus needs to be cleared—it is a good expectorant. Prepare by adding two tablespoons of leaves to one pint of boiling water, stand for about ten minutes, strain, then add one teaspoonful of honey and the juice of a quarter of a lemon. Drop the squeezed lemon into the drink also.

Roasted dandelion root coffee (some people call it dandelion tea) is an excellent liver tonic. One to three cups each day are well worth considering. Boil or percolate as for normal coffee, then strain. Add honey or a suitable "milk" if preferred.

Sea Vegetables

Sea vegetables are an important source of iodine, a common deficiency in many soils and hence the food grown on them. It is wise to use sea vegetables regularly, including kelp powder for stews, and nori for salads and rolls.

Sprouts

Sprouts are recommended as an integral part of the diet. We use them regularly in our programs and they are easy to prepare—see Appendix K.

Broccoli seed sprouts are available in many supermarkets these days and have very strong anticancer properties.

CONDIMENT RECOMMENDATIONS
- Add no salt to food unless you're hot and sweaty!
- Use pepper but not chili on the Wellness Diet. Avoid both on the Healing Diet, especially if having chemotherapy or you have a sensitive bowel.
- Most culinary herbs and spices are suitable.
- Use ginger, garlic and turmeric (with black pepper) regularly.
- Use sea vegetables (seaweeds) regularly.
- Consider the regular consumption of sprouts.

SPECIFIC CONSIDERATIONS

Fresh vs. Stored

One of the quickest, most effective ways to improve your diet rapidly is to eat meals that are prepared from fresh, raw ingredients. This means avoiding processed foods. Doing so will save you and your family many potential problems, but then raises the questions of cooking, convenience and storage.

For convenience, the solution is to develop a core group of simple, quick whole-food, plant-based recipes that can be varied easily and endlessly by altering the raw ingredients. So, whether salads or cooked meals, you have your basic recipes that you eat most of the time, and the more elaborate recipes you trot out on special occasions. One problem I find with many recipe books is that they focus on the "party food," what you would prepare for honored guests, and not the day-to-day stuff. On my blog are a group of very simple recipes to get started with that take twenty to thirty minutes maximum to prepare, and all good and very tasty. *The New Gawler Foundation Cookbook* contains many well-tested, easy-to-prepare, tasty recipes.[19]

Regarding storage, of course the refrigerator is very useful and OK. Ideally, and especially when facing active illness, it is best to start every meal with fresh, whole and vital ingredients. When you are really well, that is the ideal to aim for, but most people have occasions where a particularly quick meal is convenient or longer storage is necessary. Sun drying works well for things like apricots, sultanas and currants. Freezing is also an option and good details are available on the BBC's Good Food website, as well as stilltasty.com. Cans of precooked, organic chickpeas, other legumes and tomatoes can be useful to have on hand for when time is at a premium.

Avoid artificially preserved foods thoroughly. This may come under the heading of too much information, but undertakers say that just a few decades ago, dead bodies left in the heat would begin to deteriorate within a matter of hours. Now, due to the high content of preservatives in our food, commonly they last for three or four days, sometimes even more! That cannot be good.

Cooked vs. Raw

On the Wellness Diet, a balance of cooked and raw food is recommended. This balance is influenced by climate, availability and personal metabolism. In a tropical environment, a largely raw diet can work well all year round. In a cold winter, many people struggle on raw food and require a much higher level of cooking. In broad terms, for healthy people, a significant proportion of the diet is raw, the rest cooked. This statement is deliberately vague, as the diet does vary greatly depending on individual circumstances.

When it comes to those dealing with cancer, many Western practitioners who have focused intensively on treating this disease nutritionally recommend an all-raw diet. By contrast, most practitioners of traditional Chinese medicine (TCM), which has a history going back thousands of years, recommend a mostly cooked diet. In my experience, people are different. Some do well on cooked food, some on raw; many are best suited to a mixture. How to solve this and what to do on the Healing Diet will be addressed in the next chapter.

Cooking

For utensils, use stainless steel, cast iron, glass, tin, enamel or earthenware. Do not use aluminum or plastics, and avoid nonstick materials like Teflon.

To cook your food, use steaming, dry baking, a wok, or sautéing in water only. Boil rice and other grains, bake bread and slow stew on low heat. Do not cook with oils, especially avoid deep-frying and do not use microwave cooking.

Prepare your food with love and joy. Enjoy!

Organic Produce

We live in polluted times. Choosing organic produce wherever possible is good for us and good for the environment. Go organic and consider establishing a vegetable garden—or delight in the one you have!

If commercial food is used, most surface pollutants can be washed off in a 1 percent solution of white vinegar.

If juicing, chemicals and pollutants have been shown to concentrate more in the fiber of fruits and vegetables, so juicing actually helps remove some of them. Therefore, if you need to make a choice, eat the organic produce and juice the commercial produce.

Chemical Additives

There are a myriad of artificial colorings and flavorings used these days. It is said that around a hundred years ago, there were only about two hundred food chemicals in use around the world. Now the figure is put at more than eighty thousand! The average person is estimated to have more than a thousand food chemicals in their body at any one time. It begs belief that this is not a major problem. It makes sense to avoid chemicals whenever possible and to consider the detoxing principles we will cover in the next chapter.

> Wellness Rule 16: Read the labels of all commercially prepared food and use a chart that explains the number codes for the additives. Wherever possible, prepare food from natural, organic ingredients and minimize exposure to, or intake of, chemicals and additives.

Plastics

Plastics have been a mixed blessing. With so many uses, their pollution issues are beginning to become overwhelming. Of real concern is that some of the chemicals in plastics, particularly some of the plasticizers used to soften and mold plastics, mirror female sex hormones. These can accumulate in the fats or oils we eat and then build up in our own fatty tissue. There is suspicion this may aggravate breast cancer.

> Wellness Rule 17: Keep plastic out of your kitchen, do not buy or store food wrapped in plastic, especially the plastic cling wraps. Go back to simpler times. Use wooden spoons; ceramic, wooden or stainless steel bowls. Keep plastics away from your food!

Supplements

These will be addressed in the next chapter.

Food Allergies and Intolerances

Food allergies are acute, often severe reactions to food, whereas food intolerances lead to more common, low-level chronic reactions. So someone who has an allergy to seafood may eat an oyster and have an acute reaction that requires hospitalization. Almost always, people know when they have a genuine food allergy, and happily not many people do have them.

Far more common, however, are food intolerances. These can be associated with physical symptoms such as irritable bowel syndrome (IBS) or simply reduced efficiency in digestion. Some individual foods can be identified as causes of intolerance, quite a number of artificial chemical food additives and colorings are well-known problems, while some chemicals that occur naturally in foods are closely linked.

Cow's milk is an example of a food that has a strong capacity to produce both allergy (usually not severe), as well as intolerance (more common), while MSG is a chemical that can produce mild to severe reactions. Significantly, as well as being a common additive in Chinese cooking, MSG occurs naturally in small amounts in many foods.

Of the chemicals that occur naturally in foods and are known to cause intolerances, salicylates pose the biggest issue. Salicylates occur to some degree in nearly all foods, although there is not much in the high-protein foods. Salicylates are linked with flavor; generally the more flavor, the more salicylates, and they are intimately linked with the plants' self-defense systems. Common major sources of salicylates are strawberries, tomatoes (where concentrating the tomatoes into juice, paste and sauce leads to large increases in the salicylate content), fruits (citrus particularly), berries and wine.

Symptoms of food intolerances can include itchy skin, abdominal pain, bloating, diarrhea or constipation, swelling in the face particularly, but also the hands and feet, headaches, hyperactivity, poor concentration, depression and fatigue. Inflammatory processes including chronic ear infections, cystitis and tonsillitis have been linked by many people. Quite a list!

What to do? If you have a chronic history with the symptoms listed above, be aware that food intolerance may be the issue. In mild cases, it may be enough to simply avoid the major known causes of intolerance and eat their substitutes—(see the chart below). Accurate testing can be carried out by medical specialists in this field and involves using elimination diets and food challenges. However, over the years, many participants in this program have solved food intolerance issues by developing their own food

Foods associated with significant food intolerances	Alternatives
Wheat	Use other grains.
Cow's milk	Goat's milk may be suitable.
Hens' eggs	Duck eggs may be suitable.
Chocolate	Use carob.
Shellfish Pollen Strawberries, tomatoes, citrus	Avoid if necessary.

sensitivity and awareness. Further discussion of how to do this will be found in the next chapter.

On Eating Itself

Avoid processed and refined foods such as white flour, white rice and margarine. The diet needs to be low in salt, sugars, fats and proteins. Concentrate on fresh vital foods, primarily vegetables, fruits and grains. Wherever possible, use foods that are in season and grown within approximately 800 kms (about 500 miles) of where you live.

Aim to prepare and eat your food with a sense of joy and the expectation that it will help you back to total health. Take a short time before you eat to be still, relax and be thankful.

Do not overeat. Do chew your food well—to the consistency of mashed ripe bananas. Digestion begins in the mouth and is aided by a happy, positive disposition. Smile!

Recipes

Once you are clear on what you will and will not eat, studying recipe books becomes easier. Some recipes can be easily modified—leaving out, adding or substituting where necessary.

The best recipe book to begin with is the *New Gawler Foundation Cookbook*.

Binges and Breakouts

If you are basically fit and mostly eat this way, you have some leeway. When you are well, what you eat mainly is most important, what you eat occasionally is not such an issue. When your health is fragile, what you eat all the time is important.

THE WELLNESS DIET • The Final Word

In the next chapter we will be considering the Healing Diet. Charts containing recommendations for a large range of foods from asparagus to zucchini will be presented for you to consider and use as the basis for your personalized plan.

Remember, the Wellness Diet aims to establish healthy boundaries. The intention in this chapter has been to provide enough information to give you clarity and confidence to begin to establish a sound, accessible and healthy pattern of eating.

The Healing Diet aims to examine the prospects of using nutrition therapeutically and to help you to individualize your choices. So read on, consider the information in the next food chapter and then put your plan together.

CHAPTER 14

Nutrition 4

Eating for Recovery: The Healing Diet

THE INTENTION OF THE HEALING DIET IS TO NOURISH OUR BODY WITH THE best possible combination of foods. Eating for recovery aims to use nutrition therapeutically and as such offers considerable cause for hope, a very real means of activating our own personal resources, and the prospect of making a significant contribution to recovery from cancer.

On the Wellness Diet what you eat mostly is important. On the Healing Diet what you eat all the time is important. The crucial point of the mind, however, emphasizes that we choose to enjoy what we do, and so we need to monitor stress, be clear on our motivation, overcome any destructive emotions or habits and cultivate a sense of optimism, joy and delight in being able to use our nutrition, what we eat, to powerfully affect our chances of becoming well and staying well. Therefore, on the Healing Diet:

> Wellness Rule 18: Be particular about what you eat. Eat for recovery and enjoy it!

There are two ways to take up the Healing Diet, the gradual approach and the rapid approach.

THE GRADUAL METHOD FOR ADOPTING THE HEALING DIET

This is a systematic approach that will suit the needs and disposition of many people. The aim is to progress steadily, taking the big, obvious steps first and then attending to the finer details. These general guidelines are based on existing research and the clinical experience I have developed over thirty years working with many people who have taken their nutrition very seriously.

This gradual method involves six steps:

Step 1. Adopt the general guidelines of the Healing Diet.

Step 2. Add regular juices.

Step 3. Regularly consume foods with known anticancer properties.

Step 4. Create a cancer-unfriendly environment in your body by eating foods that positively manipulate your metabolism.

Step 5. Consider the uses of supplements and other natural products.

Step 6. Once the above five steps are in place, progress to develop your awareness, to experiment and establish a personalized pattern of eating for recovery.

THE RAPID APPROACH TO THE HEALING DIET

This is an option for those who are keen, who maybe have more severe disease, and those who like to dive headlong into things that are good for them. This rapid method is similar to the gradual method, but begins more intensively.

Step 1. Heighten your awareness, meditate, start the process with a detox, then adopt the Healing Diet and be vigilant regarding what food agrees with you and what does not.

Steps 2–6. The same as steps 1–5 above.

First we will elaborate the gradual method, then the rapid method.

THE HEALING DIET, OPTION: THE GRADUAL METHOD

Step 1. Adopt the General Recommendations of the Healing Diet

We need the very best nutrition to fuel recovery. So where there are foods that have reservations raised about them, and which on the Wellness Diet we might eat occasionally, on the Healing Diet we leave them out altogether.

Examples of this are meat, dairy products and eggs. Also, we are more thorough in avoiding salt, sugar, refined foods and so on.

Full details are provided in the following lists. The lists build on, and in many instances, summarize what was explained in the previous chapter.

Do be reminded again that these lists are offered as an introductory guide only. Each person needs to pursue their own research, using these lists as a starting point.

What to Avoid and What to Do

	Avoid	What to Do
1	**Unhealthy Fats**	**Use Fats Wisely**
	(a) Saturated fats, omega-6 fatty acids and rancidity	1–2 tablespoons of cold-pressed vegetable oil (use linseed [flax], oil or olive oil) per day is maximum to add to diet. Avoid sources of saturated fat (e.g., animal fat, palm and coconut oils). Store and prepare oils carefully.
	(b) Oils overheated in cooking	Avoid cooking with oils. Preferably sauté with water instead of frying and only use those oils that are most stable if you do choose to cook with them (e.g., olive oil).
	(c) Oils used for repeated frying	Avoid deep-frying, especially with the same oil.
	(d) Unshelled nuts and seeds	Ideally, buy nuts in shells. Do not use shelled sunflowers seeds, which have had long storage times (see Nuts in the previous chapter). Do not cook seeds or nuts.
	(e) Wheat germ oil begins to go rancid one week after processing.	Do not use it.
	(f) Flour begins to go rancid three days after milling.	Use your own home flour mill or obtain flour freshly ground at health food store, co-op, etc.
	(g) Vegetable oils stored in clear containers	Buy them in amber glass or tin containers. Flaxseed oil needs to be refrigerated.
2	**Unhealthy Proteins**	**Eat Modest Amounts of Protein**
	Meat and dairy products are better avoided on the Healing Diet (minimized on the Wellness Diet).	There are many low-protein sources in the diet that add to the overall total, the most notable of which are the grains. Add to this a maximum of 3 pounds, 3 ounces, in total per week of high-protein foods.
		On the Healing Diet, vegetable proteins are the best to use. On the Wellness Diet, there is a hierarchy, vegetable = best, down to fatty meats = worst. Revisit all the details in the last chapter and choose wisely.
3	**Unhealthy Sugars**	**Keep Sugar Intake Low**
	White sugar and refined carbohydrates provide empty calories and should be avoided.	About 1 teaspoonful of natural honey or pure maple syrup is daily maximum. Use whole-grain products.

	Avoid	What to Do
4	**Added Salt**	**Adopt a Low-Salt Diet**
	No extra is needed in cooking or at the table. (Possible exception being people who work very hard in hot weather and sweat profusely.)	Leave it out and watch your taste buds redevelop. Or, substitute by using vitamin C (only the sodium ascorbate version of vitamin C) in equivalent amounts.
5	**Alcohol**	**Little or No Alcohol**
	Best avoided on the Healing Diet as it stresses the liver, but a small amount on the Wellness Diet is OK.	On the Wellness Diet, stick to social drinking and have regular alcohol-free days.
6	**Caffeine**	**Go Caffeine Free**
	Is in coffee, tea, chocolate. A controversial area but, in balance, we prefer to avoid caffeine.	Use herb teas, fruit juices, etc. It is also wise to avoid other artificial soda drinks.
7	**Tobacco or Marijuana**	**QUIT! (If Necessary)**
	These are self-destructive habits—find a better one! Thirty percent of all cancers are directly attributable to smoking.	Stop! Find a more appropriate way of gaining pleasure and dealing with stress. Marijuana is hard on the immune system and is associated with mental illness.
8	**Aflatoxins**	**Be Careful with Peanuts and Mold**
	Aflatoxins are a fungus that can contaminate peanuts especially, and other carbohydrates—mostly in tropical areas and are linked with liver cancer.	Restrict the use of peanuts unless aflatoxin levels are known. Peanuts are also high in oil and are probably best avoided or kept for special occasions only. Avoid any part of food with signs of fungus or mold on it anywhere. (Such growth may not be aflatoxins, but it can be dangerous.)
9	**Ionizing Radiation**	**Avoid Sunburn and Minimize X-Rays, Especially CAT Scans**
	(a) Excessive exposure to sunlight (ultraviolet rays are the problem and cause skin cancer).	Refer to the section on vitamin D. Cover your skin, wear a hat. Use sunscreen lotions sparingly. Fair-haired, pale-skinned people in the tropics require extra caution to avoid excess sun contact.
	(b) Excessive X-rays. Any X-ray is associated with a risk—the more X-rays, the more risk.	While modern X-rays have low exposure, their benefits need to be weighed against the risk. Pregnant women and young children need to be extremely careful. CAT scans have very high radiation levels and need to be used very wisely.
10	**Pollution**	**Go Green**
	Particularly the end products from the combustion of fossil fuels are suspect.	Be aware of caring for your environment.

Problems and Solutions—What to Do

	Problems and Solutions	What to Do
1	**Start Your Meals with Raw Ingredients**	
	Processed and convenience foods commonly have food preservatives, additives and colorings and they lack vitality.	Learn to prepare quick, simple and tasty whole-food meals from raw ingredients; the benefits will be immediate.
2	**Use Healthy Cooking Techniques**	
	Smoked food, charcoal broiling and barbecuing can all cause pyrolysis and lead to production of dangerous polycyclic hydrocarbons.	Use steaming, dry baking, Chinese-style wok cooking, or cook over a low heat with minimal water that should not be discarded. Do not eat food that has been burned black.
3	**Combine Foods Wisely**	
	Imagine your stomach trying to sort out lobster bisque, beef Stroganoff with a side salad, watermelon, all washed down with coffee, then cheese!	To avoid internal warfare consider the food combining chart—Appendix L.
4	**Maintain High-Fiber Levels**	
	Fiber hastens elimination and its bulk protects the bowel from many problems.	Always use whole-meal grains. Avoid peeling vegetables; merely wash and scrub with brush.
5	**Use Chemical-Free Foods**	
	Some artificial colorings are still used in Australia despite being removed from U.S. markets because of possible associated risks. Flavorings such as monosodium glutamate (MSG) are suspect, as are some preservatives, particularly the nitrites. There are too many doubts about chemical additives. It is practical to avoid many of them.	Read labels. Aim to eat fresh, whole unprocessed food. If not always possible, it is preferable to avoid chemical additives but make sure the food has been properly stored or preserved. There is good evidence that adequate use of preservatives and refrigeration actually decreases the incidence of stomach cancer. Use suitable herbs and seasonings, but avoid regular use of hot spices, chili, commercial mustards and sauces.
6	**Use Chemical-Free Products**	
	We live in such a polluted environment that it is wise to avoid whatever chemicals we can. Many chemicals are low-level toxins or carcinogens. Together they become a formidable cocktail.	Do all you can to minimize the chemicals in your environment. Use natural health care products and chemical-free products in the kitchen, home and garden.
7	**Go Organic**	
	A huge range of chemicals is used in commercial food production and it is not possible that the effects of all of them are fully understood.	Seek out organically grown food and encourage its supply. The less chemical unknowns in your diet, the better. Wherever possible, establish your own veggie garden.
8	**Drink Pure, Clean Water**	
	Fluoride is helpful for children's teeth but questionable for cancer patients. Chlorine is definitely best to avoid.	Preferably use spring water or rainwater. Consider a purifier for your main's water.

	Problems and Solutions	What to Do
9	**Keep Aluminum and Plastic Away from Foods**	
	There is no clear-cut evidence, but many questions and doubts persist concerning aluminum cookware and deodorants—some may contain up to 20 percent aluminum. Plastic is a real problem.	Use stainless steel, glass, enamel, cast iron, earthenware or tin cookware. Keep plastic away from your food, including avoiding buying food wrapped in plastic. Use aluminum-free deodorants. Read labels.
10	**Aim for a Lean Weight**	
	The overweight develop more cancers than lean people. Being lean may aid recovery. As so many people are overweight, losing some weight can be healthy.	Be on the lean side. Better to undereat than overeat. Most people on this type of diet tend to a lean optimal weight. Exercise regularly.
11	**Sex Is Fun, Avoid Excesses!**	
	Too much or too little is a problem! Late age at first child's birth or little or no breast-feeding is associated with an increase in breast cancer for women, while there is an increased risk of cervical cancer if a male partner is promiscuous.	Moderation in all things. Mothers are recommended to exclusively breast-feed their babies for the first six months of life, if possible.
12	**Enjoy Life, Minimize Stress**	
	An inability to cope with stress appropriately is a common factor in the lives of many people who develop cancer.	Avoid stress where possible, but also learn how to cope with it. Meditation, contemplation and positive thinking work wonders.

The Use and Preparation of 39 Vegetables and 28 Fruits

Here are detailed charts that set out the recommendations regarding what vegetables and fruits to use and how to prepare them. The recommendations for the Healing Diet and the Wellness Diet are included. Under the Healing heading, vegetables that need to be cooked for easy digestion are identified, and, of course, if you were on an all-raw diet they would not be eaten unless raw.

List of Vegetable Uses

*J = juice   R = raw   S = steam   B = bake   Sa = sauté in water, wok

Vegetable	Healing	Wellness	Preparation*	Comments
Artichoke—Globe	Yes	Yes	S	Good for diabetics. Low-allergenic food.
Artichoke—Jerusalem	Yes	Yes	S B	Highly recommended—be careful with bloating—try a little first if they are new to you.

Vegetable	Healing	Wellness	Preparation*	Comments
Bell peppers	Yes	Yes	J R S B Sa	Red has more vitamin C than green. Juice good for sore throat.
Beetroot	Yes	Yes	J R S B	Good blood builder. Combines well with other juices. Anticancer folk remedy.
Beetroot tops	Yes	Yes	J R S	Do have a little oxalic acid, but a good source of potassium.
Broccoli	Cooked	Yes	R S Sa	All brassicas are associated with cancer-protecting factors.
Brussels sprouts	Cooked	Yes	S Sa	Brassica.
Cabbage	Yes	Yes	R S Sa	Brassica. Small amount of cabbage juice is good for ulcers and upset stomachs. Is acid forming. Can be gas producing, especially for older people—not so bad steamed.
Carrot	Yes	Yes	J R S B Sa	Excellent juice. Highly recommended. Source of vitamin A. Combines well with other juices.
Cauliflower	Cooked	Yes	R S Sa	Brassica. Caution with gas, if raw. Good source of calcium.
Celery	Yes	Yes	J R S Sa	Good source of potassium and excellent tonic for urinary system. Avoid the tops.
Chayote	Cooked	Yes	S B Sa	
Chicory	Yes	Yes	R S	Steam in other greens.
Chili	No	No		Too stimulating.
Cucumber	Yes	Yes	J R	Juice aids treatment of kidney and gallstones. Avoid "apple" varieties—too acidic. Lebanese or Burpless are best, more alkaline.
Eggplant	Caution	Yes	S B Sa	Can aggravate arthritic conditions and may be unhelpful on Healing Diet.
Garlic	Yes	Yes	R S Sa	Good condiment, flavoring, dressing. One clove of garlic in carrot juice works well. Worm treatment. Blood cleanser. Can be pickled. Sauté leads to less aromatic acids. Chelating agent for heavy metals. Recommended for chemotherapy patients. Regulates blood pressure. Has anticancer properties.
Ginger	Yes	Yes	J R	Use regularly and preferably fresh. Excellent addition to vegetables, particularly for vegetarians. Good to stimulate stomach acid and spleen function. Can add to carrot juice. Use for flavoring.
Horseradish	Yes	Yes	R	Aids lung conditions, emphysema. Condiment.
Kohlrabi	Occasional	Yes	B	
Leek	Cooked	Yes	S B Sa	

Vegetable	Healing	Wellness	Preparation*	Comments
Mushroom	Occasional	Yes	R Sa	
Okra	Cooked	Yes	S Sa	
Onion	Cooked	Yes	R S B Sa	High in aromatic acids. Good for helping with weight reduction. Better cooked than raw.
Parsnip	Cooked	Yes	S B	High calcium source.
Potatoes: Common	Yes	Yes	S B	Skins good for potassium. Baking especially recommended.
Potatoes: Sweet	Yes	Yes	S B	
Pumpkin	Yes	Yes	R S B	Easily digested.
Pumpkin seeds	Yes	Yes	R S B	Excellent for zinc.
Radish	Occasional	Yes	R	Stimulant—use moderately.
Rutabaga	Cooked	Yes	S B	
Spinach	Yes	Yes	J R S	High oxalic acid content—use 2–3 times per week at maximum.
Squash	Cooked	Yes	R S B	
Sweet corn	Yes	Yes	R S B	Can be baked in husk (475°F).
Swiss chard	Yes	Yes	J R S	High oxalic acid content—use 2–3 times per week at maximum.
Tomato	Yes	Yes	J R S B Sa	Solanum. Excellent source of vitamin C. 1 gram per large naturally ripened tomato. Less acidic varieties are the cherry types and Roma.
Turnip	Cooked	Yes	S B	
Watercress	Yes	Yes	J R	Good for arthritis.
Zucchini	Yes	Yes	R S B Sa	

List of Fruit Uses

Fruit	Healing	Wellness	Preparation*	Comments
Apple	Yes	Yes	J R B Sa	Cook in juice or water.
Apricot	Yes	Yes	J R Sa	Good sun-dried (soak before eating). Kernels can be source of B_{17}, eaten with fruit. Start with 5, add 1 each day up to 15, or, if headache occurs, decrease.
Avocado	Occasional	Yes	R B	High fat content. Tastes terrific!
Banana	Yes	Yes	R B	Excellent source of potassium. Gentle on upset stomach. Common allergen. Eat when ripe.
Berries:				
Strawberries	No	Occasional	J R Jam	Make into jam with honey. Blood builders. Acidity can be a problem and very high in salicylates (major cause of food intolerance).

Fruit	Healing	Wellness	Preparation*	Comments
Blueberries, Raspberries	Yes	Yes	J R	Raspberries have powerful anticancer activity.
Cherry	Yes	Yes	J R Sa	Good source of iron.
Citrus fruits	Yes	Yes	J R	Grapefruit, limes, mandarins, lemons. Good to start day with. Oranges require care with their acidity.
Fig	Occasional	Occasional	R S	High sugar. Excellent laxative.
Grapes	Yes	Yes	J R	Very good blood cleanser. Excellent tonic. See "The Mono Diet" later in this Chapter. Red grapes build blood, white cleanse intestines.
Mango	Yes	Yes	J R	Very palatable!
Melons	Yes	Yes	J R	Cantaloupe, watermelon, honeydew. Good kidney tonics. Eat on own—not with other fruits, foods (see food combinations Appendix L).
Nectarine	Yes	Yes	J R S	
Papaya or Pawpaw	Yes	Yes	J R	Excellent source of papain, a potent digestive enzyme.
Passionfruit	Yes	Yes	R S	
Peach	Yes	Yes	J R S	
Pear	Yes	Yes	J R S	Juice is a gentle laxative.
Persimmon	Yes	Yes	R	Must be ripe.
Pineapple	No	Occasional	J R	Contains bromelain, an enzyme reputed by some to take the outer layer off tumors. But require care with acidity.
Plum	Yes	Yes	J R S	
Pomegranate	Yes	Yes	J R	Powerful anticancer properties.
Prune	Yes	Yes	J R S	Laxative. Improves blood iron.
Rhubarb	No	Very occasional	S	High oxalic acid content.

Step 2. Add Regular Juices

Eating a lot of fresh, vital food gets the healing process in motion. It is accentuated by the use of freshly prepared juices.

JUICING 101

Juices are an ideal source of easily digestible nutrients in a well-balanced package. Freshly made, they are also full of oxidative enzymes. Authorities like Gerson believed they could help reoxygenate cancerous tissue and revitalize the rest of the body. Gerson advocated drinking juices on an hourly basis, twelve each day—hence the time commitment for those on his diet. I would recommend the need for moderation, depending upon the individual situation.

In my experience, most people on the Healing Diet find that seven per day is manageable and effective.

Wellness Rule 19: Drink seven juices daily.

The general recommendation is seven 200ml (7 oz.) juices to be taken daily.

Start the morning with citrus, preferably one-third lemon juice in two-thirds water. Other citrus may be OK, but be careful with oranges, particularly because they are quite acidic and people with brain tumors have reported them to be problematic over the years.

Next, have apple, grape, carrot, beetroot (one-third each of beetroot, carrot and celery) and two green juices. Two good options to consider for use when available or for variety and good effect are pomegranate juice (that is very good against prostate cancer and is protective against radiotherapy side effects) and the Australian blend of anticancer juices called Dr Red's ginger punch (order via the Internet).

Apple and grape, along with pomegranate juice, can be bought if pure, organically grown juices are available, while the others are best made fresh. The green juices can be made from a combination of celery (not the leaves), green pepper, lettuce, a little cabbage, beetroot tops, Swiss chard or spinach and a little parsley.

The recommendation is that ideally you do make all the green juices freshly. However, for convenience you can use commercially prepared barley juice that comes as a powder, prepared by the rapid dehydration of the juice of young barley shoots. This powder is excellent to take traveling—all you need to do is add water.

Most juices have an acceptable taste, and some are positively pleasant. Orange, apple, grape and carrot are all old favorites. The taste of green juices requires more explanation before they can be relished. Gerson claimed that the oxidative enzymes in these juices were able to enter into the bloodstream and exert a direct effect. Certainly the chlorophyll molecule, the main constituent of green plants, is very similar in structure to hemoglobin, the main constituent of red blood cells. Chlorophyll has a central magnesium molecule, hemoglobin iron; otherwise they are identical.

Wheatgrass

Wheatgrass is a special green juice that may be a great aid to restoring the degenerated metabolism of people affected by cancer. Freshly sprouted wheat is cut off when the shoots are four to five inches high and juiced. This juice is hard to extract without a specialized juicer, but a good alternative is to chew the shoots, swallow the juice, and spit out the fiber—delicately, of course.

Liver Juice

Gerson also placed great value on raw liver juice. This may sound a trifle revolting, and the taste is certainly nothing to rave over, but again, it makes sense especially if your blood count is down or you have other blood disorders. The liver is recognized as the best nutritional source of the components that build the blood. Based on its nutrient content, dietitians would certainly rate it as one of the best individual foods. So, why not cook it and eat the whole lot? Why the need to have it as a fresh raw juice? Cooking can affect the vitamins, enzymes, cofactors and other suspected, but as yet unidentified, beneficial substances in liver. Also, the fiber in it is very tough and the digestion of a person with cancer is often incapable of dealing with it well. It could undergo delayed passage through the bowel, putrefy and then add to the toxicity of the body. So, the juice avoids the fiber while saving all the goodness.

Liver juice, like wheatgrass, is hard to make, and chewing the liver in pieces, swallowing the juice and leaving the fiber is a possibility. Chewing raw liver is even less joy than drinking liver juice, so a minimum of cooking—thirty to sixty seconds grilling each side—is a fair compromise. Still, spit out that fiber! Combining the lightly cooked liver with well-grilled tomato improves the taste, while sucking a lemon afterward clears the palate if you feel the need.

Juice Machines

The normal commercial juicer uses a centrifugal action that shreds the food, then spins it at high speed. This is a fine way to separate the pulp from the juice, and the juice is packed with nutrients, vitamins and minerals. However, it is claimed that the centrifugal action of these machines creates static electricity that destroys some of the oxidative enzymes in the juice. Gerson asserted this and claimed he saw better results when using a machine that had no static in it. He recommended a machine that separately grinds and then presses the juices out by hydraulic action. Fine in theory, but expensive in practice. The Norwalk machine he preferred now costs around $2,400! The Champion juicer seems like a reasonable alternative, costing around $550 and is like a mechanized meat-mincer in its action. These machines do also extract more juice from the same amount of ingredients than the standard machines and are easy to operate and to clean. So, if you are serious about juices, the Champion is well worth considering.

Step 3. Focus on Foods with Known Anticancer Properties

Over one thousand chemicals possessing anticancer properties have been identified in the foods we eat. Of course, some of these chemicals are quite mild in their action, but fortunately some are quite potent. It makes obvious good sense to identify and regularly consume the potent anticancer foods.

First, however, let us be clear, a diet that is rich in fresh, organic and judiciously cooked vegetables and fruits will contain a myriad of anticancer agents. While these agents are being researched more (often with the motivation of identifying the active ingredient and marketing that), it is quite probable many are synergistic. That means they could support each other's benefits and create a sum total of benefit far above their individual merits. The opposite effect of this is well researched in the causes of cancer. For example, as we will discuss further in the next chapter, smoking tobacco and drinking alcohol together create a far greater risk of developing cancer than the sum of the risks associated with one factor on its own.

> Wellness Rule 20: Consider your Healing Diet as a whole to have general anticancer properties. On top of this, take advantage of the potent anticancer foods and consume them regularly.

Traditionally, folk medicine in Europe highly recommended asparagus and beetroot for their anticancer properties. Asparagus is known to be a good antioxidant and high in vitamin C, folate and potassium. Beetroot is also rich in antioxidants, vitamin C, magnesium, potassium, boron and betaine. Older beetroot produces betanin, especially in its roots, and this is unpleasant to taste (bitter) and causes red stools and urine, which can be distressing if you do not know what caused it! Despite all this, there are no scientific studies supporting the known anticancer properties of asparagus or beetroot, but I ate a good deal of both while recovering, and continue to do so.

Anticancer Food Recommendations

1. Eat at least one generous portion of brassicas daily.
2. Consume half a medium Chinese or ordinary green cabbage every few days.
3. Eat one or more of raspberries, pomegranates, tomatoes and beans daily. Make sure one of these four is in the daily diet and rotate them around.
4. Use turmeric and/or garlic and ginger daily. Rotate their use.

Step 4. Create a Cancer-Unfriendly Environment—How to Stimulate Healing via Metabolic Change

All living organisms have preferred conditions that support their life. This is very obvious in the garden where camellias, for example, thrive in acid soils but struggle and even die in an alkaline environment.

Vegetables do poorly in acid soils and thrive in more alkaline conditions, so it makes sense if we have acidic soil and intend to grow healthy vegetables that we add lime to make the ground more alkaline. The key point is that if we put vegetables in soil that is too acidic, they will die; put camellias in alkaline soil and we can kill them.

Wellness Rule 21: Make the food choices that inhibit cancer and promote healing.

One of the elegant ways we can influence cancer is to use this principle and learn how to manipulate our metabolism in a range of ways that work against the disease. Here is how we do it.

Anticancer Diet Recommendations

This is an area of great possibility. From what follows, make an action list that clarifies the anticancer approach you will adopt and delight in eating for recovery. Bon appétit!

Ten Top Anticancer Foods—And How to Use Them

Food	Main Active Ingredients	Action	Usage
1. Raspberries	Ellagic acid	Inhibits cancer cells from dividing. Powerful antioxidant.	½ cup daily. Frozen is OK.
2. Pomegranates	Ellagic acid—about 50 times more concentrated than raspberries	Same as raspberries.	A small amount of fruit or juice daily. Very good against prostate cancer.
3. Turmeric	Curcumin	Antioxidant, anti-inflammatory. Induces apoptosis. Some positive phytoestrogenic activity. Slows cancer cell division. Attacks breast cancer stem cells.	Use in similar ways and amounts as you would ginger.
4. Garlic	Allicin—antibiotic Phytoncide—antifungal Sulfur compounds Allixin—antioxidant and anticancer	Known to be highly preventative. May regulate blood sugar. Acts as a blood thinner.	Raw garlic is more potent. Use either liberally. Note: Garlic is regarded as a stimulant, so some spiritual traditions recommend not using it.
5. Tomatoes	Probably lycopene The benefits of tomatoes are known, the active ingredients are unclear.	Antioxidant. Anticancer properties suggested, particularly for prostate cancer.	Cooking does help to release the lycopene. Use raw or cooked liberally.
6. The bean family, especially soybeans	Isoflavones—the best-known and most potent of which is genestein	Phytoestrogenic activity—beneficially regulate sex hormones and metabolism generally. Mildly regulates cancer cell division and angiogenesis.	Miso has higher concentration than tofu. Use regularly. Supplements of genesteine are not recommended.

Food	Main Active Ingredients	Action	Usage
7. The brassicas— broccoli, cabbage, cauliflower, Brussels sprouts	Glutamine Anti-inflammatory Indole-3-carbinol 3,3 Diindolylmethane	Boosts DNA repair. Blocks cancer cells from dividing. Creates oxidative stress in cancer cells.	Use regularly—best when cooked.
8. Chinese cabbage and probably green cabbage	Brassinin High in vitamin C High in glutamine	General brassica effects. Angiostatin. Anti-inflammatory.	Use ½ medium cabbage every 4 days—raw, lightly cooked and/or juiced.
9. Broccoli sprouts	Sulphoraphane—this is in all brassicas but very concentrated in broccoli sprouts.	Inhibits cancer growth. Enhances tumor suppressant proteins and other anti-cancer metabolites.	Use fresh (do not cook) and liberally
10. Green tea	Epigallocatechin gallate	Induces apoptosis.	Does have caffeine but useful occasionally. Does not combine well with ellagic acid (raspberries), so is the least recommended of these ten.

Stimulate High Cellular Oxygen levels

The metabolism of cancer is anaerobic; it runs on low oxygen. High oxygen levels are cancer unfriendly. What we need is plenty of oxygen being breathed in, and then good quality, nonsticky, free-flowing blood to get the oxygen around the body. Therefore, breathing is very useful! Physical exercise, yoga and qigong all stimulate oxygen uptake and circulation.

1. Exercise three to four times per week. It has many benefits and is covered in chapter 7.
2. Strongly consider learning yoga or chi gong and practicing one of them daily. I received a great deal of benefit from daily yoga practice throughout my recovery.

Create a High-Potassium, Low-Sodium Balance in the Diet

Cancer does best metabolically with a low-potassium, high-sodium balance. This is an easy way to turn the tables on the disease. The Healing Diet generally is rich in potassium and we already know to leave sodium (or salt) out. If you are new to this diet, bananas are one of the richest sources of potassium and warrant being eaten regularly. Also, the area just below the skins of potatoes concentrates potassium, so this is another reason not to peel potatoes.

Develop an Alkaline Balance in the Body

The body has what we call an acid base balance, base referring to its alkalinity. Again, cancer is like camellias in the garden (only not so beautiful!) and prefers an acidic environment. Quite easily we can make life more difficult for cancer by alkalizing the body via an alkaline diet. The Healing Diet as a whole is highly alkaline and very suitable for this purpose.

There is much debate regarding the relative acidity or alkalinity of particular foods. It is accurate to say meat, dairy and most processed and refined foods have an acidic effect, while most fruits, vegetables and grains are alkalizing.

What is being discussed here is the effect the food has at a cellular level, which paradoxically for some foods is different to how they are before being eaten. For example, we would regard lemon juice as acidic, but in the body it has the effect of being mildly alkaline. In my view, it is best not to labor which individual foods are acidic, which alkaline; simply be confident that overall the Healing Diet is alkaline to a very useful degree.

Eat Modest Amounts of Protein
The rationale for this was covered in the last chapter.

Avoid Simple Sugars, Use Complex Sugars and Complex Carbohydrates
This also was explained in the last chapter.

Avoid Free Radicals, Eat a Diet Rich in Antioxidants
Why do we hear so much about the value of antioxidants? One of the main reasons is that they neutralize excessive free radicals. Free radicals are unstable molecules that chemically are highly reactive. Some are necessary for good health but too many can lead to cell damage and death, and cancer is linked to DNA mutation from free radical damage. Free radicals can form naturally in the body, are created by ionizing radiation and from poor nutrition.

Our intake of free radicals is reduced by avoiding fatty foods and, especially, fried foods. Microwaves create free radicals, especially when used to heat dairy and fatty foods. Both the Healing Diet and the Wellness Diet are rich in antioxidants as are some supplements. The latter will be discussed soon.

Minimize the Toxic Load on the Body
Pollutants can aggravate genetic mutation, hinder our metabolism and make life easier for cancer. Reverse this with the use of organic foods, aiming to use natural cleaners and personal hygiene products and eliminate plastics from your food cycle. Garlic is touted as being good for helping the body to detox and eliminate pollutants—another good reason to use it.

Eat Food That Is as Fresh and as Vital as Possible
Vitality is a good test for the foods you buy. If you buy fruit and vegetables that already look dead, how can they serve you well? This is a powerful bonus of the home vegetable garden—freshness and vitality.

Commit to This Highly Anti-Inflammatory, Regenerative Way of Eating
The overall effect of the Healing Diet is to be highly anti-inflammatory, highly regenerative. We know from research that cancer is aggravated by

inflammation. Researchers in this field claim that chronic inflammation is associated with the development of about one-quarter of all cancers.

Of even greater significance to any one actually diagnosed with cancer is that chemicals produced in the inflammatory process stimulate cancer growth. The clear message? Avoid inflammation. Have your teeth and gums checked regularly by your dentist, and treated if necessary, especially if on chemotherapy, which often precipitates gum disease. If you have inflammation of the skin (dermatitis), the tonsils, or any part of the body, take it seriously and have it attended to promptly and thoroughly. Then know that both this diet and the meditation are highly anti-inflammatory and actually support healing in many ways.

Step 5. Consider the Use of Supplements and Other Natural Products

SUPPLEMENTS

The question of supplements is a vexed one indeed. When considering your options, you will find that at one end of the spectrum are those who say that none are needed as "the average diet contains all you need." At the other end of the spectrum are those who recommend taking vast amounts of every known vitamin, mineral and just about everything else that can be made into a tablet and swallowed.

What is reasonable? There is good evidence that the "average" diet is frequently deficient in vital nutrients. A survey that examined the vitamin and mineral content of the diets of new patients in a Melbourne medical practice revealed startling results. The patients whose diets were examined presented for a wide range of everyday problems. They could reasonably be said to represent the average in an affluent society wherein one would expect people to lack little. Yet their diets were grossly deficient. And, significantly, the deficiencies showed up in factors directly involved in the normal functioning of the immune system, zinc being a good example.

The case for supplementation is further increased by the growing body of evidence that extra doses of some minerals, and particularly some vitamins, can be dramatically helpful for some cancer patients.

Maintain High Levels of Vitamin D

This is like a free hit. If your vitamin D levels are low, as they are for many people, particularly those living further away from the equator, your immune system and capacity to heal will be markedly compromised.

Vitamin D deficiencies are strongly implicated as a causative factor in cancer. Currently in Europe, it is estimated that one-third of all the breast cancers in women are directly linked with low vitamin D levels. The link is established with quite a number of other cancers and as research progresses in this rapidly expanding field it seems highly likely that high vitamin D levels aid in recovery and prolong survival times.

Vitamin D is manufactured in the body after sunlight, and more specifically the ultraviolet B (UVB) in sunlight, activates chemical precursors under your skin. There is a limit to how much vitamin D can be activated per day and it takes only a short while in the sun to acquire all the vitamin D you can for that day. What this means is that to develop and sustain vitamin D levels you need to get as much skin as decently possible into the sun regularly, but only for a short period of time. The more UVB when you are in the sun, the less time you need. So a hot summer's day and maybe five to seven minutes is enough; a cool winter's day, maybe twenty to thirty minutes. Clouds reduce the UVB significantly; glass and sunscreens block it out. Clothing produces a range of reduction from a little to a lot.

Vitamin D levels are easily checked by routine blood tests. Recent solid research evidence has led to the realization of just how important the role of vitamin D is for healthy immune function, as well as our health and well-being generally (it leads to happier moods and reduces depression). This has led in turn to the recommended blood levels being increased. Currently, it seems the best advice to aim for is between 100–150 nmol/l.

Many people in our groups, which are well south of the equator and experience cold, cloudy winters, record levels in the 20s, 30s and 40s. This really helps cancer! What can we do?

Vitamin D from the sun is best—if there is sunlight and warmth available. Exercising outdoors in light clothing or short periods of sunbathing (both sides) works well. The aim is to avoid the skin going red and beginning to burn. People with dark skin need longer periods of exposure to get the same amount of vitamin D compared to those with light skins. All colors of skin can burn and this needs to be avoided.

Vitamin D supplements are practical and all indications are that they work well. If you have low levels you will need significant supplementation to return to healthy levels; then you can use a maintenance dose. Check with your doctor, but with a level of 30–40nmol/l you may need 150–250,000, even up to 500,000 IU units of vitamin D to reach the recommended blood levels. While large doses can be taken in one day, it is probably preferable to only take 50,000 IU per day for five to seven days, and then after two to four weeks have another blood test.

A useful maintenance guide is 5,000 IU per day, but the ideal level is best decided in consultation with your doctor and adjusted once you experiment for a while and observe your blood levels. We have found people can create and metabolize vitamin D quite differently—some very efficiently and so needing lower supplementation or sun exposure, others not very efficiently at all and so needing good support.

Wellness Rule 22: Ensure adequate blood levels of vitamin D.

The Special Case of Vitamin C

Examining the available information on vitamin C demonstrates the controversies surrounding some supplements. While some studies say it makes little or no difference, others point to its wide range of beneficial activities. Again, Doctors Pauling and Cameron refer to an increase in the body's natural resistance in their work *Cancer and Vitamin C*.[20] They cite an improved level of well-being, as measured by improved appetite, increased mental alertness, decreased requirement for pain-controlling drugs and other clinical criteria.

Most animals make their own vitamin C. Not so we humans. We rely on our diet for all we get. It has been claimed by some authorities that an ideal, fresh food diet would provide 8 to 10 grams of vitamin C daily. Some claim this is a reasonable maintenance level, and ideally, such an amount would be obtained in the diet itself. But, in fact, most people would require supplementation to achieve this level. By contrast, the official minimum recommended daily allowance is currently 45 milligrams per day. Our Wellness Diet as analyzed (see Appendix M) contains around 560mgm per day. Gerson's diet contains 930 mgm.

Another consideration is the level required to bring the body to "saturation point." It has been suggested that, at saturation, vitamin C exerts its maximum effects. It has also been suggested that at levels below this its effect may be minimal. To explain: a person in normal health may be at saturation with a total intake of, say, 10 grams. The stress of an impending cold, however, may increase the need for vitamin C so much that 50 grams may be required to reach saturation. If the person is only getting 10 grams, the cold may develop as normal. Giving 50 grams may prevent it developing at all. Likewise, exposure to "flu" may create a need for 200 grams. Giving 10 or 50 grams would be ineffective, whereas 200 grams may be effective.

Experience tells us that the amount of vitamin C required to reach saturation varies widely with individuals and individual situations. Doctors working with this approach often use what is called the bowel tolerance test. They find that once the body is saturated, a little extra vitamin C produces a mild diarrhea, which stops once the supplementation is reduced a little. This makes the point of bowel tolerance a useful signpost to the individual's maximum requirements. So they recommend that their patients find their own level of bowel tolerance, drop the dose just a little, and keep to that, adjusting according to stress levels. Many cancer patients find this requires their adding 18 to 20 grams of vitamin C to their diet daily. Some take 30 grams or more by mouth each day. Such high levels of vitamin C are said to leach magnesium, zinc and vitamin B from the body, and so supplements of these are then required.

Often even higher doses of vitamin C are given intravenously with some good effects. A common, almost uniform, result is the lessening of pain. Some tumors also do regress. In my veterinary days, I treated confirmed cases of lymphosarcoma in cats with intravenous doses of 1 gram per kilogram of body weight on five successive days. Four out of four treated cases went into total remission. The few dogs I treated in the same manner did not respond so well.

The special case of vitamin C amply demonstrates the complex and really rather confusing issues involved with supplements.

My Own Experience

I hope it is obvious that I am only discussing the options, and avoiding making specific recommendations. Supplements pose many complex questions. Their role is not one I find easy to resolve.

My own experience with them runs the full gamut. I did take all the supplements Gerson recommended when I was using his regime. His was an integrated approach. I then dropped various factors off as I began to feel the need for them had passed—relaxing toward the Wellness Diet. At another time during my illness I did try megavitamin therapy, taking huge numbers of vitamin tablets. Apart from learning the art of swallowing thirty pills in one go, I felt it did little for me. However, for quite some time during my recovery and the ensuing years, I did continue to take a general purpose multivitamin and some extra vitamin C.

Some Cautious Suggestions

My overriding attitude is that natural sources of nutrition are the best. It seems clear to me that in an ideal world, when we are eating well, when we are happy, stress free and joyous, there would be no need for extra supplements. However, not many people with our modern, busy lifestyles seem to be in such an ideal situation. Therefore, if the diet is not ideal, if there is the hint of stress around, when we are traveling, or experiencing difficult times, it seems reasonable that basic supplements could help our bodies to cope better.

Staying with the natural is the best principle. If extra nutrients are required on top of what we eat, the next recommendation is to use juices. Juices concentrate nutrients in a form that is natural, well balanced and easily absorbed by the body. However, in many situations, particularly when facing major stress or major disease, even more help from supplement tablets may be beneficial.

A Summary of the Supplement Options

When considering the options regarding extra nutrition, consider the following choices:

- Take no extra supplements—not many people I have worked with have done this.
- Use fresh juices as a source of concentrated nutrition that is provided in a natural balanced form. This approach is highly recommended to anyone with active illness. The juices also seem to be of great help when recovering from surgery, or when undergoing chemotherapy or radiation.

- Self-medicate: Take a good quality general multivitamin and mineral supplements along with extra vitamin D and maybe vitamin C. This is what many people find helpful and it gives them the security of knowing that their requirements for vitamins and minerals are well covered. This is particularly important when preparing for, or recovering from surgery, or when undergoing chemotherapy or radiotherapy. It is at these times that the body is under an increased load and requires extra nutritional help.

- Vitamin C can be taken in the form of 500 milligrams or 1gm tablets with bioflavonoid (which help its function) after each meal. If, along the lines we discussed earlier, you choose larger doses of vitamin C, use sodium ascorbate powder dissolved in water or juices, and again, take it after meals.

- There is a real caution regarding vitamins A and E, which have been shown via large meta-analysis studies to shorten life span in people who are basically well and have taken them over long periods of time. I know of no studies being published regarding the long-term use of vitamins A and E by people affected by cancer, and maybe they are OK short term, but the caution needs to be stated.

- Seek expert advice. Take larger, therapeutic doses of individual vitamins, minerals and/or other dietary supplements. This appeals to many, and if you choose to do this, I strongly recommend that you seek the personalized help of a suitably qualified practitioner. Many doctors are now well trained in nutritional medicine and some naturopaths can be helpful. As always, you are well advised to seek out the qualifications and experience of anyone you are considering consulting. Particularly in this field, it is wise to obtain personal recommendations and feedback from people whose opinions you value and who can help to guide your choices.

COFFEE ENEMAS

The stark reality is I found these really helpful and know many, many others who experienced equally positive benefits. Often I wish this was not so! The notion of using coffee as an enema always seems a little weird and I like my credibility. Of all the things I have ever been criticized for, this is the easiest to understand as a source of mirth.

However, I am committed to sharing what works, so here we go.

I thought coffee enemas to be the funniest thing I had ever heard of when it was suggested that they could help me. I am sure Spike Milligan's crazy genius could not have produced a more comical idea. But, like everyone else I know who has tried them, I felt an immediate benefit from them, and amid some hilarity, persisted with them. What do they do, and how do they work?

Coffee Enemas Stimulate Liver Function

Gerson named the liver as the major organ of detoxification and placed great importance upon restoring and maintaining its efficient activity. He believed liver juices aided liver function and he also recommended the use of liver extract injections.

His main method for stimulating liver function, however, was through the use of coffee or caffeine enemas as they are sometimes known. Caffeine introduced into the rectum by enema is absorbed by the rectal veins and then passes into the portal vein, and on directly to the liver. There it stimulates liver function, including bile flow. Bile is a major means of eliminating toxic material from the body. Coffee is a readily available source of caffeine, and it also makes a convenient enema, therefore, it is coffee enemas that are recommended.

Coffee Enemas Provide Significant Pain Relief

Coffee enemas are remarkably effective in combating and relieving pain. When pain was a problem for me, I found them more useful than the narcotic analgesics I was having. Dr. Meares told me that he believed they have an effect because to hold an enema for ten to fifteen minutes while the caffeine is being absorbed requires quite a degree of relaxation—relaxation in an area you might otherwise not relax so well. I believe this is an added benefit, but they certainly have an immediate physical effect as well.

For many years, I have encouraged researchers I know to investigate why and how coffee enemas work. Perhaps not surprisingly, there has been little enthusiasm for such a project! However, Dr. Candace Pert, a famous researcher in the field of mind-body medicine and author of the wonderful book *Molecules of Emotion*,[21] told me of a distinct possibility.

Dr. Pert published much of the pioneering research on neurotransmitters or messenger molecules—those chemicals that the body produces in one part which, when released, influence how the body functions elsewhere. She has been particularly interested in how our state of mind affects the production of these chemicals and how they in turn affect our immune system and health generally. Dr. Pert was the first to discover that white blood cells, the front line defenses for our immune system, have opiate receptors on their surfaces. The brain is capable of producing natural opiates, such as endorphins and releasing them into the bloodstream. When this happens, we feel pain relief and well-being, as if we had had an injection of morphine. As well, these opiates attach to the white blood cells and enhance their activity, improving the effectiveness of our immune system.

Now the link to coffee enemas. Not only are these natural opiates produced in the brain, they are also produced in cells that line the bowel. It had always puzzled me why coffee enemas produced such good pain relief and such a heightened sense of well-being. Dr. Pert suggested that it may well be that this happens through a direct interaction between some component of the coffee enemas, probably the caffeine, and the endorphin-producing cells lining the bowel.

Again, if the explanation of how they work is inadequate, the pragmatic fact is that many do find them helpful (see Appendix F for details of preparation and administration).

Of all Gerson's treatments, this is the one I kept on with for longest. In the early days I used to try stopping them and I would become obviously jaundiced in one or two days. A coffee enema would clear the yellowness from my skin in about fifteen minutes.

Alternatives to Coffee Enemas
Dr. Alex Forbes, who pioneered the Bristol Cancer Help Center in England, told me that they obtained just as good results using herbs that stimulate liver function. As these herbs can be taken "down" rather than "up," they have a greater esthetic appeal! I have no personal experience of using such herbs, but Dorothy Hall, Australia's leading herbalist, feels that individual patients require individual treatments. She recommends seeking personal advice from a qualified herbalist if you are considering this type of assistance.

Roasted dandelion root coffee has been recommended for centuries as a safe but useful liver tonic, and we have found it to be a gentle and reliable aid for improving liver function—a useful but probably less potent alternative to the enemas. However, I do recommend its regular use at up to three cups per day.

The principle to reaffirm is that generally the liver will profit from active support and it becomes a matter of determining the most appropriate way of providing this assistance.

COMPLEMENTARY AND ALTERNATIVE THERAPIES (CAM)

The intention of this book is to focus on lifestyle medicine—what we as individuals can do for ourselves. There are many options in the CAM arena and some may well be useful. It can be very helpful to locate a doctor engaged in integrative medicine and who sees people with cancer regularly, or a sound naturopath. We are all unique and CAM treatments are similar to conventional medical treatments—they need to be prescribed individually in full knowledge of the individual's situation and preferences. Both conventional and CAM options will be discussed more in chapter 19 on healing.

Step 6. Move from the General to the Specific

Now we need to advance from the general recommendations to the specific needs we have as individuals. We need to personalize our way of eating. Once steps 1–5 are in place, we can proceed and begin to develop a pattern of eating that is tailored to our particular needs and conditions.

Here is how to do it.

STEP 1. DEVELOP YOUR FOOD KNOWLEDGE

It makes good sense to read, study and learn more about nutrition. It is a vast subject and, when dealing with cancer, one needs to prioritize. So if you feel what is in this book meets your needs, study that. Reread each section, put the principles into practice, and come back to the book's theories again and again. Rereading this main text over and over will make good sense.

> Wellness Rule 23: Study nutrition but avoid fixating. The need is to decide on an approach, a dietary plan, and to stick to it for a while; observe the results and readjust if necessary.

STEP 2. HEIGHTEN YOUR FOOD AWARENESS

Our mind is a great ally when we harness its knowledge and its awareness. We have talked of this regularly—meditate and we become more aware.

Practice mindfulness specifically and we do notice more clearly what works for us and what is unhelpful.

> Wellness Rule 24: Meditate, be mindful, and respond to what you may have once called intuition or a "gut feeling."

STEP 3. LET YOUR BODY BE YOUR GUIDE

Helping your body to become more sensitive to the foods you eat heightens the prospect of reliably being able to determine what foods suit your needs best. This can be achieved using one of three methods.

Simply Meditate

Over months or even years, meditation will clear your mind and you are highly likely to make more appropriate food choices. In theory this will work, although I know a significant number of people who have meditated for years and still eat poorly.

Meditation can involve the body or it can be more of a "head trip." People who meditate in their bodies, who consciously relax their bodies and feel integrated with their bodies, are much more likely to notice what goes on in that body and to treat it well. This is another reason why we emphasize the relaxation phase in MBSM meditation.

Follow the Wellness Diet

Put bluntly, the Wellness Diet eliminates the junk from your diet and adds the good stuff! With this, a gentle detox and transformation takes place over weeks to months and heightens and enhances the body awareness we have been advocating.

Thoroughly eliminating salt, sugar and chili from the diet greatly accelerates this process as those three overwhelm the taste buds and severely impair our capacity to discriminate.

This approach is very reasonable for people who are well and are seeking a really sound, personalized diet. It is also very practical and manageable for those dealing with cancer and other diseases who choose to take their nutrition seriously, but elect to move steadily into a better way of eating.

Actively Detoxify the Body

If our car is overdue for a service, we are highly likely to become nervous, maybe even anxious. We know we are not treating it well and fear mechanical trouble. Detoxing the body is a bit like changing the oil in our car. The notion of detoxifying the body recognizes we live in a polluted world and especially if our diet has been below par, the body may well be carrying an inordinate toxic load.

THE DETOX PRINCIPLES

Detoxification has been a major principle in many cultures over many years and is highly valued among modern-day naturopaths. Modern medicine is more equivocal but surely it makes sense. If our body carries a toxic load, its general metabolism and capacity to regulate healing will be impaired. Also, to develop our individual food sensitivity, we are asking our body to measure the value of the foods it consumes. If we are attempting to use a ruler covered in mud to measure a distance, the result will be highly suspect. We need a clean instrument. We need a clean body.

As explained in the last section, detoxifying will occur slowly and steadily over months on the Wellness Diet. However, what we have found most effective for those who want a more rapid process that will produce results in days or weeks is the mono diet.

The Mono Diet

A mono diet is where just one simple, low-allergenic food is eaten consistently for a fixed period of time. It is preferable to fasting on water (a traditional method for purification and detoxifying), as the mono diet does provide some basic nutrition. Clearly, a mono diet is not a complete dietary package, but that is the point. The gentle metabolic stress induced by eating just one food over a period of time triggers the body to shed its toxic load.

However, the partial nutritional content of one food means that the body is not too stressed as it may be during a more rigorous water fast. At the same time, any food that we may react adversely to is cleared from the body. It is as if the body is returned to a clean, uncomplicated state.

What we do after completing a mono diet is to gradually reintroduce a broader range of foods. By having the patience and the willpower to do this gradually, it becomes relatively easy to establish which foods agree with you and which do not.

We can tell when a food is suitable—we feel fine! When we eat something we may be better to avoid, our body will let us know. We may notice an obvious digestive upset—feeling like we ate something that was "off"— biliousness, nausea, even diarrhea. However, commonly the signs are a little more subtle. Feelings of tiredness are common, sometimes headaches or joint pain, sometimes flu-like symptoms, or with dairy products particularly, inflammatory reactions like tonsillitis, sinusitis, bronchitis—even cystitis.

When we are prepared to respond to these signals and modify our diet appropriately and when we do take time to sort out any internal influences that may be affecting our choices, then we will find that we will be free to make the fine tuning to our diet and develop what is a truly individualized nutritional program.

It is worth noting that several people have recommended that a mono diet may be helpful for people with cancer if carried on for an extended period. In her book, *The Grape Cure*,[22] Johanna Brandt recounts how she used a mono diet of grapes, backed up by periods on raw foods, as the basis for recovering from her own cancer. Macrobiotics, the Japanese style of cooking based on their philosophy of balance, recommends that a mono diet of whole brown rice helps people with cancer to rebalance their system.

Consistently I have found that people who do follow a mono diet for a relatively short period receive a good deal of benefit. They invariably experience what they describe as "feeling lighter," their taste buds clear, and their food begins to taste better. Eating the one thing for a few days certainly works to focus the attention on dietary considerations. It doubles as a good exercise in willpower. This is a major benefit as once you have done ten days eating just one food you can achieve just about anything you put your mind to! Many also find that it does develop the sensitivity we are seeking.

Mono Diets Are Not Advised While Having Chemotherapy
If having chemotherapy, it is best to wait about two months after the treatment is finished and energy levels are reasonable before starting a mono diet. Doing so at this time may well help to rid the body of any residue from the treatment. I did a ten-day mono diet on grapes about a year after completing chemo, and despite being on a good diet and meditating regularly during

that intervening period, on days six and seven, I passed the same color and smell in my urine as I did when I was having the chemotherapy. I then did ten days on rice in the winter and ten days on grapes in the summer for several years.

There is new research emerging that suggests actual fasting for a day or two around the time when chemotherapy is administered has a significantly beneficial effect. It seems while the cells in the human body can manage fasting for a while quite well, cancer cells do not manage at all well.

When Considering the Mono Diet, There Are Two Variations:

The Summer Mono Diet

In summer, when it is warm and fruit is in season, the ideal is ten days eating organic grapes only. Ten days has been recommended as a good aim but this can be a struggle for some. A minimum of three days is required to experience tangible benefits. I suggest it is best to set your goal in advance—from three to ten days—and then stick to it.

While doing this, eat as many grapes as you want. Use whatever variety you prefer, but do not mix varieties at one sitting. Drink as little as you feel comfortable with, and when you do, take only pure water or grape juice (which may be diluted fifty-fifty with water).

If grapes are not available, then do just three days using one pound of only one fruit at each of three meals, or one half-pound at each of six meals. Again, drink only pure water or fruit juices and do not mix different juices and fruits together. Eating only three pounds of fruit in a day has more of a fasting element than eating unlimited amounts of grapes, but the former is only recommended for three days.

The Winter Mono Diet

In winter, the ideal is ten days on organic brown rice. The rice needs to be cooked by the absorption method. One volume of rice plus two volumes of water is slowly boiled until the water is absorbed. The rice will then be tender. It should be chewed thoroughly—to the consistency of mashed ripe bananas. This may take up to thirty, even up to fifty chews per mouthful, so do not be in a hurry! Do eat as much as you want, without adding anything else to the rice.

Again, keeping fluids to a minimum is recommended, and only water should be taken.

Generally, the rice is relatively easy, but if you do struggle, some vegetable broth could be added. Exercise needs to be kept well within your limits and many people find it best to stay close to home, concentrating on the task in hand. If the cold of winter is a problem, warm baths are the best way to warm up thoroughly.

Coffee enemas are recommended during a mono diet to assist the cleansing process. Again, appropriate supervision is highly desirable. The more thorough you are, the better, but never overlook the need to keep within your physiological and psychological limits.

Challenge Yourself by Reintroducing Foods Slowly

Following a mono diet, the way to reintroduce foods is important. You can just go back to eating as before and hope your sensitivity can manage the variety. While this is an option, it is not so effective. To be thorough, to really give yourself the best way of fine-tuning your diet, it makes sense to reintroduce foods individually.

This process is quite similar to the elimination diets used in mainstream food sensitivity and allergy testing. There, where people are suspected of adverse food reactions, they are put on very bland low-allergy diets from three to fourteen days. This is how long it can take for reactive foods to clear the body. Then foods are reintroduced one by one—the "challenge."

If you have the motivation, the energy, the time and the support to do this it is highly rewarding.

So, in warm weather, after the transition on grapes or fruit, begin by starting with other fruits. At first stick to the one new fruit at each meal. It only takes a few days to try each of the fruits, and then go on to add the salad vegetables. Then add grains and other things until a total spectrum emerges.

In cold weather, after a rice transition, add in steamed or baked vegetables first, other grains, then raw vegetables followed by fruits. Follow the scale of cooked grains, cooked vegetables, raw vegetables, cooked fruit, and raw fruit. Steadily test all the elements of the Healing Diet. Soon a daily program will emerge.

An important tip here is that chewing our food really well enhances our sensitivity to its suitability. When we do take the time to chew food to a really fine, watery consistency, it does seem to make it easier to have the inner knowing of whether it is good for us or not. Try this, you may be surprised how helpful it can be.

Then what one does is to continue to be aware of the foods you eat and any changes in your situation. Maybe for a while you feel the need to eat lots of carrots and go off eggplant altogether. Then broccoli seems really attractive, or beetroot. As you pay more attention to your body and respect its needs, this way of eating becomes more and more natural, effortless and effective.

Speaking Personally

As I came off the Gerson Therapy I experienced a range of sensitivities. I only had to look at eggplant to know it did not suit me. Then I noticed an even stronger reaction to raw onions and avoided them completely. However, once cooked, the aromatic acids in onions are altered and I could eat the cooked form happily. With hens' eggs I experienced a powerful physical reaction—I became liverish and sometimes even showed signs of jaundice, and also my state of mind was affected and I became quite grumpy and felt miserable. Cow's milk was tricky as I quite liked it, but I had to notice every time I ate any dairy products I experienced an inflammatory reaction that usually centered on my throat, so I was better off not eating it. Of course there are good theoretical reasons to avoid cow's milk anyway.

So perhaps my own experience helps to demonstrate how our personal awareness and sensitivity to what we eat can develop.

Recommendation

Seriously consider taking the time and effort to follow the mono diet for ten days and then gradually reintroduce individual foods and test your sensitivity. The reward is you will know what is good for you and what is not, and you will have a very personalized diet that will be well suited for recovery.

THE HEALING DIET, OPTION 2: THE RAPID METHOD

This is simple. You begin with step 6, the detox and then follow through with steps 2–5 as above.

For most people, establishing the Healing Diet first using steps 1–5 in the gradual method is very manageable. Maybe after several weeks, once you have become familiar with the basic Healing Diet, then it makes sense to fine-tune and personalize the diet by using the mono diet and food testing.

Certainly it is wise now to make a plan and consciously seek the foods and the support you need to put your plan into action.

Sample Menus

These are very broad guidelines intended as examples only.

Wellness Diet

The juices are optional, depending on your situation and preferences.

Summer	Spring/Autumn	Winter
On Arising		
Glass of lemon juice (1/3 lemon juice, 2/3 water)	Glass of lemon juice	Orange juice
Breakfast		
Unlimited amount of one fruit, (e.g., watermelon, cantaloupe)	One or more well combined fruits plus 2 tablespoons yogurt and 10–20 almonds, maybe dried fruit like currants or sultanas	Hot porridge—any combination of rolled oats, rye, buckwheat, millet, rice, barley, triticale, (possibly wheat) or homemade muesli
	1–2 pieces toast with natural jam	**PLUS**
		2 tablespoons yogurt, 10–20 almonds, 1 tablespoon currants or sultanas, 1 stewed apple or equivalent
		1–2 pieces toast with natural, sugarless jam
		Cup herb tea
Mid Morning		
Piece of fruit	Piece of fruit	Piece of fruit
+/- almonds	+/- almonds	+/- almonds
+/- juice	+/- juice	+/- juice
Midday		
2 salad sandwiches with 4–6 vegetables and sprouts	2 salad sandwiches with 4–6 vegetables and sprouts	Soup—miso or vegetable broth
		Salad of 4–6 vegetables with bean spread
And kelp powder	And kelp powder	+ /-bread
Mid Afternoon		
Juice	Dandelion coffee	Dandelion coffee
	+/- whole-meal cookie or cake	+/- whole-meal cookie or cake

	Summer	Spring/Autumn	Winter
Evening			
	Juice	Juice	Juice
	Salad of 4–6 vegetables and sprouts, and sea vegetables (e.g., nori and tofu or beans or a hot meal)	Side salad of 3–4 vegetables and sprouts, followed by dry-baked veggies and rice or pasta dish	Hot meal (e.g., 50–50 steamed vegetables, plus tofu and rice, or whole-meal pasta and veg/tofu sauce, or veg pie and rice)
			Use your flair! Be creative!
Before Bed			
	Juice	Juice	Herb tea
May substitute herb teas or equivalent for juices.			

Warm-Weather Healing Diet

AM	
7:00	Arise
	1 tablespoon lemon juice in lukewarm water
7:10	Breathing exercises (e.g., yoga or chi gong)—preferably barefooted on grass (glasses removed if normally worn)
7:30	Breakfast: fruit
	Any one fruit—I frequently used watermelon or fruit salad with appropriate combinations.
8:15	Meditate. Ideally, one hour.
9:15	Juice. Then, exercise in open (e.g., walking for 30 minutes). Smile!
10:30	Juice or piece of fruit or almonds plus herb tea
	Then meditate, ideally one hour before lunch.
PM	
12:00	Juice
	Then prepare lunch.
12:30	Lunch. Salad featuring 4–6 salad vegetables, or as a sandwich, or with a rice/pasta salad, almonds, sprouts.
1:15	Exercise, gardening, reading, free time
3:00	Juice
	Then free time
4:15	Breathing exercises (e.g., yoga or chi gong)—check you are still smiling (optional if done in the morning)!
4:30	Meditate. Ideally, one hour.
5:30	Juice
	Then prepare dinner.
6:00	Dinner. 4–6 salad vegetables, plus rice, pasta or baked potatoes, sprouts.
Before bed	Juice or herb tea
	Physically relax in bed and go to sleep with a prayer and/or a positive thought.
	Jump out of bed the next morning feeling that little bit better!

Cold-Weather Healing Diet

The same basic program is used but extra cooked food is included with an emphasis on rice. Half the evening meal can be rice, the rest steamed or baked vegetables. Breakfast for the first week can be porridge, for the second week fruit, third week porridge, and fourth week fruit again.

Recipes

To repeat, the best available recipe book to begin with is the *New Gawler Foundation Cookbook* and the recipes in it will fit nicely into the programs set out above.

A FINAL WORD ON DIET

I have always enjoyed ice cream and gelato. You could almost say that when I was young, I was addicted. I am just about cured of ice cream as it has so many additives, but I still do delight in gelato. I am happy to indulge in something that pleases me.

There was a time when I felt I was so ill that I needed to concentrate 100 percent on everything that I ate. I did not have ice cream or gelato for over two years. Now I seek out natural ice cream, or preferably gelato. I recognized that it is probably full of sugar, and perhaps other things that are short of ideal.

I know, however, that the way I eat at home is close to what I regard as ideal. We have a large organic vegetable garden and orchard. The bulk of what I do eat is homegrown or bought having been organically or biodynamically grown.

I know that what you are wise to eat when you are well really is different compared to when you have active illness. When you are well, it is what you eat "mostly" that is important. Eat well most of the time and the occasional gelato is fine! When you are dealing with major illness though, what you eat all the time is important. So now that I have been so well for so long, I feel well blessed, and as I savor my gelato, I give thanks for its wonderful taste and swallow it with a smile.

Wellness Rule 25: In your own mind, be clear about what you will eat when, and enjoy doing it! Use the three principles of positive thinking with your nutrition.

Set Clear Goals

On the Wellness Diet, be clear about your boundaries. Be clear about what you will eat when; when you are at home, when you are out, when there is a special occasion. Remember, when you are well, it is what you eat mostly that is important.

On the Healing Diet, be clear about what you will eat when. Remember, when you are eating for recovery, what you eat all the time is important.

Do Whatever It Takes

Ensure you have a collection of tasty recipes that convert your choices into delightful meals.

Choose to Enjoy Doing It

Bon appétit!

CHAPTER 15

The Causes of Cancer

It Is All in the Mind—Or Is It?

WHILE NUTRITION AND FOOD ARE OFTEN PROMINENT IN THEIR THOUGHTS, ask most people diagnosed with cancer the question that first went through their mind after they accepted their diagnosis and you are highly likely to receive a common answer:

"Why me? Why did it happen to me? Why have I got this thing?"

The question is always there. Sometimes it is voiced out loud with anger. Often it remains inside, unexpressed but smoldering with an attendant sense of injustice.

This response is understandable, for there is a popular misconception that the causes of cancer are not known. Therefore those who are diagnosed frequently feel as if they are the victims of a random, vindictive fate. Invariably they find themselves looking around and making comparisons.

"Why not him? Why not old George down the road? He smokes like a chimney, drinks like a fish. Never got a kind word for anyone, never helps anyone; but there he is, eighty years old and still going. Well, I mean I know that I'm no saint, but I sure have been trying to do my best all these years. Why *me*?"

Those who are brave enough to express this vital question out loud to their doctors or friends often hear in response: "I am sorry, we don't really know the causes of cancer." Or, worse still, they are told: "It's just one of those things. Bad luck, I suppose."

IS IT BAD LUCK OR DOES IT HAVE A CAUSE?

Bad luck! Can something as serious as cancer be just "bad luck"? The whole of the universe as we know it is governed by laws. A fundamental one is that for every action there is an equal and opposite reaction. Everything in the physical world is ruled by this law of cause and effect. The investigative skills of modern technology probe from the smallest atoms to the largest stars and find no exceptions. Can man, the central figure in our universe, be excluded from a similar governing law? Can cancer really be the product of mere chance?

If the causes of cancer are not identified, then cancer patients are hapless victims of external influences beyond their control. People who feel this to be the case inevitably regard themselves as victims. Such victim-consciousness is probably the most negative emotion in which we can indulge. It allows us to feel as if we had no part in the development of the disease itself, as if the disease just happened and we had nothing to do with it.

Worse, it leaves us feeling helpless, powerless to resist an external force that we can neither understand nor deal with.

To call yourself a "cancer victim," or to be described as one, conjures up all the worst negative images associated with cancer. Those words, "cancer victim," must be avoided totally. "Cancer" itself is not a dirty word and we need to feel free to use it. "Cancer patient" is fine. Being a patient—someone undergoing treatment—is fine. In another sense, being patient and showing patience, the calm endurance of a situation with attendant perseverance, is a fine attribute. Being a "victim" is totally inappropriate. Perhaps you would rather be described as a "person with cancer" or a "person living with cancer." I was quite content to be a "cancer patient" although these days being someone who "had cancer" is even better!

However, the exciting fact is that there is no reason for using the word "victim." Most of the causes of cancer can now be identified.

For years it seems as if everyone has been looking for the one cause: the one agent, the one food, one chemical, one virus. One anything! Just let there be one thing to blame for the whole problem. It is now obvious that it is not so simple. Cancer has many contributing factors.

This is the exciting fact. If we are prepared to broaden our horizons and take account of the full spectrum of possibilities we can understand the nature of cancer. There are many factors, not just one, which are involved in producing those final physical symptoms we describe as cancer.

To understand the causes of cancer we must explore our physical, emotional, mental and spiritual realms. Not one factor, but many, combine to produce cancer.

CANCER IS A CHRONIC, MULTIFACTORIAL, DEGENERATIVE DISEASE

Like the camel's back, the body must be laboring under the weight of many burdens before one final straw can break it and allow cancer to develop. This is probably the best news that people diagnosed with cancer can have. For once the causes of the problem can be identified, it makes it so much easier to take the appropriate action to rectify the situation. If we remove the causes, lift the load off that broken back, then we have gone a long way toward creating a healing environment. It may be challenging but it can be done. Virtually all the known causes can be remedied.

Cancer is a dynamic process. It is responsive to the influences acting upon it. It is not a one-way, downhill street. It has causes, and those causes produce effects. Remove the disease-producing causes and replace them with health-promoting influences, and recovery is under way.

It is as if there were a set of scales with influences that create health and influences that create disease hanging in the balance. When one side prevails—health results; when the other is down—disease. Once the disease scale is down with cancer, it requires an intense effort to tip the balance again. Attending to the sheer physical realities can often require top priority. But by understanding the disease process we can set about a rational self-help program based upon removing the cancer-producing causes and replacing them with health-promoting factors.

THE KNOWN CAUSES OF CANCER

The starting point is recognizing that there is such a process involved, and understanding what set it in motion. Professor Gabriel Kune, one of the world's leading authorities on the causes of cancer claims that nine out of ten cancers are due to noninherited causes—or, in other words, only 10 percent of cancers are related to inherited factors. This may be in conflict with what many people assume or fear, but it is thoroughly confirmed by modern research. What also comes from the research is the clear fact that the majority of the known causes of cancer relate to lifestyle issues. Kune's book, *The Home Health Guide to a Cancer-Free Family*,[23] is an excellent and readable resource for anyone wanting more detail on the known causes and how they relate to particular cancer types.

Professors Sir Richard Doll and Sir Richard Peto were two of the earliest and most highly respected investigators of the physical causes of cancer. Their research, published in *The Causes of Cancer*,[24] established that it is reasonable to attribute the causes of cancer (excluding cancers of the skin) as follows:

- 35 percent to dietary factors
- 30 percent to smoking nicotine
- 10 percent to infections
- 4 percent to occupational hazards
- 3 percent to alcohol
- 3 percent to geophysical factors
- 2 percent to pollution
- 1 percent to medicines and medical procedures

Less than 1 percent of all cancers are attributable to each of food additives and industrial products.

Doll and Peto's research is now over thirty years old and their figures have been confirmed by many more studies. The one major new causative factor that has been identified and needs to be highlighted is the lack of sunlight and vitamin D. In Europe these days, it has been estimated that around 30 percent of all new breast cancer cases in women are directly linked to lack of sunlight and its related vitamin D. This deficiency has also been associated with an increased risk of colorectal, prostate and pancreatic cancers.

STATISTICS AND INDIVIDUALS

What these statistics mean is that if there were one hundred cancer patients in a random group, we could expect thirty-five of them to be the products of an inappropriate diet. However, exactly which thirty-five may be difficult to determine. Being more specific, we do know that a high-fat diet is associated with an increased risk of breast cancer. But for an individual woman who does happen to have breast cancer, it is not so easy to say her breast cancer was caused just by a high-fat diet, even if she happened to have been on one.

The high-fat diet is just one identifiable, and of course very easily rectifiable, factor. However, that particular woman may also have been eating a lot of other "junk" food, drinking alcohol, been emotionally uptight, financially insecure and so on. The high-fat diet may have been the final "straw" that precipitated her breast cancer. For another woman with the same background burden of risk factors, but without a high-fat diet, being a smoker may have been the final straw, or "trigger factor," that meant she developed lung cancer instead of breast cancer.

RISK FACTORS ARE OFTEN SYNERGISTIC

Another significant issue we need to be aware of is that many physical factors known to cause cancer interact with each other and in combination produce greatly increased risk factors. This is amply demonstrated by the research on smoking tobacco. Someone who smokes 30 grams of tobacco or more per day has about eight times the risk of esophageal cancer compared to someone who does not smoke. Drinking 40–80 grams of alcohol per day results in seven times the risk of esophageal cancer compared with someone who does not. Now if a person does both, what is their risk? Eight plus seven, or fifteen times greater? Unequivocally no! The evidence is clear-cut. The two risks do not simply add together—they are synergistic—the effect is more like multiplication. The combined risk of smoking and drinking together, at that level, is put at thirty-six times that of doing neither.

Similarly, asbestos workers who smoke are diagnosed with ten times more asbestosis when compared with those who do not. Cigarette smokers in the cities have twice the lung cancer of their country counterparts. What extra synergistic factors are involved here? Pollution? Stress?

The basic contention is that cancer is a chronic, multifactorial, degenerative disease. The causes of cancer are often subtle, usually multiple, frequently synergistic and generally build up over a long period! So a person may have a "background" of low-level cancer risk factors that are present in the way they live their life over many years. Then there may be the one more obvious, more identifiable trigger factor, like the high-fat diet or the smoking, which is like the final straw that actually precipitates the specific type of cancer.

But there is still more to all of this.

THE SYMPTOMS AND THE DISEASE

The end point of cancer, and the physical symptoms that go with it, is not so subtle. Once it becomes apparent, cancer is generally very obvious and often acute. Some cancers, once they do appear, are very fast moving and potentially life threatening. Faced with this crisis, the temptation is to regard cancer as a purely physical problem, to focus on treating the symptoms and to overlook or neglect the underlying disease and its collection of causes. While this is understandable, it makes no sense to continue to smoke or to continue to eat badly if those things have contributed to the cancer's onset. At the very least, by adopting a healthy lifestyle we remove a large part of the burden of the cause—but also, by doing so we are creating the basis for recovery.

NOT ALL SMOKERS GET CANCER • What Else Is Going On?

We all know the "old George" type who smokes and drinks and does not get cancer. It seems fairly obvious that just one trigger factor, such as being a smoker, or having a high-fat diet, is not enough on its own to account for the great majority of cancers. Even the cumulative and synergistic effects of the known physical factors do not explain them all. Also, we need to go beyond the "Why me?" question to "Why now?" Why has the cancer developed at this particular point in my life? Why now?

Now we need to go beyond the obvious physical risk factors and take account of the possible role of the psychological and even spiritual aspects of life. While it may be that some people do have a poor diet as a major precipitating factor, others may have a large psychological component; for others, conflict in their spiritual life may be a real issue. We need to consider other possibilities.

Do not despair! The more causes we identify, the more we can do to overcome them by taking appropriate action. Cancer is a dynamic process. When we replace destructive tendencies with constructive ones, we immediately begin to tip the scales back toward health.

THE CANCER-PRONE PERSONALITY

In my experience, psychological factors are important in the causation of most cancers. There is a typical psychological profile that occurs in more than 95 percent of the many thousands of people affected by cancer with whom I have discussed their disease. This profile, this cancer-prone personality, was first expounded by Dr. E. Evans in 1926! It has gained increasing attention over the last few years, especially through the work of Dr. Lawrence Le Shan,[25] as well as Dr. Ainslie Meares, Dr. Carl Simonton and Stephanie Matthews,[26] and Dr. Lydia Temoshok.[27]

This increase in attention is important for if the psychological factors are identified and treated appropriately, then a major driving force that has been keeping the cancer going is immediately removed.

Most people diagnosed with cancer recognize this psychological profile. For some it comes as a shock to hear their basic life history so accurately recounted.

HOW THE CANCER-PRONE PERSONALITY DEVELOPS

Childhood Stress

In childhood, a cluster of stresses build up over a period of time. The stresses often relate to the child's interaction with their parents or peers, the prime influences acting in their life at this time. The key component of this stress is that there is a sense of a lack of approval from the important people in their lives. They feel unappreciated, or more specifically, unloved for what they do, for who they are.

This stress may come from parents and others who are downright physically or emotionally violent, or more subtly from those who are actually quite loving but emotionally nonexpressive or even abusive in ways they do not realize. The end result is that the child begins to feel they have little worth because they are receiving little encouragement in their endeavors, or because they are not feeling adequately loved. Their self-esteem suffers and they become increasingly concerned by what they believe other people think of them.

Climactic Event

Next, usually around seven to nine years of age, there comes a major traumatic incident which, again, is like the final straw that breaks the camel's back—its psychological back. This event seems almost unbearable, and through it, the feelings of lack of self-worth, lack of self-respect, lack of self-love threaten to become overwhelming. They know that they cannot endure this type of stress anymore. The child cries, "Enough." Something has to give. They need to find a new way of relating to their world, a new way of coping. No longer can the child react in a free, uncomplicated manner.

Premeditated Pattern of Behavior

Now interestingly, the cancer-prone personality types do not become aggressive, rebellious or difficult at this point. Quite the opposite. They determine that the way out, the way back to feeling good about themselves, is to win back the love, to win back the approval. So while something does snap inside and the emotional shutters go down, they determine to become "nice," successful, likable people. They decide to adopt a rigid pattern of behavior in response to stress. They begin to actively focus on pleasing other people and winning their approval. By doing so their stress becomes manageable; life becomes tolerable again.

The key point here is that in the cancer-prone personality this rigid pattern of behavior revolves around attempting to be as other people want them to be, rather than as they personally feel they should be. This commonly leads to trying to please other people, to doing what others would want them to. There is often an overtone of passive subservience. The cancer-prone personality types are not the ones to become outwardly aggressive or antisocial. Maybe they become manipulative, but they want to be liked. They seek approval.

So cancer patients are frequently "nice people." When diagnosed, their friends often say, "Why her? She's so nice, always trying to help other people. How awful this has happened to her. Why her? Why not that old creep George down the road?"

The fact is, of course, that trying to please other people is a fine ideal. It is the motivation behind it, however, that creates problems for the people who develop cancer. For them, this begins as a conscious means of coping, a defense mechanism, not a pure motivation. It is taken up as a premeditated defense mechanism and means they become reliant on factors outside of themselves, outside of their control, for their fundamental happiness and their sense of self-worth. This personality type relies on external approval.

Rigid Response Becomes Automatic

This conscious effort as a child to be a particular type of person is soon repeated so often that it becomes an automatic response. Now all stress is handled in the same basic, rigid way.

As this involves putting other people first, this pattern works well and these people are liked and usually successful. They frequently seek out positions where they can gain their gratification through the approval of others. It is not easy for them to do things based simply on their merits and to be satisfied by them. They find it difficult to develop a good self-image, and frequently rely on the approval of others for their own self-esteem. This need for outside approval is very real, if not always consciously expressed. Outwardly, their rigid pattern of behavior can produce a confident and assured air, but all the time they are seeking to cover this lack of self-esteem. Deep down, there can lurk a marked lack of self-confidence with a tendency toward self-negation, almost self-destruction. Deeply bottled inside is the feeling that all is not well. True reactions, emotions especially, are often suppressed. There is a continual effort to block out basic feelings. It is like trying to push the truth from the conscious awareness, like trying to keep the lid on a constantly bubbling pressure cooker.

Inner tension is established and maintained. There is a limited range of responses possible when it comes to dealing with stress.

Another Major Climactic Stress

In later life, another cluster of stresses is followed by one major event that changes the person's whole life circumstances. For example, we see this happening with people who have put all their emotional security into one relationship. Then if that relationship fails through death or separation, the sense of loss can be profound indeed. This can involve relationships with parents, lovers, spouses—or even with a devoted mother whose children leave home. The same effect can occur when a "workaholic" retires or is put out of work. Suddenly there is no outlet. Their whole life pattern is upset.

Financial difficulties followed by a foreclosure may be enough to tip the balance for some people. Betrayal by a partner at work has been the precipitated factor for many in business.

Inability to Cope

This change in life circumstances threatens the person's very source of self-worth and purpose. There seems to be no way their rigid pattern of behavior can deal with it. Their very life has been undermined. The person feels to be a victim of circumstances beyond their control and they can see no answer to this new situation. They feel as if life has dealt them a bitter blow, often one they half expected to occur. Life no longer has any meaning for them. Because they do not feel they can change their way of coping, they can see no viable future.

Feelings of Hopelessness and Helplessness

Faced with an unsolvable problem, an underlying feeling of hopelessness develops. But there is even more to this. People with a cancer-prone personality have a strong need to be liked, to gain approval. So faced with what they perceive to be a hopeless situation, they are also helpless. They feel bound to appear well and cheery. Becoming angry, or even sad or grief-stricken has the perceived potential to upset the family or friends.

So on the outside, their rigid pattern of behavior keeps these people going. Often they carry on with their rigid, cheery, helpful front. They are often unable to express their loss, their feelings of hopelessness and helplessness and outsiders often remark how well they seem to be coping, how little they have changed, despite their adversity.

The Body Mirrors the Hopelessness

However, potentially, this style of coping comes with a high cost. The inner sense of hopelessness is soon mirrored by the body itself. It is as if the body, too, gives up. It is as if the body also loses the will to live, it loses the ability to defend itself. The effect is a significant drop in the effectiveness of the body's own physical defenses, the immune system.

Again, this concept ties in so well with the idea that cancer involves a basic fault in the body's own natural function. It is as if this stress is so major that the body is laid open to having a self-destructive disease like cancer to develop.

Another straw, another major cause, becomes apparent.

In my experience most people diagnosed with cancer can observe this scenario in their life. Most recognized a climactic stressful event three months to two years before their symptoms first appeared. The most common interval by far for the people that I have worked with has been around eighteen months. It is as if it takes this long for the body to produce the external symptoms of that internal state.

The key factor here, the key problem, is the long-held pattern of coping with major stress in a particular, rigid way. It is important to realize this fact because, as we know, most people during their lives will be confronted by events involving major stress. These stresses are an inevitable part of life. However, not everyone who experiences major stress has a cancer-prone personality. Clearly, not everyone who experiences major stress will develop cancer. Those who do develop cancer tend to respond to stress in a common but very particular way. So next we will review stress itself, then reexamine what we can do to reverse it.

QUANTIFYING STRESS

Dr. Richard Rahe has done interesting work quantifying the effects of life-changing stress on our lives. Initially with the help of his colleague, Thomas Holmes, Rahe developed a Social Readjustment Rating Scale that placed a relative figure on a range of potentially stressful events. First published in 1965, the scale has been reevaluated and updated in 1977 and 1995.[28]

Back in 1965, Holmes and Rahe identified loss of a spouse as being the event having the highest potential for stress. They rated it as 100 Life Change Units (LCU), and then identified a range of other events that might occur in our lives with potentially stressful consequences. Importantly, events we may perceive as "positive" such as marriage or retirement, figure prominently—as do the obvious "negatives."

When you study the Life Changes Scaling Across Time chart, you realize that the relative impact of some stresses has changed over time. However, overall, the general impact of stress using this assessment is calculated to have risen 43 percent in the years from 1965 to 1995. This validates what many people are feeling—life is becoming more stressful. Who is not in need of learning to cope more effectively so that stress affects us less? No wonder meditation has such wide appeal!

The chart can be used to assess the total amount of stressful events you may have experienced in a given year. Identify the events, add the 1995 LCU score (see the following table) and check your total! A score of more than 300 from the table in any one year produces a 40 percent change of developing illness, while a score of fewer than 200 produces less than 10 percent of risk. This demonstrates the direct link between stress and illness: the more stress, the more illness produced.

HOW WE REACT TO STRESS IS THE ISSUE

The emphasis with all these factors is the changes they produce in our life circumstances. What is at issue is the ability to adapt to change—and for people with cancer, the particular way they go about doing it.

The fact is that many of us do seek to preserve the status quo and do find change a hard thing to manage. However, when it is unavoidable, most people do manage to pass through challenging periods of change and while they may be stressed for a while, life goes on. While more significant or dramatic clusters of stress may produce more of a setback, even some level of related physical disease, most people still do manage to bounce back and do not develop cancer. Many people have their own ways of coping or find new ones, and are able to adapt to new circumstances. They do not feel hopeless for any lasting period.

For those who do go on to develop cancer, it would seem it is not so much the nature of the challenge that is the problem, but their rather rigid pattern of reacting to it. This is most important. Everyone is subjected to challenge. Everyone is likely to be faced with some major life-changing events during their lifetime. Whether it be the death of a loved one, the need to change jobs, a move to a new city, whatever, such events are inevitable. Certainly many of the lesser challenges in our lives actually give it zest and flavor. Many challenges work to extend and develop us, and life would be pretty dull without them.

Life Changes Scaling Across Time (1965–1995)

Life Events	1965		1977		1995	
	Rank	LCU	Rank	LCU	Rank	LCU
Death of spouse	1	100	1	103	1	119
Divorce	2	73	4	62	2	98
Marital separation	3	65	8	52	4	79
Jail term	4	63	6	57	7	73
Death of close family member	5	63	2	73	3	92
Major personal injury or illness	6	53	16	42	6	77
Marriage	7	50	10	50	19	50
Fired from work	8	47	3	64	5	79
Marital reconciliation	9	43	17	42	13	57
Retirement	10	43	11	49	16	54
Change in health/behavior of family member	11	44	9	52	14	36
Pregnancy	12	40	5	60	9	66
Sexual difficulties	13	39	12	49	21	45
Gain of new family member	14	39	14	47	12	57
Major business readjustment	15	39	21	38	10	62
Change in financial state	16	38	16	48	15	36
Death of close friend	17	37	15	46	8	70
Change to different line of work	18	36	22	38	17	31
Change in number of arguments with spouse	19	35	24	34	18	51
Mortgage or loan greater than $10,000	20	31	18	39	23	44
Foreclosure on a mortgage or loan	21	30	7	57	11	61
Change in responsibilities at work	22	29	32	30	24	43
Child leaving home	23	29	36	29	22	44
Trouble with in-laws	24	28	25	33	29	37
Outstanding personal achievement	25	28	25	33	29	37
Spouse begins or ends work	26	26	23	37	20	46
Begin or end school	27	26	28	32	27	38
Change in living conditions	28	25	19	39	25	42
Change in personal habits	29	24	30	31	36	27
Trouble with boss	30	23	20	39	33	29
Change in work hours or conditions	31	20	27	33	30	36
Change in residence	32	20	26	33	26	41

Life Events	1965		1977		1995	
	Rank	LCU	Rank	LCU	Rank	LCU
Change in schools	33	20	39	28	31	35
Change in recreation	34	19	33	30	34	29
Change in church activities	35	19	35	29	42	22
Chance in social activities	36	18	40	28	38	27
Mortgage or loan less than $10,000	37	17	42	26	35	28
Change in sleeping habits	38	16	31	31	40	26
Change in number of family get-togethers	39	13	41	26	39	26
Change in eating habits	40	15	38	29	37	27
Vacation	41	13	37	29	41	25
Christmas	42	12	*	*	32	30
Minor violations of the law	43	11	29	32	43	22
Mean LCU value for all events	–	34.5	–	42	–	49

Note: LCU—Life Change Unit

The problem for many people who develop cancer is this inability to cope with a major challenge, particularly when it involves a fundamental change in their life. The inability to react appropriately and find release from the situation produces the changes in body chemistry we know as stress. This in turn affects the body's metabolism and lowers the immune system, so adding a significant factor to the list of causes of cancer. The more I talk with individual patients and groups, the more I am convinced of the importance of this factor.

Being able to recognize this in their nature is a great asset for a cancer patient. By accepting that this did contribute to their situation, they can make a great deal more sense of it. It is then relatively simple, in principle at least, to learn to cope with these psychological aspects of stress. By dealing with it appropriately, patients can contribute greatly to their own well-being and return to health. We shall explore in more detail the means available to do this in the next chapter.

WHY ME? THE SPIRITUAL QUESTION

Finally, however, having considered the physical and psychological causes of cancer, we need to go one step further. We need to be brave enough to ask, "Why me?" once more.

Why do some people have this cancer profile, and not others? Why do only some people find themselves in those complex childhood situations that lead on to particular attitudes and a pattern of behavior that, in turn, predisposes them to cancer? Why are some people drawn to smoke, to eat potentially harmful foods, to work in dangerous environments and, as a consequence, be faced with disease?

Unless we can answer these harder questions, we will remain unsatisfied and still be tempted to wallow in victim consciousness. Again, is it just chance that these circumstances develop? Surely not! We are now faced with a basic philosophical question that must be tackled.

A PERSONAL ACCOUNT

I consider myself fortunate. Right from the time my cancer was first diagnosed, I recognized that there was a spiritual thread running through and connecting all the events in my life. Moreover, prior to the cancer, I felt that I had been living with disharmony between my inner spiritual attitudes and my outer physical actions. There was conflict between what I felt I should do and what I actually did.

Basically as a young and rather impecunious veterinarian, I had put my interest in spiritual matters on hold while I focused on making money and establishing myself in the material world. While I was not doing anything illegal or dishonest and while I was actually working very hard, I felt I was not being true to my own inner aspirations. I felt that this disharmony was another major factor in the development of my cancer.

Now, clearly I am not suggesting this existential problem I held inside by focusing on making money was the sole cause of my cancer. I did have a type C personality, I did have major issues courtesy of my diet and so on. However, I am confident this more deep-seated, more spiritual dilemma was a significant cause—for me. More important, recognizing this problem provided me with a basic stimulus and raison d'être for seeking harmony in my spiritual, psychological and physical nature. I saw the three as interwoven and interdependent. Because I could see the interrelatedness of my past actions and present circumstances, I felt confident that justice would prevail. If I could make the necessary changes and find the right techniques, health may well be reattainable.

Now it is relatively easy to talk of psychological and physical things. These issues are relatively straightforward and not too emotionally charged. It is not so easy with things spiritual. However, knowing the important stimulus it was to me and having seen so many others gain strength and direction from their own spiritual endeavor, I feel it appropriate to delve into these deeper areas.

I hesitate for one moment as I do not want to be simplistically and unhelpfully labeled, nor do I want to run the risk of having good, straight-forward techniques like meditation labeled. All these techniques do stand independently in their own right and are quite free of spiritual bias. They can all be judged on their own merits.

At the same time, I feel that any life is rather facile without some spiritual loading. Most people diagnosed with cancer are interested—in fact, they are often preoccupied—with the quest for answers to spiritual questions. Many people do flavor their life with spiritual concerns and it is appropriate to rec-ognize this. Being raised as a Christian in the Anglican Church, I grew up with an earnest desire to know the Truth. There was an ever-present feeling that behind the mysteries of life, beyond the basic teachings of religion, lay a profound, unshakable Truth. Truth with a capital T.

In searching for this Truth, I have been deeply blessed to read many great books and by meeting and studying with many great spiritual masters from all traditions, particularly the Tibetan Buddhist Lama Sogyal Rinpoche who for many years has been my main teacher.

So while I continue to value greatly my Christian heritage, the answers I found that helped me through my illness, the answers that helped me to find more meaning and purpose in my life, were not limited to the orthodox Christian ones.

It seems worthwhile to present these views as a means of provoking dis-cussion in this vital area. It is for each of us to search out the meaning, to make sense of our own situations, our own lives.

So, why should any person be placed in that combination of conditions that eventually lead to cancer? While people do seem to learn best and develop most through adversity, is it really necessary to go through cancer? And why should young children get it? There must be some reason why.

There really is a clear-cut, basic choice to make at this point. There is either order or there is not. Either we have to say life is meaningless and harsh in the extreme as no loving God could allow such things, or we say there is some order, some reason for it, some logic behind it all. I confess to not being able to make sense of what I see happening around me just on face value. Why do some people get it easy, others apparently hard?

I have an undying faith in the basic structured order of the universe. There has to be an explanation. The only one that satisfies me is provided by the Eastern philosophy of karma and reincarnation, the spiritual laws of cause and effect. Karma is a concept that says every action we take produces consequences to match. As we sow, so we reap. Good action, good consequences and the opportunity to benefit by them; bad action, bad consequences and the need to face those consequences and learn to get it right.

We can certainly see this principle operating in current life circumstances. Most of our current situation is the product of events we can easily identify. But it is often difficult to see justice or order in all of our own life patterns and certainly it is easy to judge some others harshly. Some people seem to face impossibly difficult odds in life, while on the surface they appear blameless. Some appear to do terrible things and get away with them. I am drawn, therefore, to widen my frame of reference to include the concept of reincarnation, the notion that we have a series of lives, rather than just one. If we do pass from life to life and carry over basic traits and blemishes, it makes sense of many seemingly inexplicable events. The child genius, the congenital birth defects, the hopelessly poor, the uncaring rich, all assume explainable stations in life.

For me, these concepts provide a framework into which I can comfortably fit and feel confident working within. Regarding successive lifetimes as opportunities for spiritual evolution provides a reason to strive for ethical conduct in all situations. It also means that no effort is wasted. Every attempt we make to reach a greater degree of harmony in our lives will eventually bear fruit. Any effort, be it in the physical, psychological or spiritual realm, if made with a positive, harmonious motivation, will be to our benefit.

Recognizing this spiritual thread to life and its ongoing nature was a great comfort for me as I battled the odds. It helped me to understand my situation, even if I could not relate my present predicament to definite events of a previous lifetime. Also, it made me feel the efforts of attempting to get well were worthwhile. Death lost its sting as final arbitrator. If life went on and my attitudes and actions had effects on my future circumstances, it meant I would be sensible to give 100 percent in every situation. Anything more I could not do, but anything less would be totally inappropriate. Finally, I had to realize that I had to do my 100 percent and then be prepared to let the results take care of themselves. I had to learn the need to avoid being attached to the results of my actions and not to view them as win or lose situations.

Similarly, I came to recognize and accept that at the most fundamental level I was responsible for my own condition. It is relatively easy to accept our role in disease through our patterns of eating and thinking and the environment in which we live. I feel it even more satisfying to consider disease as an opportunity for spiritual growth through learning and endeavor. Our spirit has put us in this position to test our reactions and give us the opportunity to learn the lessons we need in a very intense way. We never get more than we have the potential to handle! Remember the people who say, "Cancer has taught me so much—much more than I could have learned without it."

THE CAUSE AND EFFECT OF RECOVERY

It is vital to recognize in all this that cancer is a dynamic situation. It is good to identify what causes you can in your own life, as then you can act, make changes and get well again. This thinking gives a rationale for a total approach for treatment.

On the physical level, the actual symptoms certainly need to be attended to. Appropriate, direct therapy must be considered for them. However, do not overlook the real possibility that the lumps and bumps are only symptoms. Do not forget to tackle the underlying causes. Again, on the physical level, it makes good sense at least to adopt the organic Wellness Diet or to be more thorough with the Healing Diet. It also makes sense to avoid any sources of pollution and to utilize any treatment that increases the body's natural defenses.

Psychologically, the big need is to change. If we recognize that a particular pattern has aided in creating the disease, then obviously a new pattern is required. Changing to that new pattern can be done through conscious action based on the desire to get better.

However, often it will just flow on as a result of the disease itself. The disease creates the excuse for change. It produces a new situation or insight that allows the patient the space to change their rigid patterns.

Hope is the key here. It may come from within with a change of attitude or be built by inspiration from without. Once that hope is revived, then the rebuilding process is under way. The attitude becomes positive and focused upon living well again. The sense of being a victim gives way to a feeling of being responsible and in control.

Many find that they no longer feel guilt about their past. Their new perspective sheds fresh light and allows them to seek forgiveness for errors of the past. Now they feel free to concentrate upon building a new future, to concentrate upon loving life and everything around them.

One step leads on to the next and the physical condition soon reflects this improvement. While there may be ups and downs, the healing process gathers momentum. Frequently, meditation takes the bumps out of this path. Having benefits on all levels of our being, it both smooths out and intensifies the healing.

For many people, the end result is a health that is described as "weller than well." Having recovered from such an illness, they have a new zest for life. Just getting well from cancer is cause enough for a boost in self-esteem. Add to this all that is learned along the way and people frequently portray a new confidence and a quiet but genuine regard for themselves and all around them. The joy they feel enhances their own lives and infuses joy into those with whom they come in contact. It is a process of self-discovery and self-fulfillment.

MOVING ON TO FIND SOLUTIONS

While considering the spiritual issues around disease and its causation may be somewhat esoteric for some, there can be no doubting the immediacy of the role played by our psychology and especially our emotions. Again to be clear, cancer is a chronic, multifactorial degenerative disease. So while I am not saying the psychological component is *the* cause of cancer, I am sure that it is another major contributing factor.

On the psychological level, the reality is that once the cancer is actually diagnosed, for many a seemingly hopeless situation will exist. However, what if the person diagnosed with cancer had previously lost the desire to live in the manner we discussed above, and now the diagnosis gives them the opportunity to not expect to live? A rather blunt friend, a fellow cancer patient, once described cancer as a socially acceptable form of suicide for people who found themselves in an intolerable position.

I can hear people yelling in protest, "It's not me! That's not me!" However, it is usually the families, not the patients, who protest most. Many patients recognize the sequence readily, are relieved to understand what is going on and are happy to set about correcting the situation.

To restate it, hope is the starting point. To re-create hope we need to bolster the desire to live and the expectation that a continuation of life is possible.

Now another curious fact. The desire or will to live can often be rekindled by the diagnosis itself! Having cancer can change a person's life dramatically and totally. Suddenly they become the center of attention. Friends and family rally, work may be avoided, a ready excuse is available for that long-put-off holiday, all manner of new possibilities present.

Some patients become very good at it—at being patients. While they may have a flourishing victim consciousness, under all the attention they rally. Life becomes enjoyable and worth living again, and the body responds to this new surge. Many then find new ways of coping and do get back to leading healthy lives again.

However, some do come to that difficult point where they are getting so well that their friends no longer call, the family returns to its own normal pursuits, and the need to work reemerges. A difficult choice: to be sick and happy, or well and miserable. This may well be funny if it was not real. It would be foolish to oversimplify the complexity of this problem, but very frequently psychological trauma is a major consideration for cancer patients.

A CRY FOR LOVE

The cry of anguish that creates disease is a cry for love. It is a genuine need that needs to be met. Love is the appropriate response and it works 100 percent every time.

In my experience, emotional factors do play a major role in cancer. People who are diagnosed with cancer are frequently emotionally tight. Many prefer to keep their emotions to themselves and they have difficulty in expressing them even if they want to. It has taken me years to feel comfortable telling people how I feel about them, particularly if I want to express my feelings of love.

When we recollect the stress response and the psychological profile involved in cancer, we see the challenge in that profile is frequently emotionally based. The fear that turns the challenge into a stress is usually one of not being loved, of being rejected, or of being emotionally hurt.

For cancer patients it is most frequently emotional challenges that produce the bodily reaction with its accompanying changes in body chemistry. For them, there often seems to be no adequate action they know of that can be taken to resolve their situation and so gain relief.

Emotional fear fixes them in a state of altered body chemistry. The contention is these biochemical changes can be so profound as to reduce their body's potential to heal and sustain itself in good health. Then, when a cancer begins—as might be prompted by a high-fat diet, cigarette smoking, some bodily malfunction, or whatever—the body no longer cares, it no longer recognizes it has a problem. It allows the cancer to develop and life-threatening symptoms can follow.

This being so, it is vital when we are seeking recovery from cancer to work on our emotions too—to "let go" emotionally, to heal the emotions as well as the body. Most people enjoy this part of it, once they get going! Everyone wants to feel love in their life and feel capable of giving it freely. So in the next chapter we consider the healing power of healthy emotions. How do we transform destructive emotions into healing emotions?

CHAPTER 16

Healthy Emotions 1

Feeling Well, Being Well

IT IS VERY USEFUL TO THINK ABOUT THE POWER OF THE MIND: TO ANALYZE, contemplate and plan how we train the mind; get the most out of its vast potential; use it as a key ally for healing.

By contrast, emotions need to be felt. And emotions have a powerful role in the healing process. So give yourself a moment or two to feel this.

If in the past you have felt resentment toward another person, or say you feel resentment for someone in current time, imagine you suddenly and unexpectedly meet that person.

Imagine they were in front of you now.

What happens in your body? Most people when face-to-face with resentment notice their muscles tighten up pretty quickly. Teeth clamp down harder; perhaps there is a grimace, the stomach contracts, maybe even fists clench and the arms draw close in to the body. Contact with the other person is avoided.

Now, maybe you have learned to mask all this, to sublimate the feelings and appear neutral from the outside. But if you go into the feeling, into the body, it is all about contracting, tightening, withdrawing. The feeling is of curling up or hunching over. The feeling is cold and hard and tight with a pervasive agitation.

What place has healing among that collection of feelings?

Now relax. Then bring to mind someone who delights you—maybe someone you have not seen for a while or someone whose company you really enjoy. Maybe you would say they love you, you love them. But now, just imagine meeting up with them again, suddenly and unexpectedly.

What happens in your body? Exuberance. Your arms probably go out and up. A smile breaks into happy laughter. If you were to check you would probably notice a feeling of gentle warmth and relaxation, maybe even a tingling in your body. Contact is welcomed. Maybe you hug, embrace, kiss.

What place has healing among that collection of feelings? Everything. While resentment almost feels like cancer itself, when it comes to the joy and delight of meeting an old friend, it is as if every cell in your body sings. That is a healthy emotion. That is a healing emotion.

THE STORY AND THE EMOTION

Now the crucial point. Emotions do not exist in their own right. You do not just feel angry, feel sad, feel joyful for no good reason. Emotions need to be produced by something and we can call that something "the story." So you feel angry because of the story relating to what he did. Or you feel sad because of the story relating to what happened in the past. Or you feel apprehensive based upon the story relating to what might happen in the future.

Simple is it not? There is "the story" and there is "the emotion." The emotion follows the story.

Of course, there is compelling logic in the way we link the emotion and the story. "Of course I am angry; let me tell you what he did." "Of course I am happy; let me tell you about my child's success." Etc., etc. But do you notice what it is like to be around someone who is miserable all the time? Complains all the time? Speaks badly of others all the time? Then remember what is it like to be around someone who recognizes the good in all they experience, who brings a sense of humor to all they do; a person who has warmth, compassion and love. Which person would you prefer to be with? If they were sick or needed help in any way, who would you be more likely to make time for?

So back to the crucial point. Just as we can decide how we will respond to our circumstances, we can decide to regulate our emotions. Now, if "regulating your emotions" sounds a little dry or calculating, or you have some other aversion to the notion, pause for a moment and consider the practical realities.

My old friend Jazzer comes to mind. Jazzer had a difficult form of leukemia many decades ago. He had chemotherapy off and on, actually more on than off, for over twelve years. These were in older times and Jazzer would vomit relentlessly and uncontrollably for hours and hours after each treatment. His reaction was so consistently bad he needed to be hospitalized for each treatment. Yet rather than develop an aversion, Jazzer welcomed the help he received. He would greet everyone in the hospital with genuine warmth, acknowledge even the smallest kindness, thank everyone for everything and, above all, use his natural humor to make light of his fairly extreme difficulties.

One of Jazzer's favorite ways of enduring the convulsive vomiting he was confronted with was to make his way to another ward in the hospital, get down on his hands and knees, and pretend he was a barking dog. Some probably thought he was barking mad, but we would crawl around on the floor, moving from bed to bed and alternating between making noises like a barking dog, making his involuntary noises associated with the dry retching, and pretending to lift his leg like a dog urinating on his fellow patients' beds. His smile and his manner was infectious and laughter accompanied his regular stunts.

Some will know of Dr. Patch Adams, another old friend who was portrayed by Robin Williams in the film *Patch*. Patch uses humor and clowning as a way to move past people's pain and into their hearts. A very skillful doctor and therapist, Patch is a living example of the healing power of laughter.

SCIENCE SUPPORTS HEALTHY EMOTIONS

In mentioning the medical profession again, let us consider another good reason why regulating our emotions makes good sense. There has been a great deal of research completed in recent years investigating how our emotions impact upon our health. The science is very clear. What commonly but perhaps unhelpfully are described as "negative" emotions generally weaken our health and well-being, they make us more prone to disease and adversely impact on our capacity to heal. Negative emotions are bad for us. No surprise there! Happily the converse is true—what we call "positive" emotions enhance our health and well-being, help to prevent disease and actively support our capacity to heal. Positive emotions are good for us, good for our recovery.

Now, what we do need to be very clear about is that our emotions are always valid. If you feel an emotion, it is real enough. So rather than describing our emotions as negative and positive, we will be kinder on ourselves and more accurate when we use the words destructive and constructive. Or life denying and life affirming. The real questions we need to address are: does a particular emotion harm or help you, and do you have the capacity to manage your emotions, particularly if you are intent on healing?

A quick answer comes with considering the scenario of living with yourself. Yes, if you were living with yourself, what would you be keen to change?

A more measured response comes by deliberately cultivating healthy emotions. Here is how:

FOUR TECHNIQUES THAT DEVELOP HEALTHY EMOTIONS

More good news. The answer to the last question, "Can I develop healthy emotions?" is a clear yes. Once you recognize the power of emotions and decide to cultivate healthy, healing emotions, there are four groups of potent yet straightforward techniques that will convert this intention into reality.

1. Meditation—has the natural power to release destructive emotions and foster the constructive ones.
2. General antidotes to destructive emotions—simple yet profound solutions for complex problems.
3. Specific antidotes to major destructive emotions—how to transform fear, shame, resentment, guilt and grief.
4. Techniques to cultivate constructive emotions—that are life affirming, healthy and healing.

We will consider the first two in this chapter; the other two in the next.

MEDITATION NATURALLY GENERATES HEALTHY, HEALING EMOTIONS

We have discussed this in some detail in the specific meditation chapters, but to recap:

When we meditate regularly and effectively, anger, resentment, depression, anxiety, fear, a whole range of unhelpful emotions simply falls away. At the same time, there is a natural rise in optimism, enthusiasm, joy and appreciation. It is natural for people who meditate to find themselves happier and more content, to be good humored and to smile more regularly and in a way that reflects a satisfaction that comes deep from within.

What meditation also does is to loosen up old habits, old states of mind. Therefore, against the background of regular meditation, the antidotes and the techniques to generate healthy, healing emotions become easier to work with.

GENERAL ANTIDOTES TO DESTRUCTIVE EMOTIONS

As with most things, there are a number of choices when it comes to managing emotions more effectively. None is better than the other per se; although the antidotes are a bit like treating the symptoms while the transformation gets at the cause. What makes sense is to consider the choices that follow and use whatever resonates with your own particular situation and needs.

The General Antidotes and the Transformation

CHANNELING THE ENERGY CONSTRUCTIVELY

Take anger as an example. There is a lot of energy in anger. The question is, how is that energy used? Many horrible things have resulted from uncontrolled and poorly directed anger. Many good things have been accomplished in the world when anger has motivated people to take strong, bold, decisive, and even prolonged action. Much that is good in social activism was inspired by anger.

Roger was caring for his wife, Beth, who had a series of difficulties associated with secondary bowel cancer. Their specialist seemed very despondent regarding Beth's case and was increasingly gruff and offhand in their meetings. Roger became increasingly agitated, increasingly angry.

Finally, with his wife complaining of pain and the doctor seeming intent on just getting them out of his office, Roger exploded.

"Look," he said, "we seem far more focused on trying to get my wife well than you are. How about you wake up to yourself and try to help us!"

Now the interesting thing is that this particular doctor had quite a good reputation for being caring, open-minded and a great communicator. To his credit, Roger's words had an electrifying effect upon him.

"I am so sorry," he said. "Please forgive me. I have been so busy, there is so much to do." Then he spent half an hour going over Beth's situation in detail and making sure her other needs, as well as her pain, were attended to.

What is important to note here is Roger channeled his anger wisely. He did not sit on it. He did not block it, he did not take it out on someone else. Also, he did not hit the doctor or abuse him! Very important. What he did was to use the energy of the anger to break through his natural reticence to speak up. He voiced the concerns he had for his wife and his dissatisfaction with the way she was being treated. And again, to his credit, the doctor took it in, realized his error, owned it, apologized and made good. As an addendum, Roger said they never had anything but the best of kind and attentive treatment throughout the time they saw that same doctor.

UNDERSTANDING HELPS

Part of what helps us to understand the difficulties people have with their emotions is to know where these difficulties come from. For example, in the cancer arena, we need to be aware that anger is a common reaction to grief. In Elisabeth Kübler Ross' classic description of the Five Stages of Grief,[29] denial comes first, anger second. Being aware that the diagnosis of cancer frequently triggers a grief reaction in patients, families and friends, we need to be on guard. Many unkind things have been said or done through anger, when actually grief was the real issue.

Jenny had six years cancer free after an initial diagnosis of breast cancer and a year of treatments. When it returned, her husband was dismayed by the way Jenny's attitude toward her teenage children changed. She began to find fault in every little thing they did or did not do. She withdrew from John, avoided contact, and yet several times John found her crying in their bedroom on her own. When asked what was wrong or if he could help, John was met with hostility and abruptly told to leave her alone.

Fortunately, John was helped to appreciate what Jenny was going through, to support her to express her anger with the relapse, and to begin to face her very natural fears of dying and leaving her family without a mother.

Supported by her husband's love and care Jenny began to be able to talk with others about her situation both in the support group where there was natural understanding, as well as with her closest friends where there was natural empathy, genuine care and love.

In my observation Jenny followed a common emotional path. Anger gave way to a lingering sadness that lay beneath a genuinely bright exterior. From time to time the sadness came out in tears or just the recognition of painful feelings. But the intensity, the heat of the early anger was gone and in the main, optimism, resolve and enjoyment of life filled Jenny's common experience. This seems natural and reasonable. Faced with a potentially life-threatening situation Jenny's disappointment and sadness makes sense. But if her emotions, coupled with fear, anger and resentment were to dominate her day, then she would both be having a miserable life and those emotions could well weaken her chances of recovery.

As it was, Jenny channeled a good deal of constructive energy into reinforcing her good nutritional and meditation habits. Given her relapse, she determined that her emotions were what needed the most attention, and focused on ways of resolving two significant, long-held resentments and becoming more loving with her family. Happily, she went into remission again and remains well.

RELEASING EMOTIONS SAFELY

People affected by cancer tend to bottle up their emotions. They feel them strongly enough, but they tend to keep them to themselves. We discussed some of the reasons for this when we addressed the cancer-prone personality type, and to repeat, blocked emotions are unhealthy emotions. For many of the people I have known who became long-term survivors, turning this around was pivotal to their success. They learned to be more open, more fluid, more authentic with their emotions.

Put simply, healthy emotions are authentic emotions. When emotions flow easily, comfortably, authentically, then health and well-being follow. Stifled emotions, repressed emotions and fabricated emotions all weaken the potential for healing as well as significantly reducing our sense of well-being. How then to change a deeply ingrained habit? How do we learn to release emotion safely?

The first thing is to recognize this is not so easy, but it can be done. This is an area where groups can play a particularly positive role. A good group leader creates what can be well described as a "safe place." Using a variety of techniques, it becomes increasingly obvious that the group is a place where people can express their emotions, be understood, be well "held"—as in supported and nurtured—and learn to be more at ease with being emotionally open.

Often it is among peers we learn best. So among other people going through similar experiences with cancer there is an inner knowing that binds the group. At first this goes unstated, but gently, as the more adventurous or "extroverted" speak up, what has been left silent, contained in silence, kept as secret, begins to be expressed.

CHANGING THE CHANNEL

This is a simple and effective technique for when a difficult emotion is really bugging you, but is not too strong. It is like turning the TV on and finding that what comes up first is unpleasant—maybe like a horror movie, and so you simply change the channels and watch something pleasant. This is a reliable method that aims to take your mind and your emotion away from something difficult and unpleasant to something comfortable and pleasant.

To change channels, all you need to do is choose to think of someone, something, or some event you enjoy. Or you could remember, reimagine your quiet place—that inner sanctuary which is reliably peaceful and calming (revisit chapter 10). This technique provides an easy short- to medium-term fix.

FEELING THE EMOTION AND DISSOLVING IT

For a longer-term solution this technique offers a wonderful possibility.

The theory is simple. The story resides in our head, the emotions are held in our body.

When we focus on the story, we continually rekindle old memories related to who said what, what happened when, and on and on. Focusing on the story can be like rerunning endless episodes of a classic soap opera where a few key players manage to recycle a never-ending list of problems. The more we dwell on the story, the more we fuel the emotions. When linked so directly to the thoughts in our head, emotions tend to become stuck, linked to their story and gone over again and again with no resolution. Left in our head, it is not surprising that emotions may well be painful and chronic and, as such, either suppressed or left uncontrolled and unpredictable.

Here then is the key point. Emotions are felt in the body. To work on our emotions, we need to turn our attention in to our body.

Often, before our awareness is brought to this and we train ourselves a little, we may well have felt our emotions as some vaguely pleasant or unpleasant feeling that we recognized as an emotion, but had difficulty really knowing what it was, or where it was. In this way, emotions remain rather abstract, vague and difficult to work with.

This antidote of dissolving emotions is based on the fact that when dealing with an emotion that is recurring, unpleasant or maybe quite painful, we can learn to use our willpower, to selectively drop any thinking about "the story," and instead go into "the emotion." By doing so, the remarkable outcome is that the emotion will actually dissolve. Here is how it works.

The solution is simple. If you have not done this before it is easy. It can be done in meditation posture, sitting casually or lying down—probably easier with the eyes closed. We simply bring to mind the emotion then notice where in the body we actually feel it. Most emotions register in our central core—abdomen, solar plexus region, chest; maybe up into the throat region, but mostly in the chest and abdomen. If you have a strong emotion, you can try this straight away. If not, and you want to experiment with this technique, you can recall one of your emotional stories for a moment, just long enough to generate the emotion, then drop the story, bring your attention into that central core area of your body, and go into the bodily felt sense of the emotion.

There are three crucial points with this technique:

Simply dwell on the feeling in your body

Avoid the temptation to think the feeling in your body needs to change or you need to fix something. Your awareness will take care of it automatically. By holding your awareness on the feeling, it will slowly, steadily and reliably dissolve.

Hold the physical feeling in your awareness nonjudgmentally

This is very important. Let go of any tendency to be critical or to analyze. Simply be interested to notice the feeling. That is all. Just notice it free of any judgment and free of any commentary or internal discussion.

To do this is the discipline, the personal kindness you need for the technique to be effective. So whenever you notice yourself becoming judgmental, simply drop the commentary and go back into the feeling. Be patient. Stay with the feeling.

Remain undistracted

Whenever you become aware that your mind has wandered or you have gone back to dwelling on the story, recognize this, be gentle with yourself (do not beat yourself up), and return to the bodily felt sense.

This technique is well described as mindfulness of emotions* and is a powerful way to actually become comfortable with, and then release, destructive and painful emotions.

DISSOLVING THE STORY

Any story that triggers an emotion lives in our mind. It is a complex construction, based on an event that actually did happen in the past, or we think may happen in the future. This event is then overlaid with our beliefs, habits, associated experiences, prejudices, knowledge, biases, preferences, hopes, fears, desires, dislikes, etc. We end up with a "story" made up of what we believed happened, or what we believe may happen. This becomes our version, our recollection of what actually did happen. The story.

However complex it may seem to be, once we have one, the story is the trigger for the emotion. So while we did learn in the last section how to dissolve the emotion, what about the story itself? There are three main techniques we can use to clear or dissolve the story:

Self-Analysis

This is possible but highly problematic. If our mind is deeply stable, then analysis of a past story may well be useful and effective; leading to perspective, clarity and resolution. However, for many of us, attempting to analyze the story tends to get us stuck in the unhelpful cycle of ongoing and unproductive thinking as described in the previous section.

---

* For more on the mindfulness of emotions, refer to the chapter of this name in my book *Meditation—An In-Depth Guide*.

Counseling or Psychotherapy

This is a real option, particularly if the emotions felt are distressingly painful and chronic.

There is a wide range of therapeutic techniques on offer, so where to go for the best help? The research is clear. When it comes to psychological change for the good, the quality of the relationship between you and your therapist is more important than the particular techniques or therapy style they use! It may be surprising, but constructive therapeutic change is most likely to occur when you have a good rapport with the health professional assisting you. So seek out a therapist you can develop confidence in and trust fairly quickly. It is always wise to regard the first visit to a potential counselor as a job interview. Is this person someone you can trust to help you with your life? If the answer is yes, make the next appointment and allow the real work to begin.

It is useful to mention that a well-run group also has the possibility to help in this regard. Sometimes I marvel at the shifts people experience in the group situation, so again, it is an option to seek out a well-led group in which you can feel confidence and trust.

Dissolve the Story Using Mindfulness and Meditation

This technique can be described as mindfulness of the story. Strange title, but great technique. This is a more advanced technique that requires some preexisting stability of the mind. Here is how mindfulness of the story works.

Preferably you take up your meditation posture, but you could do this sitting casually or lying down. Give yourself the time and space wherein you will not be interrupted. Then bring the story to mind. Being an old familiar story as the one you would work on will always be, it will only need a modest invitation. As you think over the story's details once more—who did what, what happened, what was said—allow the story to flow like a movie or a video clip in your head. And the key point again is to observe all that unfolds free of judgment. You need to avoid the running commentary of "That was good," "That was bad." You need to let go of attempting to manipulate the story, or attempting to reframe it in some way. Just let it run and remain aware, undistracted and nonjudgmental.

If you find emotion welling up to accompany the story, just observe that impartially as well. Even if tears flow or other emotions arise, simply observe them, stay with them, allow them their time, but in this technique, your focus stays with the story.

This exercise can be compared to allowing a bad movie to run through to completion, while you watch it as an impartial observer. When it is over, it is over. It is the emotion and the ongoing reflection and analysis that revives an old story. Simply letting it run under the light of full awareness allows it to reach completion and dissolve.

Now this is a powerful and effective technique but it is not without consequence. Often amidst the clarity of giving a story full awareness comes the realization that action is required. So maybe actively engaging in forgiveness is the next step. Maybe some restitution is required, some justice needs to be sought, or some personal change undertaken on your behalf.

Dissolve the Story in the View

The "view" is a word used to describe our philosophical understanding of life, coupled with the meaning and purpose we hold for it and our spiritual reality. So our view could be defined by our religious beliefs and our faith. We could hold a Christian view, Buddhist, Hindu, Islamic, Jewish view, etc. We could have our own personal philosophical view that has developed through our own experience, culture and learning. Our view may be abstract and vague, or well defined and precise. In simple terms, our view plays a major part in how we interpret and understand the world, its events and its people—and how we decide our part in all that goes on around us.

Many people find their view satisfactorily resolves past events. Things happen, you take them in, interpret them, make sense of them, act accordingly and life moves on. What we are discussing in this section is where our view fails and we are stuck with an unhelpful emotion. Maybe at such a time we can benefit from expanding our view.

Maybe resentment has been the issue. Maybe your view has accommodated holding on to resentment. You believe in your cause—"He did that atrocious thing," "She was so . . ." You believe in your right to be angry, to be chronically angry, to become angry over and over every time you recall the story. This is your view.

However, what if your view was expanded and you began to believe in forgiveness? If you did forgive, the story would dissolve!

Was Michael Leunig correct when he said:

"Love one another
And you will be happy.
It is as simple and as difficult as that.
There is no other way."

Reflecting upon this, we move on to examine specific antidotes to destructive states of mind and emotions.

CHAPTER 17

Healthy Emotions 2

Transforming the Negative, Accentuating the Positive

BACK AT THE END OF THE 1970S, WHEN I WAS BEGINNING TO FORMULATE the idea of starting a lifestyle-based cancer self-help group, it seemed clear that everyone was fully aware of the many problems associated with cancer. Virtually everyone I talked to at the time was beset with the difficulties they were facing; fear and despondency were commonplace. It was logical to conclude that a new approach was warranted.

Therefore, when the groups actually began in 1981, we concentrated on the positives. There was unspoken acknowledgment of the difficulties; we spoke of them very little, passed over them quickly and focused on the positives. So, positive thinking, positive emotions, meditation, exercise, diet. We talked about and put into practice the positive things that worked.

In the process hope was rekindled. Optimism soared, people felt rapidly better within themselves and many reported significant physical gains. Many doctors commented on the positive changes in the demeanor and the physical parameters of those attending the groups. The word spread, the numbers attending the groups increased rapidly, and all seemed wonderfully good.

OBSTACLES TO ONGOING PEACE OF MIND

Then came Barbara. Actually Barbara was there in the first group I ever ran, which started on September 16, 1981.

She had rung me the night before to tell me how difficult things were for her as a result of the advanced, medically untreatable brain tumor she was dealing with. She became more and more emotional and distressed as we talked, then she told me she was not sure if she would commit suicide or come to the group tomorrow. Then she hung up. Being new to all this, I had not yet taken her contact details so I could not get back to her. I could only spend a somewhat anxious time before experiencing considerable relief when she did turn up for the group.

Barbara was in her early forties and she came with her partner, Michael. Together they quickly warmed to the program, embracing all the recommendations, and Barbara experienced a swift, uneventful and complete recovery without any medical treatment. Barbara was a star patient—or so it seemed.

A little over a year later Michael called me. Barbara had been very well but recently was eating more and more things they both knew were not good for her. When Michael questioned her, he was told very curtly to mind his own business.

Michael and I discussed this a little but then a few weeks later he called again. Now Barbara had abandoned her meditation. Michael was increasingly worried. We discussed the situation some more. but a few weeks later he called again. Now the brain cancer was back and this time Barbara was completely opposed to meditating, eating for recovery or being positive. I went to see her in person.

Barbara was a very intelligent and articulate woman. She was reasonably open and frank with me. Barbara explained that before the cancer was diagnosed her life was in deep disarray. Problems abounded in every aspect of her life: a disturbing childhood, difficult past relationships, unhappy in work, conflict in her current relationship. The cancer diagnosis came as no surprise and she had related strongly to the group discussions regarding the cancer-prone personality. But the diagnosis changed everything.

Following the diagnosis of cancer, Michael had become more attentive and their relationship flourished. With the cancer, she was unable to go to work. With the cancer she had a ready-made, unarguable excuse to do whatever she liked. So she did. She came to know a new level of happiness.

Then she recovered. What now? She needed to face her life again. But she did not like it. The job seemed as unpleasant as ever. Now her friends were not so attentive. Her past felt as if it was crowding in on her.

Barbara put it to me quite simply: "Ian, I would rather die than go back to my old life." And despite everyone's best efforts at the time, she did die quite rapidly.

Often the stories that carry major insights or reveal key points are dramatic. Barbara's story, coupled with those of other people with similar dilemmas, affected me deeply and led to a new level of understanding. The so-called positive approach worked well as a starting point. It gave people hope and direction and nearly everyone who committed to the techniques involved improved dramatically in their health and well-being.

But over time, what we came to observe was that many people hit barriers to maintaining their peace of mind and when that was lost, the motivation to look after themselves was lost, and almost invariably, the health of the people involved suffered badly.

Now, with the benefit of many years of study and the cumulative experience of my colleagues and the many thousands of people from the groups, it is possible to categorize the barriers and to set out effective antidotes.

WHEN TO ADDRESS DESTRUCTIVE EMOTIONS?

There are five destructive emotions that people affected by cancer commonly encounter. But before we examine them, first a perspective and then the question of timing.

For any individual diagnosed with cancer the recommendation remains to focus on the way forward. By that I mean the positives—the food, the positive thinking, the healthy emotions, the meditation and so on. There is no need to go looking for destructive emotions. If they are an issue, they will find you. What is meant by this is that peace of mind is the thing to aim for. When it comes to states of mind and emotions, in broad terms it is peace of mind that will heal you. Experiencing more love, being happy, rekindling passion, experiencing joy, laughing—all these are powerful healers. So cultivate them in the manner we will discuss soon, but if you find a block emerges to your peace of mind, then that is the time to address the destructive emotions.

Some people do have fairly uneventful recoveries and experience peace of mind as an ongoing reality. Many more come up against one or more of the following destructive emotions and when the time is right, benefit from working through the problem.

How do you know when the time is right to address one of these issues? When the issue itself insists upon it. For example, an occasional fear is reasonable, rational and normal. There is no need to give attention to the occasional fear; just observe it, recognize it for what it is, a fear, and let it go.

However, if fear is with you all the time, if fear wakes you up regularly in the night, if fear takes up residence on your shoulder and whispers its message into your ear fairly constantly, then that is the time to address it.

FIVE BARRIERS TO PEACE OF MIND AND THEIR SPECIFIC ANTIDOTES

Now it is time to address fear, shame, resentment, guilt and grief. Something for everyone, really!

Fear and Its Four Antidotes

Fear is the most common emotion experienced by people when first diagnosed with cancer. Sometimes it is so strong it virtually paralyzes otherwise competent people. Curiously, in the groups' experience it is the easiest to deal with. For most people, a realistic hope and meditation combine in such a way that fear simply drops away without being addressed directly.

However, for those for whom it remains a problem, or for those who experience relapses and find fear rearing its head again, it is wise to address it on four levels.

PHYSICAL FEAR AND HOW TO FACE IT

This is the category in which we talk of the fears directly associated with the disease and the prospect of it advancing: fear of pain, fear of dying and fear of change. Each of these topics is discussed in other chapters of this book, but the actual fear is best overcome by facing it directly. If one attempts to ignore, minimize, suppress or even just take our attention off this group of fears, they simply return, commonly stronger than ever.

How to face these fears? First, some stability is needed. Denial is a common first response to grief because it puts the problem out of mind and helps to make things manageable.

Denial can be very useful short term—it just does not work well over the long term. It is helpful to understand this especially if you are supporting someone recently diagnosed. Denial can be a valid coping mechanism and people often need time to internally process their change in circumstances and support to regain the strength required to face their options with more awareness.

Rarely have I seen the benefit of dwelling on the issues of pain, death or change soon after diagnosis. However, when the time is right and if these early fears remain strong, the antidote is to "face the tiger."

Clive was a successful businessman who had lived on his own for many years. Diagnosed with advanced prostate cancer he began the program, reduced his pain, improved his health generally and stabilized his PSA. Then he found himself obsessing about his future. What would happen if the disease progressed? How would he cope? Could he manage at home? What to do? Clive became increasingly anxious, lost sleep and was heading into depression.

Acting on advice, Clive approached his GP, whom he valued for his skill and his capacity to communicate. Clive made a long appointment then explained that he was working hard toward his recovery and was essentially optimistic, but that fear for the future was really preoccupying him. He needed to understand his worst-case scenario—what might happen if all went badly and what he could he do about it.

The GP discussed the possibilities. He explained that pain was something he was very confident would be manageable medically if the need arose. He discussed how the cancer Clive had in his spine could progress and possibly interfere with his mobility, even lead to paraplegia if the possible treatment options he outlined were not successful. He pointed out that there may come a time when he would need home help or need to go into a nursing home or hospice. Then the GP described how in his experience many people die from cancer after first lapsing into a coma, and that again, in his experience, most die peacefully.

Clive recounted later how challenging this conversation had been. However, he stayed with it and at each point he and the GP made plans regarding Clive's options. He followed up by contacting the local visiting nurses' services, identifying home help options and visiting his local hospice, being pleasantly surprised by the quality of the facilities and the staff. Clive updated his will and did all he could to "put his affairs in order." Then he relaxed.

Having "faced the tiger," Clive now had a complete backup plan. Now, whenever fear for his future arose, he recognized the nature of that fear, reminded himself he had things well covered and was able to quickly dismiss the fear.

Facing death is a big enough issue to warrant its own chapter and that does come next, but the prompt here is to actually read and consider it when you come upon it.

EMOTIONAL FEAR AND ITS ANTIDOTE, LOVE

How will my relationships be affected by the disease? How will my friends react? My family? What about my work, should I tell people? Should I keep it to myself? How open and honest should I be?

First, there is no "should." Everyone is different. Every situation is unique. However, we can make some powerful general observations.

People who develop cancer tend to bottle up their emotions. They tend to "put on a happy face" and keep their distress inside. Many long-term survivors report that transforming this trait was integral to their recovery and one of the major benefits that came into their lives provoked by the harsh realities of their disease.

The simple antidote is to be more loving. Unconditionally loving. Many people these days, and many people with cancer particularly, love conditionally. I will love you on the condition that you are nice to me in return; if you look after me well, if you meet my needs. This is a neurotic form of love that is more like a deal, or a trade-off, than real love.

Real love heals. Real love is unconditional. Real love is cyclical. If you want it coming into your life, you need to be giving it out as well. The antidote to emotional fear therefore is to develop ways of becoming more loving.

The first step is to start working on reducing the conditional love. The two best ways to know this is working is when you can say no to requests, and when you can ask for help. Most people with cancer I ask—and I have asked thousands over several decades—have trouble saying no when asked to do just about anything, and similarly, most have trouble asking for help. These traits are powerfully linked to the cancer-prone personality. We can observe that these two habits are symptoms of an inner need to be liked, to be approved by those around us. The fear behind these habits is that if I do not say yes to all requests, people may not like me, may not approve of me, may not love me. If I ask for help, I may be a burden or create an inconvenience. To repeat, there is the fear people may not like me, may not approve of me, may not love me.

In my experience, revising these two ingrained habits is a very good indicator of long-term recovery. Of course, you do not want to spend the rest of your life saying no to everything and continually asking for help, but for a while, it is a very good idea! Once you have done both often enough to get over the usually acute awkwardness people feel when they first start this, once you have a free choice to unemotionally say yes or no, to ask for help or not as you really need it, then this job is done and you have taken a big step forward.

Regarding who to tell and how much to tell depends upon what type of relationships you have and what type of relationships you would choose to develop. This is a particularly important and obvious consideration for parents. What sort of model do you want to be?

Jacky had breast cancer, a difficult prognosis and was a single mother. Her two children were behaving differently. The fifteen-year-old boy was silent and sullen, the twelve-year-old girl argumentative, rebellious and obviously angry. Jacky's strategy had been to attempt to shield the children from what she regarded to be the harsh realities of her illness as well as the fears she held for the uncertain futures of herself and her children.

There is strong evidence that when children are left in the dark they "awfulize." So if important information is withheld, the truth is distorted, or worse still, if children are lied to, they tend to think the situation must be even worse than it is because why else would they not be given the accurate story?

The reality is that when given the truth, when included in a loving way, children are remarkably resilient. When this was discussed with Jacky, it brought to light another level of her difficulties. She had such a fear of what might happen to her children if she became incapacitated and then died, and struggled to face her own pain let alone share all of this with her children. She actually had a fear of the children seeing her cry.

Jacky was reassured that in her situation, tears were both reasonable and normal. She was helped to understand that how she chose to respond to her situation would provide powerful modeling for her children. Invited to consider what sort of model she preferred to provide, consciously she yearned to be open, honest and authentic. But underneath lay the habitual tendencies of nondisclosure and the emotional pain attached to all her doubts and fears.

Change begins with motivation and then comes intention. Jacky was highly motivated to do the best for her children. With the clarity that resulted from discussing and thinking through her choices, Jacky made a firm resolve, a strong intention to change her emotional habits, to share the truth of her situation with her children, along with the feelings that accompanied them.

A good intention needs a plan that results in action. Jacky realized what she proposed would take some doing. She needed help. Regular attendance at a group where other people were working on similar issues provided a good start. Then Jacky enlisted the support of school counselors for both her children as well as arranging several family therapy sessions. Finally she resolved quite simply to be more open and honest at home.

The outcome? At first Jacky was disappointed. She made a huge effort to consider how best to begin this new phase of communicating with her children. She was determined to explain to them the truth and how she was worried for them and for her; how she had thought so far it would be best to keep the details of her condition from them; and how she had been afraid of showing her emotion to them.

Jacky then made an even bigger effort to actually tell the children. Not surprisingly, it was not long before a few tears began to trickle down her face. She described how the children were riveted, paying full attention to her and what she was saying. However, they had little to say at the time, showed no real emotion themselves and once Jacky completed her spiel, they went off to their own activities.

But within weeks things were different. Regularly, each of the children came and asked her a question, one piece of the jigsaw puzzle they were trying to put together in their own heads. "What is chemo?" "What does this test mean?" "Will your hair grow back?" At school, behavioral challenges were seen and the counselor reported steady progress. Their grades improved and at home a new openness was felt. There were still times of acting out, still challenges, still issues, but a new level of ease and almost normality.

For Jacky the shift was life changing. In the groups she talked with a newfound ease and confidence. Whereas before her "atmosphere" was of tragedy and difficulty, now she had the quality of lightness and zest. Whereas before her physical situation seemed to involve one problem after another, now her reports were steadily improving, her energy up, her enthusiasm for the future buoyant.

Speaking personally, back in the eighties, a couple of years into running the cancer groups, I heard myself discussing all this with a group and it suddenly hit me. I had two children at that stage, one was four years old, the other two, and I had never told them I loved them. It occurred to me that I had never heard my own parents tell me they loved me—I did not doubt that they did, but they had never said it. I had adopted the same pattern. Simple, I thought. I will go home tonight and tell them.

Wow! It was so difficult! That was some habit to shift. Happily, what I do notice many years later is that my two children who have children of their own are very fluent with their love. They find it easy to express their love to their children and discuss the range of thoughts and feelings much more fully than I ever did in my younger days.

This is probably a good time to point out that making personal changes like these can take time. While some people become clear on what is needed and change rapidly, and while those in an effective therapeutic group may progress quickly, for many of us, changing habits takes months rather than days, sometimes even years. A helpful book to refer to is *How to Help Children Through a Parent's Serious Illness.*[30]

MENTAL FEAR

While it is true we could say that all fear is mental because fear essentially is in the mind, we have categorized it into physical, emotional, mental and spiritual to make it easy to understand and learn how to overcome fear on all levels.

There is an old maxim "knowledge dispels fear" and it holds an important truth. Just like the children who tend to "awfulize" when information is withheld, where anyone lacks knowledge there is ample room for doubt, uncertainty and fear.

The antidote, therefore, is simple—become informed.

What is needed is good information and a clear mind to assess it. This was well discussed in chapters 7–9 on positive thinking and mind training. Just one reminder: stress and anxiety also produce doubt, uncertainty and fear. Therefore, being free of mental fear is greatly assisted by our meditation. With meditation, fears dissolve.

SPIRITUAL FEAR

Why me? Why did I get this and not the person next door? Is there any rhyme and reason to my life and my illness? What is its meaning? What of its purpose? Where did I come from—before I was born? Where will I go to after I die? What is it all about?

These are the great philosophical questions. The questions that are at the heart of the spiritual quest as well as religious practice. We will go into them in some more detail in chapter 18, but for now the antidote is easy.

In the spiritual realm, when we seek answers to the big questions about life, we can begin by learning from other people's experience. It can be very helpful to read good books, to listen to authorities in this field, to discuss, reflect and contemplate these matters. However, other people's experiences or opinions can always be debated. Our own ruminations invariably have the quality of conjecture—maybe this is the answer, maybe that; maybe this is real, maybe not. No, the only satisfying conclusion to investigating the truth of major spiritual questions is direct experience. Hence the essence of meditation and its place at the heart of all the great philosophical and religious traditions.

Meditation provides a direct and reliable means to go beyond the speculation of the mind, beyond the ordinary thinking mind and to directly experience the truth of who we really are, what is in our heart's essence.

We live in a world where common, everyday truth is relative. I heard her say that, I think he did this. One authority claims this is true, but another argues the case. Is there an absolute truth? Meditation offers the way to explore that question and to experience the answer. Not to "think" we have the answer, but to "know." To know the truth of who we really are.

The value of experiencing this inner truth, this truth of who we really are, is that in doing so we find it is inherently good, fundamentally pure and absolutely inviolable. Just like the sky is never stained by the worst of stormy clouds, just as the sky is an ever-present, luminous, infinite presence, so too is this inner essence pure, whole, inviolable, unending.

To know this to be fact, to know this because we have experienced the truth of it directly in meditation, this experience leads to a deep confidence. We come to know there is a part of us that will be OK. Sure, our bodies may hurt, our emotions be fragile, our mind be troubled, but there is this inner core, this inner essence which is always pure, whole and OK. To reconnect with this essence is to find a place of inviolable refuge, a source of deep comfort and peace.

Meditation may well contribute to healing your body, emotions and mind, but even more, meditation can heal your spirit.

Shame—and Its Antidote, Self-Esteem or Self-Love

Shame is well described as the feeling of not being good enough and is commonly linked to low self-esteem.

Sally was in her late thirties, a single woman, diagnosed with leukemia. When asked why she was joining the cancer group, she replied in a very soft, fragile voice, "Oh, I was just hoping I could learn to cope a bit better."

When asked whether she could imagine any more positive, more forward-looking outcomes, it quickly became apparent that Sally was barely coping. She went on to express her deeper feelings. "I don't deserve anything more, this is the best I can imagine."

In later sessions, Sally confided the difficulties of her childhood and the troubled relationship she shared with her mother. For a variety of reasons, her mother had found it difficult to love Sally from her earliest days and gave her continual messages that she, Sally, was a nuisance and a burden. Everything she did was met with criticism. The feeling of not being good enough was deeply ingrained in Sally's psyche.

In an extraordinary, powerful moment, Sally revealed to her group that she even felt unworthy to be alive. For her, cancer made sense and on one level represented a way out. However, the group atmosphere encouraged her. She knew in her heart these really tough feelings were a product of her life experiences. They were not natural and, she reasoned, they could be changed. No doubt the warmth she felt from the group, the understanding, acceptance and encouragement helped her a good deal. In a real sense, attending the group was for Sally like attending a specific program to boost self-esteem.

Then the suggestion was made to choose an affirmation—a statement of intention to help change her way of thinking. It was suggested she consider using the word "worth," to counteract the shameful feelings of unworthiness.

Sally's first response? She came up with the affirmation "I am worthy of being here!" Quite a number in the group could not grasp its meaning and asked Sally to explain. She said she hoped that by using the affirmation she would reach a point where she felt OK to be alive, where she felt worthy to be here, as on the planet, as a living person. Several in the group were moved to tears.

Then Sally was encouraged to extend herself and to consider "I am worthy of being happy, I am worthy of being loved." Even to consider such a possibility was a real stretch of the imagination for her, but buoyed by the group and the possibilities, she embraced both and began repeating them regularly.

Sally remains clear in my mind as a woman whose life was transformed by affirmation. As she began to feel more worthy, she began to take better care of herself. She chose her company more wisely, she attended to her health more diligently, and she began to experience a new level of joy in her life.

What is of particular note is that as Sally began to feel better about herself, her meditation improved. She explained that early on when she began meditating, she often found excuses to avoid sitting quietly in her own company, finding that the meditation confronted her with her own inner feelings of inadequacy. As the feelings improved, so too did her comfort with herself. As she gradually came to experience the deeper stillness of meditation, Sally came to experience something of her inner essence. She realized the truth we talk of, that there is this pure, inviolable inner essence inside each one of us and as she reconnected with this more fundamental aspect of her nature, she felt deeply comforted, deeply at peace.

Although Sally's condition was expected to respond well to medical treatment, it was her life that was healed through her own awareness and efforts.

Resentment—and Its Antidote, Forgiveness

Resentment is well defined as chronic anger. Anger describes an immediate reaction to a person or circumstance that creates strong displeasure. Anger in the true sense of the word is a strong emotion that comes and goes fairly quickly. Resentment is when anger persists, lasts a long time, festers and stays with us. Resentment is always a destructive emotion.

Now we are all highly likely to have been involved in relationships in the past that have not turned out as we would have liked. This is quite normal, but often we get so enmeshed that the situation seems irretrievable and we can see no way around it. Such relationships can often be a constant sore point and a cause for chronic emotional stress. We need a way to let them go, a way to forgive. This can be done by using another meditation technique which, when combined with imagery and affirmations, can bring about profound and effective forgiveness.

The Forgiveness Exercise—Using Imagery and Affirmations

To begin, start as you would any meditation exercise and settle into your posture.

Relax. Take up a slightly uncomfortable position, preferably sitting in a chair or on the floor, and go through the standard relaxation.

Visualize the person you are considering. Aim to build up as clear an image of them in your mind as you can, as if they were sitting in front of you and you were looking directly at them. Some people find it helpful to begin by looking at a photograph, and in so doing, fixing the person in their mind.

Repeat the following four phrases, one at a time silently to yourself, over and over, as you would with an affirmation, until you can say each one with conviction, before going on to the next:

I forgive you.
Please forgive me.
I thank you.
I bless you.

As you begin this exercise, you will find that it takes an effort to concentrate on the person's image *and* the repetition of "I forgive you, I forgive you." Then, when you do begin to repeat the phrase, you will probably begin to think of all the good reasons why you should *not* forgive them!

"Forgive *them*? I have every reason to hate that person!" you may think. Every reason, except that the hate affects *you* more than anyone else. As you dwell on it more, a wider, healthier perspective will come.

As you keep repeating the phrase, you enter into meditating on why you would benefit from forgiving them. Think of all the reasons they are like they are, why they did what they did. You will find yourself slipping over into contemplation and a new insight developing. As you continue you *will* reach the point where, with conviction, you can say, "I forgive you!"

I found "Please forgive me" was the hard one. While at first I was beset by all the reasons why I should not forgive this person, how horrible they had been, how much they had hurt me, etc., I found that as I persevered I came to realize my role in all the problems. If I had behaved differently, the whole situation would have developed in a different, more harmonious way. This exercise led to remarkable insights and helped me to reframe my whole experience.

"I thank you" was sometimes something of a test too. Thanking someone for putting you through a hard time that finally taught you so much demands a fairly elevated perspective of forgiveness and acceptance. This exercise develops a great understanding of life and relationships in general.

"I bless you" is easy after the first three have reached the point of conviction. "I bless you" is a release, a letting go. At that point you recognized the worth in the other person. While you may agree to differ on points of view, you are now free to go your independent ways without any negative attachments.

I found it good to start this exercise with easy things, like the man who cut you off while driving home, the woman who stood on your toes, or the shop assistant who was so difficult. It is a great exercise to do regularly—choosing one person to work with each day for a while. I used to recall someone that I had met during each day and practice the exercise with them. Soon I found the whole thing happening automatically as any incident occurred. If a difficulty with a relationship looked like developing, it was as if those four little phrases whizzed around in my head, defusing the situation even before it developed. Then I worked on the hard relationships, the cluttered old ones from time gone by. The effect was considerable. I really felt freed of old attachments.

Alcoholics Anonymous takes this idea further and suggests that reformed alcoholics need to make restitution to people they have harmed. They recommend actually fronting such people, apologizing and doing all they can to physically make good any loss they caused. I do not think it is necessary to go that far unless you choose to. However, I know it works, for there was one particular person that I had been involved with in a difficult way and had not felt comfortable with since. I practiced the technique until I really could genuinely say those four statements. When I then called the person, the atmosphere between us was totally different to the usual tension. We fell easily into an extended talk, discussing our old problems in a way we had never done before. We both left feeling lighter and happier. It amazed me that the whole nature of that relationship was balanced by that exercise. Many of the people in our group have found it works for them and I recommend this exercise in forgiveness highly.

Guilt and Its Antidote, Self-Forgiveness

Guilt is when we dwell on the feeling of having done wrong in the past and feel badly about that. The obvious antidote to guilt is self-forgiveness, which can be helped greatly by developing more self-love.

So it is eminently possible to do the four-step forgiveness exercise with oneself. Doing so is easier for most people after having first used it to forgive others, and in the process becoming familiar with the four steps. Then when we come to do it with ourselves, the contemplations that result can be intriguing, insightful and freeing. What do I need to forgive myself for doing? What do I need to forgive myself for thinking about myself? For judging myself? What do I thank myself for? And then the fourth step, the blessing of self, the acceptance and the deep peace that follows.

But there is even more to this. With whom do you have the most important relationship—your wife, son, mother, or none of these? It is yourself! We all know that old maxim "Love thy neighbor as thyself." Yet we seem preoccupied with the first half of the saying. Everyone wants to be seen as loving and helping their fellows, but they overlook the ". . . as thyself" bit. This is the really vital part. If you do not have a good relationship with yourself, you can never relate openly or love honestly. You will be looking to other relationships to cover up your own seeming inadequacies, or seeking out people who show you in a good light. Only when you love yourself can you love another. This is not love in an egotistical sense, nor is it any other false emotion. It is a basic human right. You need to love yourself.

"Why should I?" you say. There is every reason. "But am I not fat? Haven't I got a crooked nose? My hair is not what I'd like and, besides, haven't I got cancer?"

You have a body that is so complex, so intricate, delicate and wonderful that if you consider it, really consider it, you cannot fail to be impressed. Your heart pumps one hundred thousand times each and every day. Can you imagine that? No mechanical pump could come close to doing it—especially without being taken out for regular overhauls and repairs, and yet yours does. No one else does it for you. Your body does it, regularly, automatically.

Think again. There was a time when you were just two cells: one from your mother, one from your father. They merged, became one, and then began dividing again. From those two cells, just two, your whole body has been created. In the process you have mirrored evolution. In the warmth of your mother you passed from being two cells through stages like a protoplasm, fish, reptile, animal to man. You have this incredible, creative, inner force that has created the body that you are in at this particular moment. There were no genetic engineers standing by to direct the process—you produced it all! You have the intelligence, the inner know-how to produce and to maintain a human body. Amazing!

Just as amazing, this same creative inner force maintains your health. It can heal broken bones with ease. Given the right conditions, it can heal or create anything. Those right conditions begin with love of self. That love is innate, a part of our natural being. Children show it perfectly. Adults often cloud it through fear. It grows, however, with reverent awe as the true wonder of the body and spirit are realized. If you have difficulty with this, I suggest you have another of those clear-cut choices. You either love yourself or you do not. It is a simple, basic choice.

If you want to reinforce that love, or come to feel it, meditate and contemplate it. Think of yourself. Think of the workings of your body, emotions, mind and spirit. As you contemplate this, you may well become aware how your outer realities are temporary ones. Your body, your personality and your environment are all changing rapidly and frequently. But in the stillness you may become aware of something more permanent, more stable and more meaningful. This, your inner core, your true self, is what you need to recognize and love. Then you will be able to accept that you have limitations—everyone has those external limits. But also accept you have strengths. Think how you can put them to good use. Come to the point where you can accept totally that "Yes, I am worthy of my own love. I have strengths. I have weaknesses and I have this inner core which is pure and true and inviolable."

Be prepared to admit your outer weaknesses in a nondefensive, nonaggressive, open way. Be prepared to put your strengths forward and to make good with them. Know that you have that inner core which is perfect. Know that you are worthy of love!

Grief

This will be covered in the next chapter on death and dying.

CULTIVATING HEALTHY EMOTIONS AND HEALING STATES OF MIND

The big three states of mind that are powerfully constructive and healing are love, hope and faith and we have covered them well already. There are two more states of mind that, while they may be less recognized, can be equally powerful agents for healing and well-being.

Generosity

When we are sick, and especially when we are fearful for the future, we tend to contract, want to hang on to whatever we have and can verge on becoming stingy. Reversing that trend, transforming that state of mind and practicing generosity can be a powerful force for healing.

What to give? Start small—a few words of praise, a small gift, maybe then something larger. If you can give knowledge you give something of great value, and if that knowledge allays someone's fear and brings them peace and contentment, now there is a real gift.

I had a graphic lesson in this. Having been an athlete, I was always conscious of "style" in running. This has something to do with poise, with balance and flair, and, dare I say it, elegance. I enjoyed watching others who had it, and while I did not speak of it, I did try to develop it myself. It gave me joy to aim to learn to run with style and happily, the more I worked at it, the faster I went. Following my amputation, I then spent a lot of time trying to move on crutches with "style." It sounds funny, I suppose, but I tried to move fluidly and easily. I never told anyone about my "training." However, one day a young man quite unknown to me came up and said to me with clarity and conviction, "It is a pleasure to watch you move. You look as if you are just floating along," and left.

Nobody else before had ever commented. Most people simply ask me what happened, why I do not wear an artificial leg and what do I do with the other shoe! Having had an amputation through the hip, I continue to find crutches more convenient and comfortable than an artificial leg. As it happens, having one leg, a kaftan is more comfortable and in my view more esthetically pleasing than wearing trousers with one leg. And I have my one shoe personally made so as not to waste the other. While I have always felt comfortable with all of this, this young man's single remark, said with genuine feeling, sticks in my mind and warms my heart.

The old saying "A word of praise is worth a thousand of criticism" is so true. You can make someone else's day by seeking out what it is in them that deserves praise. A single, well-placed, genuinely felt word can have someone else smiling for a long time.

Of course, it would be no surprise to notice ourselves beginning the practice of generosity hoping that if we give someone something nice, we will receive something even better in return. This is understandable as a starting point, but the real power comes and the real benefits flow when we let go of the "trade" mentality and go unconditional. Experiment. Can you give even a small gift with no thought of being appreciated, let alone receiving a gift in return? The challenge with all the positive states of mind is to aim to develop them to the point of being unconditional. Now there is a real challenge!

Gratitude

Take a moment to go back to the feeling that goes with bitterness and resentment. Cold, hard, tight, contracted, withdrawn. Very antihealing, very pro-cancer! Now feel into gratitude: warm, positive, open, embracing—very anticancer, very much to do with healing!

Gratitude is another state of mind we can choose to develop very easily. We mentioned in the positive thinking section that one of the best ways to develop gratitude and to feel its benefits is to remember as you go to bed each night to list just three things from your day you can be grateful for. Maybe it is as simple as the fact that you did wake up again that morning. Maybe it was a sunny day, or a rainy day and it was good for the gardens. Maybe you were given something, achieved something. Maybe you had a good laugh or a moment of real peace. Just list three things. Some people actually keep a "gratitude diary," write them down, and marvel at the list as it grows.

This simple exercise is remarkably powerful and, as an aside, good research demonstrates it to be a powerful antidote against depression.

But then take gratitude further. Get into the habit of thanking people for what they do for you. You probably do a lot of this—however, it is all too easy to take someone who is helping you for granted and to think they know how helpful they are being and how grateful you are. Maybe they are psychic, but why not tell them! It reinforces their kindness and leaves them in no doubt. Express your gratitude.

WHAT TO DO? WHAT IS EMOTIONAL HEALING?

When you are focused on recovering from cancer, there is no need to go chasing problems. Sometimes you hear people saying, "Oh, she has cancer, she must be big on resentment, or have had a big childhood trauma, or . . ."

Maybe. Maybe not. Being judgmental of others is a risky business. What is very clear from my many years of helping people and getting to know their states of mind quite well is that there is far more healing to be gained from developing healthy, constructive states of mind than by going digging for the destructive ones.

The place to start is with valuing, generating, experiencing and giving as much of the following as possible: hope, love, faith, laughter, joy, gratitude. Be generous with your emotions!

Look over the list again. Almost certainly one, two, maybe even three of the above will speak directly to your heart. "Pick me. I am the one you need right now. Cultivate me; I will get you going. Together we can heal!" So focus on developing that emotion, that state of mind to begin with. As you progress, from time to time return to this chapter and the list. What next?

And if at some point it becomes obvious that resentment is an issue, then that will be the time to give some weeks, maybe even months, to focusing upon forgiveness. If fear raises its ugly head at some point and hangs about too long, consider how to alleviate it. Is it physical fear, emotional, mental or spiritual? Use your mind to train your mind; to identify the issues you face, to reason how to respond and to motivate you to follow through and transform any destructive emotions into the energy of healing.

Above all, meditate regularly. Meditation creates balance. Physical balance, emotional balance; balance in our mind and our spirit. For some, meditation has been enough on its own. For most, training the mind, using the power of the mind, transforming destructive emotions and cultivating constructive states of mind has transformed their health and their life.

These positive states of mind have an effect that is very similar to turning on a light in a darkened room. Turn the light on and the dark, which may have been in the room for just a few moments or for eons, is immediately transformed. Moreover, with the light on there is nowhere for the dark to hide. If illness is compared to the darkness, healthy emotions are like the light.

CHAPTER 18

Death and Dying

How to Live Well, and Die Well

YOU MAY WELL ASK, "WHY IS THERE A CHAPTER ON DEATH AND DYING? Isn't this all about conquering cancer, about being positive, and getting well?"

There are two compelling reasons why considering death and dying makes powerful, positive sense. First, and perhaps most obviously, many people have enough fear about dying to not only significantly inhibit their chances of recovery, but to adversely affect the very way they live. Learning how to transform the fear of dying leaves us free to heal.

Second, consideration of death can transform your life. During thirty years of working with people affected by cancer, it is truly remarkable how many of those people have told me how glad they are to have been diagnosed with cancer. This sense of gratitude, which sometimes not surprisingly can seem perverse to outsiders, can take a while to develop. However, months or years later, many people tell me that being diagnosed with cancer was the best thing that ever happened to them.

How remarkable is that? And the reason? Because by considering their death they addressed their life. Being aware of the real possibility of dying sooner rather than later, they had the impetus to prioritize, to make changes, to do what was important, to make time for the things they really valued, to transform their lives.

So be brave. This discussion definitely has the capacity to transform your life. Read on!

LIVING IN FEAR OF DEATH OR INFORMED BY DEATH?

All of us will die one day. However, we need to be careful not to glamorize death. When we die, everything changes. When we die, there is a great deal we will lose. We lose connection with this body and this life. We lose direct connection with our family and friends. We certainly lose the capacity to work and it appears fairly clear we can take nothing with us. Alexander the Great, who ruled over more of the world than just about any figure in history, insisted on being buried in a simple white shroud with his hands left exposed and empty—to show what he took with him.

When someone we love or care for dies, we lose that direct contact with them. Their qualities, their energy, their presence, their inspiration, strength and weaknesses may stay with us and continue to influence our lives, but everything changes. We need to acknowledge death can be tough and it has the potential to be fearful.

Everyone knows this. Everyone deals with this knowledge in one of two ways. People aim to live in denial of death, or they live informed by death. One of the key points here is the proposition that the latter, living informed by death, while not so common in our society and perhaps challenging when first considered, is a better way to live and can make a major contribution to recovery.

CANCER AND THOUGHTS OF DEATH

In my cancer work, many people have told me the only reason they gave consideration to death was due to the fact of their cancer diagnosis. That was because before the diagnosis they were in denial of death. On one level, denial makes good sense. By denying death, by pretending we will live forever or at least die at some convenient time way off in the future when we are ready, we can avoid dwelling on the immediate pain of the losses death may well bring.

But denial comes with a cost. With denial of death comes the optimistic hope that we will have time to do all the things that are important in life. Later. So with denial there is often a willingness to postpone, to procrastinate, to compromise. And there is also a tendency to take life for granted, to function on automatic and to just allow life to drift along.

A cancer diagnosis can cut right through that. That is its power. That is its positive potential. If life may end sooner rather than later, what is the priority? What is really important?

Of course many consider it is the cancer that provokes these thoughts. While this is often the truth of how life unfolds, everyone who is alive will die one day and no one knows when. Back in the mid-seventies, nearly everyone who knew me thought I would be dead in a few weeks. Decades later, I have been to quite a few of those people's funerals and I remain alive and well. The point is, if you are alive, you will die one day and you do not know when that day will be. If you take that fact into account, it will enhance your life.

When we live a life informed by death, we really appreciate how precious life is, as well as how fragile it can be. So we value life; we value each moment. Once we overcome the immediate fear of death and the shock that can often result when for the first time we do contemplate it deeply, then life becomes more vivid and more focused. There comes a freshness, a vitality that seeks to get the most out of life. Almost paradoxically, by considering death, we become truly alive.

This is where the thanks for the cancer diagnosis originates from.

IS A GOOD DEATH POSSIBLE? AND IF SO, HOW?

I have known people diagnosed with cancer who were deeply scared of dying and who thought that to speak of it, or heaven forbid, shed a tear over it, was a negative thing to do and as such was to be avoided at all costs. And the costs associated with this view are high: noncommunication, bottled-up emotions, deep-seated ongoing pain and anguish, and the capacity to heal significantly impaired. What then does being positive really mean? What do we do with the natural fears that most feel, especially in the early days after a diagnosis?

Most of us have experienced the death of some of the significant people in our lives. You may have noticed how some people seem to have what we could characterize as "a good death," while others we might describe as "a bad death." Having helped many people, including family and friends to approach death, I can honestly say that after many years nearly all who died having following the approach I advocate died well. Many confirmed this for me in the lead-up to their deaths. Many families tell me after someone they love has died how amazed they were at the extraordinarily high "quality of death" they all experienced.

Perhaps the greatest revelation, and to be open, the greatest surprise to me in my many years of working with people experiencing cancer, has been how consistently people died well with cancer. Sure, many do learn to live well with cancer and it has been wonderful to witness and be a part of people surviving against the odds, but that was expected. Transforming suffering, being with people who found happiness amidst what was real adversity, seeing people die well consistently, that has been a real blessing.

And do be clear: most of these people began the groups or picked up *You Can Conquer Cancer* in denial of death. Most had significant concerns, many suffered anxiety, and the majority were deeply fearful. The common fears are fear of the process of dying, fear for the moment of death and fear for what happens after death. These fears are held for the person themselves and for those they love and care for.

The question is simple. Given we all will die one day, is it possible to have a good death? And is it possible for those who survive us to go on to have a good life? Given some people seem to have "a good death" and others not, what can we do when our time comes? Do we approach death in denial and just hope for the best, or is it wiser to prepare?

Clearly, experience points to the great value that comes from being well prepared. There are four areas to consider:

1. How to prepare for your own death
2. How to help another approaching death
3. What to do at the moment of death
   1. For yourself
   2. For another
4. Coping with grief

HOW TO PREPARE FOR YOUR OWN DEATH

The type of death you experience will be most affected by how you have lived your life, the state of your mind at the time of death and how prepared you are. Before discussing these key points in detail, it may well be useful to revisit the highly recommended "What if . . ." exercise that puts life and death into perspective and is reproduced again here:

Now, some may have seen this exercise popularized in the film *The Bucket List*. It featured Jack Nicholson and Morgan Freeman playing two characters diagnosed with cancer who shared the completion of their "bucket list"—the things they wanted to do before they kicked the bucket. We have used this exercise for decades with those affected by cancer and those who

The Contemplation on "What If . . ."

- Take a piece of paper and a pen to a quiet place where you will not be disturbed for about half an hour.
- Imagine that for the next three months everything in your life will remain basically the same as it is now; but at the end of the three months you will die. So you have the same level of health, same finances, and the same capabilities. The fantasy is that only you die and the question is, what do you do in these last three months?
- Clearly, this is a fantasy. No one knows how long they will live. However, imagine you have three months to go, with everything else staying basically the same, and now write down the ten most important things you would choose to do in those three months.
- As the list forms, you may have a sense of priorities—some things may seem more immediate than others. If so, rank them in order of importance.
- Only write down the things that really warrant being on the list. If you do not reach a total of ten, just stay with the significant items.
- Once your list is complete, consider how much time you are giving currently to each item on the list. If there are items that are being postponed or unattended to, consider what it would take to get them done.
- Use this list. Refer to it regularly. Maybe you have been doing it somewhat already courtesy of a cancer diagnosis. Do it formally and continue to review your list. This list can transform your life. This list is particularly useful for people who are well. It is how they can obtain the benefit of a life-threatening illness—without needing to get sick!

are well. Do take time to review it regularly. It is one of the most useful techniques I know.

A Good Life Leads to a Good Death

This is a powerful generalization. The experience here is clear. The great majority of people who have lived to the fullest, done all they could, used their lives to help others wherever possible, minimized the regrets, forgiven others and themselves, developed a good heart with generosity and gratitude. People who have lived well invariably die well.

Now of course, unless we were fully enlightened from birth, there are things we will look back on with regret. So most of us will benefit from checking our guilt, shame, blame and resentment levels. Maybe this is a good time to be reminded that we can always change our mind, retrain our mind, reconcile the past and learn to be happy in this present moment.

Our State of Mind at the Time of Death

People who approach death in an unpremeditated way rely on their life experience to determine their state of mind. So for people who arrive at the end of their life full of fear, bitterness and resentment, it is easy to imagine things will not go so well.

This is where death can be like an ally to our life. In this sense, death can be a valuable friend, as it reminds us to live well, to develop what we call a positive state of mind, to address our fears, to forgive wherever necessary and to cultivate a sense of joy and gratitude throughout our life.

There is no doubt that a good state of mind is closely aligned with a good quality of death.

Be Prepared for Death, Be Free to Live Well

What follows is a fairly comprehensive list of the major items to consider when preparing for death. Many people find it useful to write this checklist out, complete it and then share and clarify it with the people they are closest to, so they understand the preferences.

This is a list that warrants regular review; maybe an update once a year is ideal.

End-of-Life Checklist

THE PRACTICAL MATTERS—GETTING YOUR AFFAIRS IN ORDER

- Prepare or update your will.
- Attend to your financial affairs and ensure your partner can access joint accounts and other key financial and legal matters if necessary.
- Create an enduring power of attorney (a simple power of attorney ceases if you become incapacitated).

- Consider establishing a living will or enduring power of attorney—medical treatment form. This will set out your preferences and directions for end-of-life treatment options. These directions would provide guidance to medical staff and family if you become incapacitated, are not likely to recover, and choices need to be made regarding being left to die naturally or to have major interventions. You can also mention the levels of pain medication desired (maximum or minimal) and whether you would elect to have CPR (cardiopulmonary resuscitation) if your heart were to stop in this end stage of life. You could also nominate who you might want present (or absent) at the end of life and indicate a preference for being at home, in hospital or a hospice.

- Consider your possessions. Do you prefer for some items to go to particular people? If so, make sure this is clear. Maybe consider giving some things away while you are alive.

- Designate who you wish to look after any children, parents or other dependants if you and/or your partner were to die. Make sure the designated people know and agree.

- Complete as many of the tasks in your life as possible. Give priority to your bucket list. Aim to die free of regret for things left undone—either do them or let them go.

COMMUNICATE. DO NOT DIE LEAVING PEOPLE WONDERING!

- Express your love. You may think they know, maybe they are psychic, but tell them anyway!

- Consider leaving messages for significant people to be read or viewed at significant times. This can be particularly useful and comforting if you have young children now. Ideally, write or record your messages and deliver them in person on the eighteenth birthday or at the wedding; but if you are not there, the message will have real meaning.

- Consider documenting your life. You could simply create a photo album from childhood on, or collate any old videos or DVDs. Or you could be more personal and specifically record your insights, reflections, regrets, passions, etc.

- Forgive. Forgive. Forgive. Resentment is like a cancer in itself. Forgiveness heals the heart and sets us free. Review the forgiveness section in the healthy emotions chapter and do it! Forgive others. Forgive yourself.

IMMEDIATELY AFTER DEATH

- What preferences do you have for your body? Should it be left undisturbed for a while, and if so, for how long? In hospitals especially, there is often a need to clear beds for the next person (a tough reality), but family and friends may find great value in being able to sit quietly with the body after death. Also, some spiritual traditions indicate there is real benefit for the person who has died if the body is left undisturbed for even up to three days after death. This length of time may not be practical, but you may choose to indicate your own preference.
- What procedures do you want carried out with your body? Have you registered for organ donation? Embalming is a highly invasive procedure and only legally required if the body is being transported internationally. Have you a preference for who should wash the body and what clothes it will be dressed in?
- Have you a preference for a particular type of coffin or casket?
- Burial or cremation? Where?

FUNERAL SERVICE

- Do you want one? If so, will it be closed to include only the immediate family, or open for everyone who wishes to attend? Be reminded a funeral can help those left behind a great deal and consider wherever possible what will help them.
- Where will the service be held and who will officiate—a civil celebrant or a member of your religious tradition?
- What style of service? Traditional according to your religion? Themed such as New Orleans jazz? What emphasis will there be on the celebration of life and the grief of loss?
- What music, poems, readings to include?
- Who will speak? Who gives the main eulogy? Will others reflect on your life, offer readings, etc.?
- Are there particular interest groups to include and feature, such as sporting or service clubs?
- What about after the funeral? Will there be a wake? If so where, who organizes it and how will it be financed and provided?

ANYTHING ELSE IMPORTANT?
If so, add it to your list.

A Healthy Lifestyle Makes for a Good Death

A surprising number of people make the mistake of approaching death in an unhealthy way. Some people tell me, "I tried the diet and the meditation. It helped for a while, but now I am approaching death I am going back to my old way." This is a crucial point. Eating well makes it easier to die well. Why? Because heavy foods and junk foods add a burden to your system. High-fat diets make for sticky blood and lead to higher risks of embolism, stroke and heart failure. Bad diets promote inflammation that is both uncomfortable and is likely to aggravate any health issues you have. Bad diets are degenerative, whereas our healthy diet is regenerative and anti-inflammatory. Meditation is also anti-inflammatory and regenerative, while it also clears the mind, reduces anxiety and pain and helps us connect with who we really are.

If I thought I was really closer to dying rather than just the fact of knowing I could die any day, I would be even more particular about what I ate and drank, and I would meditate even more than the average one hour per day I do currently.

Be gentle on yourself. Live well and die well.

HOW TO HELP ANOTHER APPROACHING DEATH

Be involved. Communicate. When a question occurs to you, such as "Do you still think you can recover or are you ready to die?" be brave and ask it. Ask it skillfully (we will discuss how to soon), but do communicate. Feel free to express your emotions. Be authentic. Be real. Do recognize your own needs. Look after yourself so you can be of most use to the one you love and care for. Here are some guidelines.

Clarify Your Role

Are you the key caregiver? Or are you a close member of the family or close friend, someone who supports both the person with the illness and their primary caregiver? Or are you a more casual friend who is intent on being as useful as possible, or a casual friend who has little time? It is wise for you and all involved if everyone is clear on your role as well as the roles others are contributing.

Is the Focus on Recovery or Dying?

Tricky question. Challenging to ask and often challenging to answer. In my experience, most people with cancer know the answer to this question within their own hearts. However, when someone reaches the point where they are ready to die, it is often difficult to express it. Close family and friends often attempt to dissuade them. "Don't talk like that. You'll be OK. Here, have another carrot juice."

Having the next carrot juice may make good sense, but so too does honoring the person you are helping. Many of the things that help people to recover, help them to die well. But if someone has accepted they are ready to let go of the intention to recover or even the possibility of recovery, they may well choose to focus their attention on different things.

The way to get the answer to this question is to do what is often quite difficult, to put your own preferences aside, to be open and nonjudgmental, and to ask. Sometimes these words help: "I can imagine that some people in the situation you are in at the moment would be focused on getting well. But maybe others might be at a stage where they would rather let go of that and accept they are ready to die. Where are you in that spectrum of aiming to recover and accepting death is becoming the more likely outcome?"

Adjust what you do and how you are to the intentions of the person you care for.

Be Aware of Intentions

Use the suggestions and checklists in the previous section, How to Prepare for Your Own Death, to clarify what your loved one has decided to do. Talk through the options. If you are the principle caregiver, it is highly recommended to work through the lists together. It may be emotional. Tears may flow from time to time. It may take a while, it may take several sessions, but then you have clarity.

Clarify What Sort of Friend You Are to Be

What happens if the person you are helping falls short on their intentions? For example, what if they say they will have seven juices a day and balk after three? Or they say they will meditate three times a day and only manage one?

It is wise to discuss this possibility in advance, when things are warm, friendly and rational. Does your person want you to remind them of their intention? Is it helpful and desirable for you to provide the proverbial "kick up the backside"? Or are you meant to be passive and watch quietly as they do their own thing. Plan for this, as many couples have suffered badly if the scenario unfolds where there is a disparity between good intentions and actual actions. Aim for peace of mind and accord. Work as a team.

Recognize Your Grief—Be Gentle on Yourself

For many caregivers, the diagnosis of cancer naturally triggers a strong grief reaction. Recognize this may affect you, and see the later section on coping with grief.

It is OK to express your grief as long as you do not get stuck in it. It is very normal for couples to share their grief at first diagnosis. Shock is common. Numbness, tears, even feelings of injustice or rage are common enough. There is a time for that. Then when the initial storm passes, there is a time to gather your energies, make plans and set about the task of recovery.

Balance Your Own Needs

Some people become so dedicated to providing full-time care they exhaust themselves. Illness can follow, as can a general level of grumpiness, resentment and disinterest.

There is a need to nurture yourself so you can best nurture the one you care for. It makes sense to take some time out. To give yourself permission to enjoy hanging out with friends, to go to a movie alone or with someone else, to play golf—to do something that provides a real break. Doing this is another form of kindness to the one you are looking after. Rather than the common feelings of guilt people initially feel taking time out, pat yourself on the back and be grateful you can balance things as best as possible.

Be Aware of Overconcern—Balancing Care and Trust

Just because someone has cancer does not mean they are completely incompetent. Obviously, I hope! But some caregivers do feel they need to do everything and go into full-on sympathy mode. This can be really counter-productive, really obnoxious.

While it can be a delicate balance to strike, the need is to communicate. Talk about what is easy, what is challenging, what requires help, what can be left to the person with cancer. Many patients clearly value their independence and struggle with the notion of being a burden on those they love, so they may well need to address this sensitive issue too and jointly develop a strategy you are both happy with. Talking is the key.

For the Immediate Caregivers

If you live with a person with cancer, there will be a cycle of routines with meals, treatments and other activities. Be on guard that life does not move into automatic. It is easy to get caught up in the routines and miss the moment. So do remember from time to time to be more intimate and to check on feelings, hopes, fears and aspirations. Do take time to go out of your way for fun, enjoyment and meaningful time together. You may need to put these events in the diary too—make sure you include time for life as well as healing (even though so much of healing is about living well).

If You Are an Occasional Visitor

Whether you are a family member or a friend, if you only visit occasionally, also be on guard. Occasional visitors often make a real effort to visit. They come from overseas or interstate, they give up time, and they feel the natural urge to have an impact.

Here is the caution: you do not have to fix everything in a visit of an hour or two, or a day or two. As an occasional visitor, the real job is to express your love and concern and to support the primary caregivers. Relax. Trust that those who are there the most are best placed to provide the active support.

Do feel free to enter into intimate conversations. Again it is fine for you to acknowledge and express your own feelings. When with someone who is close to dying, the two key areas of interest are entered into by saying something like, "Let's talk about your life and what you have come to know of love. Who did you really feel loved by? Who did you love? What did you love? What were you passionate about?" And second, "What did you learn in your life? If life was like going to school to learn lessons, what were the main lessons you learned?" These questions will take you directly into the heart of what most people are interested in toward the end of their lives—love and wisdom.

If You Get Frustrated

What about if you realize that you wish the person you care for was different, did things differently, and more fully agreed with you regarding what they should be doing?

For your own integrity and the one you love, it is wise to express your preferences rather than bottle them up for risk of confrontation or offense. The aim of course is to avoid discord, but if there are differences, you have a right to express an opinion, just as the person with cancer has an even stronger right to choose their own path.

Do your best to strike an accord. Use this book, use the lists, enlist professionals and friends; explore the options and aim for agreement. If conflict emerges, remember grief commonly produces anger and commonly people find it easier to express anger with people they are close to and trust. In an almost perverse sort of way, people can be angriest with those they love the most, so do what you can to be understanding and keep a perspective. Of course, unreasonable behavior is always unreasonable and so everyone needs to keep cool. If the atmosphere remains difficult, counseling, especially family counseling with an experienced therapist, can be very valuable.

The reality is there may be a need to accept the one you love is different to you, does make different choices, and through your love you need to acknowledge this, accept it and do what you can to support their choices.

By aiming to be attentive, present and nonjudgmental, at least you will know you are putting your compassion and love into action—you will do no harm and, who knows, maybe in that atmosphere a miracle may happen.

WHAT TO DO LEADING UP TO THE MOMENT OF DEATH

The moment of death is one of the most important moments in our life. Think of this. When we die we will get to find out the answers to the really big questions. If nothing happens, we simply die and that is the end of everything, well that will be OK. But if something does happen after we die, the chances are it will be really extraordinary. So while I am keen to live as long as possible, I look forward to dying and to finding out what happens. It should be truly amazing!

So how to die well? How to lead up to a good death? What to do at the very moment of death? And what about afterward?

Leading Up to Death—for Yourself

Ideally, all the issues raised so far in this chapter have been attended to. If not, there is a lot of homework to do! As well as using the "be prepared" guidelines, here are some other major issues to consider.

LOSS OF CONTROL

As people draw closer to death, particularly through an illness like cancer, it is common for their physical body to weaken. Weight loss is common, mobility can be reduced and, for some, there will be loss of control of bodily functions.

These changes deeply disturb some people, particularly those who are fiercely independent or proud. It is curious to me. No one balks at changing a baby's diaper or carrying them around. For many, these changes at the end of life are just as natural as the limitations we all experienced at the start of our lives. At the end of life, there is the challenge to let go, to accept things as they are and to be grateful for the people who love and care for us, or for those who are paid to look after us.

PERSONAL CHANGE

If we approach death gradually, rather than as an accident, we are bound to notice an array of personal changes. As well as loss of control, our body can change dramatically, our energy levels drop, and our range of interests narrow.

For some, the range of emotional expression also narrows and it is common that people's true nature emerges. Happy people emerge as basically happy, the grumpy ones grumpy. At the same time, intellectual capacity and interests can wane but then there is the good news. What we have talked about so far is all to do with our ego. As we approach death, our ego tends to dissolve somewhat. If we are aware of this we can free ourselves more from this aspect of our lives. We simply let it go. At the same time, almost invariably as the body and ego diminishes, our spiritual awareness and presence will strengthen and come to the forefront.

This is why many people choose to work in palliative care or hospices. Many people at the end of their lives come more fully into their spiritual nature. It is there for all to see. When someone is close to or at the point of dying, you will feel this presence, this spiritual quality. This goes beyond the intellect, even beyond emotion. It is the presence of the person's fundamental nature, their spiritual essence. It is real and it is tangible.

So when your time comes to die, it is a good time to consciously let go of the things to do with the mundane aspects of life and your ego. Focus your awareness on what you have learned, what you know, what you love and what you aspire to in the spiritual aspect of your life.

PAIN CONTROL

Refer to the chapter of that title but then think seriously about what pain, if any, is being felt and being addressed. Obviously, loss of control and personal change can be painful. No doubt some people appreciate being "bombed out" on heavy analgesics so these more emotional issues are dulled out of their awareness.

I recommend you to be as aware as possible at the moment of death. While the essential part of our nature is unaffected by pain medication, a conscious death is a real possibility and may have great value.

INCLUDE CHILDREN

Do not shut them out. Be prepared for their questions, which are often profound, often mundane; often come at odd and unexpected moments. Answer what you can, being confident and clear about what you do not know.

It is really helpful to offset children's main fears by repeatedly telling them two things. First, if you are coming to the end of your life and you have young children, assure them regularly that you really do love them, and that you have done and will continue to do all that you can to live as long as possible and to stay with them. Children, especially young children, can feel abandoned when a parent dies, so this needs regular repetition.

Children also commonly feel that they are at the center of the universe and as such are responsible for everything. While this may not be rational, they commonly feel responsible for their mom or dad's cancer. Therefore, the second thing to tell them regularly is that the illness is not their fault.

As with other crucial needs, if you are worried about how children are managing, seek professional advice. Judicious and skillful counseling can transform a lifetime of difficulties into a well-managed major life change.

CONFESSION, FORGIVENESS AND LETTING GO

As the prospect of death becomes real, what might help to clear the conscience if necessary, and allow us to die at peace? In the old melodramas, this was the time when people were advised to "make their peace" or to "make peace with their maker." It was good advice.

Maybe you have not been near a church or a temple for ages past. But anytime is a good time to return to your homeland or your spiritual roots. The Catholic Church has excellent rituals of confession and absolution and, when done meaningfully and authentically, these rituals can bring great peace. While other religious traditions have their own rituals, some people I have known developed their own personally meaningful rituals and techniques that enabled them to let go of guilt, shame and resentment. (Refer to the previous chapter on healthy emotions.)

Some leave it to their deathbed to forgive. Sure, you can make a case for doing it earlier, but it is never too late.

What would you benefit from letting go so that you are in a better state of mind to die?

Leading Up to Death—for the Caregivers and Friends

TRANSFORMING SUFFERING

As a caregiver, your first challenge is to maintain some stability—within yourself. Particularly if the person you care for feels that all is falling apart, stability provides an anchor, something to hold on to and something to be supported by.

If you find yourself overwhelmed by your own emotion, take it elsewhere—it will not help the one who is dying. Balance your own needs and, if necessary, seek counseling or share your emotions with others you are close to.

THE TWO GIFTS—FROM THE PRIMARY CAREGIVER

As a person draws near to the moment of death, there are two things that make dying much easier when they are heard to come from the person who is closest to them. Both usually take quite some preparation before that caregiver is able to say them in a heartfelt way.

First comes: "It is OK to die." This is like a permission. It is best said after explaining how much you love the person, how they know how much you would prefer them to live, and how you would do whatever possible to bring that about, but if it is their time to go, "It is OK to die."

Second: "We will be OK." Again, with the death of someone so close to you, and if families are involved, everything will change and clearly life will never be the same again. But life will go on for those left behind and while there may be difficult and challenging times to manage, if you can have the confidence to authentically say, "We will be OK," it can be deeply reassuring to the one who is close to death.

Preparing to say these two phrases can be deeply emotional. It may require some resolve to first contemplate and think them through, and then to be able to genuinely give voice to them. However, doing so can produce profound comfort for the dying person, allowing them to relax, be assured things will be OK and to let go into the process of dying. Also, for anyone who says these things authentically, there is immediately a very real and major step forward in resolving their own grief.

WHAT TO DO AT THE MOMENT OF DEATH

Ideally, all we have covered so far has been taken care of. What follows next is a sequence that in a conscious death you may remember to follow, or perhaps it could be spoken to you at the time of death by whoever is closer to you, as a reminder and as a guide.

Instructions for the Moment of Death

- Remember, it is OK to die. Dying is a natural process. We will all do it, and we will all do it successfully! When the time comes, all you need to do is breathe out and when you do not breathe in again, it is done. It is very easy. There is nothing to fear. Relax and go with it.
- While you can, remember the good things about your life, maybe dwell on what wisdom you learned, what love you experienced.
- Generate a sense of gratitude for this life and for the people who were a part of it. Know that they too will be OK.
- When you are ready, consciously bless those whom you are leaving behind, thank them again and let them go.

- Turn your mind away from the world you have known in this life and the people in it and bring your attention to your spiritual essence.
- Imagine whatever symbolizes or embodies your own spiritual truth as if they or it were in the sky above you. So it may be Christ, Mother Mary, a particular saint, the Buddha, Krishna or a beloved teacher. Or it may be a more abstract image—a ball of light like the sun that symbolizes the universal energy that runs through all of life. Even if you have a particular religious or spiritual view, this ball of light may be easiest, representing as it does all that is good and all that has your own best interests at heart.
- Generate whatever devotion you feel and direct it to that figure or ball of light. This is like the longing you might have felt as a small child to be with your parents. If you are comfortable with prayer, quietly repeat whatever prayer comes to mind.
- Imagine that this feeling is received by the focus of your attention and returned to you. There is an outpouring of love that streams toward you and that you imagine, that you see as a stream of luminous white or golden light. This light flows from the heart of the figure you see in the sky before you, or from the very center of the ball of light.
- As this luminous, loving light reaches down and touches you, you feel it drawing you magnetically toward its source.
- Consciously letting go of this life and being intent to remain undistracted by either pleasant or unpleasant diversions, allow the flow of light to carry you into the very heart of your spiritual figure or the center of the ball of light.
- When you do this, they say that dying is as easy as running into your mother's arms.

What to Do Following the Death of Someone You Love

- Hold the atmosphere of peace, love and reverence for as long as possible. Grief is natural. Tears may well flow. If necessary, move away from the body while emotions are really strong, then aim to sit quietly with it.
- It can be very helpful to repeat in your mind or speak out loud to the body the instructions for the moment of death.
- Most people have their own knowing of when it is time to leave the body, to move away and do whatever comes next.

- If possible, do not move the body for an hour or two—many prefer longer if it can be done.
- Ensure any specific religious or spiritual practices chosen by the deceased are carried out.
- It is really helpful if there is a designated "minder" who can protect the atmosphere, keep unthinking staff away if necessary, regulate visitors and monitor everyone's needs, especially those of the key people.

What if I Was Not There at the Moment of Death?

First understand this: I have been a part of family vigils that went on for days. Then, in the few moments when everyone left the room, dear old Grandpa died. Or other times where defying all expectations, someone held on to life for days, even weeks until a particular person arrived by their side, at which point they died almost immediately.

The reality is some people are very private, some really seek company. Whatever the fact of this, I know how some people find it deeply disturbing when they are unable to be there when someone close to them has died. What can you do?

- If you know someone is dying and you cannot be there, stop whatever else you are doing. Pray, meditate or just hold that person in your mind. Imagine the instructions for dying as if they are happening. Project with your mind as if you are with the person and guiding them. Take comfort that the mind can do this—the mind can transcend space and time.
- If you find out after someone has died, allow yourself to grieve. Once you are reasonably calm and clear, draw on prayer and meditation and project the earlier instructions even though the person has died—there is value in doing this hours, even days after the death.
- If there has been a long delay before you learn of a death, you can still be very helpful. What has been useful for many is to meditate and imagine in your own mind a place where you feel particularly peaceful and comfortable, just as you do when going to the inner sanctuary (see chapter 10). Then invite the person who has died to join you in that place. You imagine them joining you in that place, imagining all this to be as real as you can. Once you feel the connection with the person who has died, you can say what you need to, what you feel. Maybe they will say something

back to you or for you. Many people have found this exercise profoundly helpful in resolving the mixed feelings that commonly go with being apart from someone you love when they die.

COPING WITH GRIEF

For many people, a diagnosis of cancer triggers a major grief reaction. Some resolve this grief in such a way that the moment of death is experienced quite differently to the powerful grief reactions many feel at that time. What is normal? What is reasonable and OK? And what may require attention?

The Five Stages of Grief

Elisabeth Kübler-Ross identified five now-classic stages that dying people pass through. These are explained in her book *On Death and Dying*.[31] In my experience, it needs to be stressed that these stages overlap considerably and people can travel back and forth between them. Also, I see a secondary pattern emerging in people who are better prepared for death, and this pattern has some quite different elements. It is very useful to be aware of these stages as they help to make sense of our experiences.

DENIAL

"It's all a mistake. This cannot be true! The X-rays were mixed up in the lab." I remember thinking this one myself—for about two seconds! And then I accepted it was for real. Some people become stuck in denial and go from place to place seeking a new opinion. Others just refuse to believe that they have a potentially life-threatening illness.

ANGER

"Why me?" "Why did I get it, why not old George down the road?" Again, some people take this emotion to its extreme and go through a particularly difficult time.

BARGAINING

"If I go back to church regularly, then perhaps I will live another six months." The thing about bargaining is that it involves a fantasy. You may well go to church, find ingredients missing in your life, make changes and recover completely. No sense of bargaining there—just taking appropriate action. Any self-help techniques could be regarded as being bargaining unless the motivation was right.

The point about bargaining techniques is that they are not sustained. Because they are based on fantasy they are not carried through. Genuine self-help techniques are sustainable because they bring results, even if those results do not change the physical situation. It is important with cancer particularly not to view healing as a game of winners and losers with death the end point. Cancer is an intensification of the game of life. In one sense it is a game of winners and losers, but success is marked by wholeness, peace and harmony. This is not a cop-out or rationale to justify death.

I see people who accept their situation and work with it. Incredibly, they often feel death is of far lesser importance than what they are gaining through the process. For most in our groups, this third stage, then, is one of acceptance and commitment and it leads on to taking appropriate action. The acceptance is sustainable and it carries them through getting well or through dying. They can accept life and they commit to doing all they can to live well and to die well.

DEPRESSION

"I don't want to know anyone." People close to dying can go through periods of deep depression where everything is "wrong." In this state they can be very difficult to help and very insular. I feel depression happens when people are beset by the physical reality of their situation and preoccupied with thoughts and fears of their lack of immortality. Often, however, this can be interspersed with moments of great clarity when their spiritual realities appear more real and comforting.

ACCEPTANCE

"It's OK to die." People in this stage may be insular or not, but they are characterized as being at peace. Nearly everyone, it seems, unless they are absolutely overwhelmed by fear or anger, passes through this stage before dying. Physical pain often melts away and there is a great sense of calm. For people who work at it, this stage can be a wonderful peak experience. If shared, it can offer families and friends an experience they are unlikely to get in any other way.

It is as well to realize that friends and relatives can also be involved in this five-stage process. A little of them is dying too as they lose someone near and dear. They, too, can need help to get it right before death. People who exhibit love and faith have death marked by kindness and compassion. People who express bitterness and fear often find confusion and loneliness.

The art of dying well lies in the art of living well.

What Emotions Are Normal?

A wide range. It is common for people to fluctuate between the deep despair of loss and the exalted highs of the spiritual atmosphere that commonly surrounds death.

Most of us find it challenging to help another through a period of grief. It is always an emotionally charged time. What should we say or do? Faced with indecision it would be easy to do nothing. However, by using some simple principles we can be very helpful indeed. The aim is to communicate, to give the grieving person the opportunity to express their thoughts and particularly their feelings, and for you to communicate your care and empathy.

So if someone needs to talk about death do not try to change the subject. Do not make light of it but share in the difficulties it can produce. By being prepared to talk of the person who has died and the situation they face through the loss of that person, you give them the opportunity to express themselves. Often only emotions and feelings will come out and logic may not be a part of the conversation.

Quite often surprising negative emotions may come out. Guilt, anger, despair, even rage, are just as likely to appear as gratitude, acceptance and love. Do not develop an argument by trying to counter negative feelings with positive ones. What is being expressed is an emotional response and if it is not released in the early days after the death, it will remain. Repression of such emotions and feelings may cause bitterness and disillusionment. Frequently this means that your role is to say very little. It is certainly harder to be a listener than a talker and often the grieving person will say the same thing over and over. Often they will be expressing feelings, not logic. Given the opportunity to do this, the feelings will gradually settle, and at the next meeting a more logical discussion of the situation may well be possible. Sometimes the initial talks will lead to tears. Have the courage to let this happen if it is needed because it allows the person to "let go" of their inner tension, and that in turn leads to release.

Honoring the One You Love

There are many ways you can honor the life and memory of someone you love after they die.

- Prayer is common to all traditions and naturally is highly recommended.
- Planting a tree, particularly a deciduous one, both honors the person and reminds us of the cycles of life. Planting many trees is another option.
- In some traditions, freeing fish or animals that were destined to be eaten is valued.
- You can dedicate the merit of projects, or kind acts, or even simply the good thoughts you have to the benefit of the person who has died. You can make donations on their behalf, or simply meditate and wish whatever benefit comes from you doing something useful goes to them.
- If you come from a tradition that believes in reincarnation, these actions are considered to enhance the deceased person's chance of achieving full enlightenment after death, or of experiencing a better rebirth in their next life.

What Can I Do?

Action reinforces your own feelings, so find something to actually do for the grieving person. Whether it be taking around a prepared meal or accompanying them on a day's outing, the physical act shows you really do care. Remember that at the time of a funeral there is always a lot to do and a great deal of support comes forward. However, four to six weeks later, everyone is getting back to their own immediate concerns and it is at this later stage the loss will be most noticed by those closely affected. Make a note on your calendar to call on them and to help your friend to find new interest and directions. Helping them to do things for themselves is a start, but once they are helping others, life is well under way again.

Other Dimensions

One of the more fascinating aspects of dying is the work that has been done on the near-death experience. Raymond Moody in *Life After Life*[32] was one of the first to write of his experiences with people who had been revived after being clinically dead. Their experiences were remarkably similar. These near-death experiences are not only recalled by people with a yen for spiritualism, but by ordinary everyday people. A later study showed that 40 percent of all people who have been clinically dead recounted some or all of these experiences.

First, people who recount these experiences comment on how they were struck by their feelings of calmness and lack of fear. Even people who were involved in severe accidents and suffered serious physical injuries were aware at the time of the accident that they felt no pain. They felt like a calm observer—yes, an observer—standing to one side or, more commonly, looking down on the scene surrounding their physical body. People who have been on operating tables and lapsed into clinical death have often been able to recall the words spoken by the doctors and what was done to revive them. One of our group who experienced this recalled her exasperated doctor saying in the middle of intense efforts to revive her, "Don't give up on me now, you bitch—breathe!" It was a red-faced doctor who verified using those words.

Many have then experienced the sensation of leaving the vicinity of their body and passing down what seems to be a tunnel. It is often a tunnel of light, or there is a light at the end of this tunnel. Again, the feeling is one of comfort and security—not fear. Frequently, there is someone known and loved by the dying person at the other end as if to greet them. It is then, as if they reach a threshold—to pass over it would be irreversible and death would occur. Obviously, people telling these stories came back and usually they felt a compelling reason to do so. They either had unfinished business or a sense of mission. So one of our group, a devout Catholic, got to the end of her tunnel to be met by her deceased grandfather. "You're too early, lass. You have to go back for the children." She recovered from surgery and now has a profound knowing that death is OK.

This is the exciting thing. People who have this near-death experience are left with a feeling of comfort and peace. For them, death is transformed. It is no longer a thing to fear. In fact, it is described as a very pleasant process.

I had an experience like this following my amputation. It seemed to be triggered by an adverse drug reaction and it began with a weird feeling. It was as if my awareness became out of time with my body. I felt like I was outside of my body and that I was watching myself call for a nurse. Then it was as if I was watching someone else trying to explain what was happening, only that someone was me! Then I lost awareness of my surrounds altogether.

I recorded in my diary that I felt as if I was being propelled along a hose in a stream of water. If you have ever pointed a stream of water to the sky on a sunny day and seen the stream break into beads of sparkling light, you will know how I felt. It was as if I reached the end of the hose and had a glimpse of a glorious array of cascading beads of light in an infinite expanse of space. I felt strongly that if I kept going with those beads I would not return. It was a beautiful sight. I took one glimpse and said to myself, "No thanks, not yet," and I actively retreated. Soon my awareness returned to the hospital room.

At the time I wondered if I had hallucinated or had experienced something more. However, the experience having been so real, I felt sure I had been through a genuine experience. It left me knowing that death was OK. It is all very well to rationalize and talk about it, but after an experience like that, you have this inner knowing that death will be OK.

This positive view of death is backed by a philosophy that regards death as an integral part of life. Meditation has enhanced that feeling by adding to my appreciation of spiritual reality. So I would like to think that just as I can celebrate all the other life events, birth, marriage, child rearing, maturity, so I am able to celebrate death. While I accept that remorse, anguish and grief are real and need to be dealt with, I give thanks for life and wish people well in their new phase of it after death. I try not to cling to old memories and so bind people who have new directions to explore. I seek to avoid complications by communicating well with people before they die, seeking to explore the practical issues as well as feelings, thoughts and attitudes.

FINALLY • An Approach to Death

It is well to have the courage to develop a concept of what you think will happen when you die. You might like to meditate and contemplate it. This is not a ghoulish thing, but a useful prerequisite for approaching death in an open way. Again, you do not need a life-threatening illness to gain enormously from this. You will probably find fears well up and it is good to analyze them and use the techniques to let them go. Letting go of attachments is the key.

It is also good to discuss the practical details concerning any preferences you might have for when you do die, especially in case you die unexpectedly. What schools would you prefer the children to attend? Is it intended that outside help come into the family? What about remarriage? And so on. Remember the benefit of sharing the checklist.

Whatever else you do, talk about this vital area. It is probably one of the hardest conversations to get started, but everyone is amazed at how well it flows once it begins. Such sharing leads to increased bonding between families and friends, heightened peace of mind and does a great deal to enhance quality of life. Remember, if you are alive, one day you will die, and none of us know when that will be. So you do not need to have an illness for these conversations to be useful—you just need to be alive and to be interested in living well! In the words of the great impressionist painter Paul Gauguin:

How brief this life,
So little time to prepare for eternity.

Perhaps one of the most beautiful comments around death came from four-and-a-half-year-old Anna. When asked by her mother what she thought had happened when her grandmother died, Anna paused to reflect for a moment and then replied, "Well, Mommy, just the *living part* went out of her."

It occurred to me recently how many people dread the prospect of death. Yet so often the fear of dying inhibits both healing and life itself. To reconcile death, to face it, to integrate it; to be ready to die, is to be ready to live fully. Perhaps this is a feature of survivors—they have faced death, moved through its domain and reemerged to celebrate life. So we aim to become confident, confident to be able to live well and to die well, but not so confident with death that we become blasé and forget how precious this life is— instead we continue to do all we can to make the most of it.

On top of all this it may well be that the moment of death is a moment of delight, filled with mystery and magic—so here is what occurred to me:

The Clear Moment of Death
The moment of death may be the greatest moment of your life
It may be better than the best chocolate sundae you ever had
It may be better than the best orgasm you ever had
It may be better than the dearest, happiest moment you hold in your
   memory
For in that moment of death

The spirit separates from the body
And in that moment
It is free—totally free
If you can grasp that clear moment of death
Recognize it for what it is and experience it fully
Then you will experience fully who you really are
And unite with the mystery and essence of life itself
The only thing that scares me about the moment of death
Is that I may come to it unprepared
To be prepared for the moment of death
I would need to feel that I had lived fully
Loving and learning as much as I could during this lifetime
And feeling free of regrets
To be prepared
I would need to feel that those around me would be all right
That I could let go of my worldly attachments
And that they could release me
To be prepared
I would need to be free of fear
And to have had some glimpse of my own true nature—
Perhaps through the introduction of meditation
Being prepared for that clear moment of death
Then it may well be
That I would be able to recognize what I have been searching for always—
The heart and essence of who I really am.

CHAPTER 19

Your Healing Choices

Principles, Practicalities and Spirituality

HEALING IS ANOTHER INTEGRAL PART OF THE PROCESS OF LIFE ITSELF. IN seeking to understand the healing process we can compare it to a journey between two great cities—one called Disease, the other Health. Disease is known by suffering, separation and restriction; Health by joy, interconnectedness and authenticity. The journey between the two is that of healing.

It would be tempting to say the journey was on a purely physical level and that being free of physical symptoms assured a place in the city of Health. Experience tells us otherwise. We see people of sound body beset by emotional distress and mental anxiety. We see people of no purpose wandering the byways with no direction. We see others racked by physical disease whose inner light shines strong and pure. So, this is a metaphorical journey indeed—a journey of personal evolution.

The paths between any great cities are many and varied; the routes people take between Disease and Health are diverse indeed. It is as if we are born somewhere along that route with our own particular inborn level of health and our own range of talents with which to work. As we grow, we respond to the environment around us. Some of us, it would seem, pass our days being merely bumped along by the external events of life. In what appears to be a waste of a grand opportunity, these people make little progress as their life passes by. Others do move off in search of a better clime, but find no compass to guide them. Often they stumble deep into the city of Disease before realizing they are on the wrong track. Then comes the test—to change direction, to learn to read the map and to head back to the security of Health.

Those brave ones who do dare to tread the path to Health, unprovoked by such a stay in the compelling city of Disease, are the ones in life I admire most. Those who value life and its opportunities, who respect their deeper nature and their body, and work to better it have really grasped the purpose of their life. They are the ones who when you meet them along the path, exude the joy of the search and uplift all they encounter.

The paths between the two cities are as varied as the travelers. There are narrow, winding lanes for those who wish to dally, and wide, direct highways for those with purpose and perseverance. And for some, although few it seems, there are the airports where, spreading wings, it is possible to fly direct to the destination. All along these routes are towns and places of interest. Some are unrewarding, mere dalliances and distractions along the way, while other stops add quality and enrichment.

As the travelers move along the separate routes, their paths often cross. When they do, it may appear to the passing individuals as if they are heading in opposite directions. Without the benefit of a grander map they might be tempted to say the other was wrong in pursuing such a course, exclaiming, "You are going in the wrong direction. Follow me. My way is the right, my way is the best, my way is the only path to Health." However, those with a grander vision acknowledge their fellow seekers and bless them as they move on their way, for direction comes with discovering that this is more than a physical quest.

Disease: "dis-ease." The word says it all—lack of ease, lack of balance, lack of harmony. Health is harmony and the purpose of life is to seek harmony on all levels of our being—physical, emotional, mental and spiritual.

The further we journey, the more we realize that we are responsible for our own position on the map of life, and that we must accept this responsibility. We see that life has a pattern and we are an integral part of it. We are intimately involved with the complex pattern of events that has resulted in us being in our current situation. Maturity comes with finding our position on the map and accepting that position. Then, if we are strong enough not to indulge in looking back with guilt or regret, we can chart our own course and take the first steps toward Health.

Some of us find it hard to accept responsibility for being in our present position. Particularly if physical disease is evident, it is far easier to blame something or someone else for our own misfortune and so to feel a victim of circumstances. But some time, somewhere, the realization dawns and we appreciate that the pattern of the life we have been leading has determined our current circumstances. We *are* responsible, just as we can be in control.

If our past pattern has produced the symptoms of disease, and now we are seeking to reestablish health, we must be brave enough to look for a change in direction. Change is required to establish the pattern that leads to Health. Some can make that change almost instantaneously. With the speed of jet travel they can relocate themselves in new and happy surroundings. For most, however, the journey becomes a process, the healing process. It develops as a series of changes that gradually lead to the place of their dreams. Commonly, the first steps are superficial ones and there is a preoccupation with the obvious physical steps that need to be taken. So, people with illness journey to places of physical treatment, change their diet and begin to exercise. These outer things are easy to start with, easy to work on. As they come under control, the effort becomes more profound. The inner work begins. The need to change fundamental attitudes and direction becomes apparent. To change just one really basic trait for the better is a major accomplishment for any lifetime.

So, where is the map? Where is the compass? What can guide us through this maze? In essence it really is very simple. Once our basic course is realigned with harmony, once harmony is the prime motivation, then healing is under way. The more harmony in our actions, attitudes and spirit, the better our quality of life and the closer we move toward that wonderful city of Health.

Harmony comes with peace of mind, so as we seek peace of mind, we seek Health. If, at every step along the way, peace of mind is the basic criterion that must be satisfied, then each and every step will be a good one—one that takes us in the right direction. To begin with, the physical may lag behind, but in terms of inner development, once harmony is the aim and peace of mind the governing principle, then progress is surely under way.

In fact, once we are free of physical symptoms we often discover that the journey has only just begun. While many find that healing their physical ailments does bring great personal spiritual growth, they soon realize that the true aim of the process of healing is really synonymous with the aim of the process of life itself—to seek harmony on all levels. Their spirit leads the way and often aspires to journey beyond the place where their physical and psychological reality dwells and works.

So, often this journey takes us out of familiar territory, out of our comfort zone. This journey has the potential to produce tension, a tension of growth, as the spirit leads the personality toward its goal. If this tension is creative, the path runs smoothly. If the personality lags or resists, then bumps abound. When the prime motivation is peace of mind, the journey to Health is steady indeed.

The means to Health, the paths of healing, run on many levels and are extremely varied. To clarify the map a little we can summarize some of these many varied routes.

YOUR HEALING CHOICES

When we seek healing for ourselves or someone we love, what are our options? It must be obvious that a book like this can neither give specific advice, nor should it even attempt to do so. Sorting out your own particular needs requires specialized advice. What follows is merely an introductory overview of some of the possibilities. If you feel drawn to a particular area, then seek help from the appropriate qualified practitioner.

Let us review the choices systematically. There are three main areas of treatment and support we need to consider. Please note that it is important to use the right words to describe the specific area of treatment or support you are engaging with. Unfortunately, these descriptive words are often used loosely, with little attention to their real meaning. In my opinion there is a compelling need to use the words more accurately; particularly to know that what is advocated in this book is not "alternative" medicine, it is not even "complementary" medicine (although it does complement all other forms of therapy)—it is lifestyle medicine.

In the sections that follow, we will examine the three main avenues for healing, define our terms, clarify the concepts and discuss the options.

CONVENTIONAL MEDICINE

Conventional or orthodox medicine generally describes medical interventions that are taught at medical schools, are generally provided at hospitals, and that meet the requirement of peer-accepted mainstream medicine and standards of care. The main focus in the conventional treatment of cancer is on:

Surgery

Surgery is the first line of mainstream treatment for the majority of cancers and is associated with many people returning to their normal life expectancy. Surgery may well be crucial and directly lifesaving in some cases, as in the case where a bowel cancer may be causing an obstruction. But surgery also takes a load off the body, immediately reducing the burden of the cancer, freeing the body to regenerate and providing a better opportunity to prevent recurrences. Surgery is best used when tumors can be removed en masse, leaving nothing behind. When surgery is supported by a healthy lifestyle, it seems to have little significant adverse effect on the immune system. Surgery makes good sense for many cancers, especially where it is relatively straightforward.

Chemotherapy

The side effects need to be weighed against the benefits. In some situations chemotherapy can be effective, but quality of life can suffer and the balance needs to be watched. Many people these days have an inflated notion of how helpful chemotherapy actually is. There is good evidence that chemotherapy improves five-year survival rates for twenty-two of the major cancers by an average of less than 3 percent.[33] More detail of this is available on my website,[34] but this well-documented, evidence-based information comes with a word of caution. While chemotherapy can be quite useful for some childhood cancers and some of the less common adult cancers, and while there is more positive science regarding the potential benefits of what you can do for yourself, it is worth observing some people find some of the statistics relating to chemotherapy distressing and prefer not to know about them.

To my mind, if chemotherapy offers real benefit compared to any side effects, then it makes sense to consider it seriously. But the question should be "Why would I have chemotherapy?," rather than "Why wouldn't I have chemotherapy?" In other words, you need to be convinced it is in your best interests.

Radiation

This is often used to reduce pain and can do so, particularly when bone is involved. It is effective as a treatment in a limited number of situations, but personally, is my least favored form of treatment due to the potential long-term side effects. In recent years, radiation treatments have become more localized, more targeted, and so are relatively safer than they used to be.

Immunotherapy and Other "Biologically Elegant" Therapies

This is a rapidly developing area in conventional medicine. For example, monoclonal antibodies that aim to stimulate the immune system can be helpful in some cases. Angiostatins are new drugs that have the potential to halt the development of new blood vessels and starve the cancer.

Hormonal Therapy

Some tumors can be hormone responsive; for example, some breast cancers and prostate cancers.

NATURAL MEDICINE • Three Main Components

Complementary Medicine

In the United States, the National Center for Complementary and Alternative Medicine (NCCAM), defines complementary and alternative medicine (CAM) as a group of diverse medical and health care systems, practices and products that are not presently considered to be part of conventional medicine, as defined by medical peers.

The diversity of these therapies does make them difficult to categorize as a group, yet they are often collectively referred to as complementary, alternative, lifestyle, integrative, unorthodox, unconventional, unproven, natural, traditional and holistic medicine, and are contrasted with conventional, mainstream, allopathic, orthodox and scientific medicine. Hence the need to define our terms.

NCCAM classifies CAM into five categories or domains.

ALTERNATIVE MEDICAL SYSTEMS

Alternative medical systems are built upon complete systems of theory and practice such as homeopathic and naturopathic medicine, traditional Chinese medicine and Ayurveda.

MIND-BODY INTERVENTIONS

These interventions include patient support groups, cognitive-behavioral therapy, meditation, prayer, spiritual healing and therapies that use creative outlets such as art, music or dance.

BIOLOGICALLY BASED THERAPIES

These therapies include the use of herbs, foods, vitamins, minerals and dietary supplements.

MANIPULATIVE AND BODY-BASED METHODS

These methods include therapeutic massage, shiatsu, chiropractic and osteopathy.

ENERGY THERAPIES

These therapies involve the use of energy fields, They are of two types:

- Biofield therapies such as qigong, Reiki and therapeutic touch.
- Bioenergetic therapies involving the use of electromagnetic fields, such as pulsed fields, magnetic fields or alternating current and direct current fields.

You will notice how some of the above modalities such as nutrition and meditation are what we will define soon as lifestyle therapies. Also, unlike in America, where complementary medicine and alternative medicine are linked and the acronym CAM is used all the time, in Australia, the term "alternative medicine" is used by many in the medical profession in such a negative way that complementary medicine and alternative medicine tend to be spoken of quite separately.

Specifically then, complementary medicine has been defined as any therapeutic practice that does not satisfy the standards of the majority of the orthodox medical community, that is not taught widely at medical schools, and that is not generally available at hospitals.

However, even this definition creates some difficulty as these days many medical schools—both in Australia and overseas—offer courses in complementary medicine and many hospitals provide complementary therapies.

Although there is growing evidence that a number of complementary therapies can be safe and helpful in cancer management, particularly in the area of symptom control, there are a number of legitimate concerns regarding the use of CAM among cancer patients.

These concerns include:

- Heightened concerns for vulnerable cancer patients and families
- The suggestion of false hope
- The potential for monetary exploitation
- Delayed use of effective conventional treatments
- Little scientific evidence for some therapies
- Potential dangers, interactions and side effects
- Poor training and regulation of some practitioners

Of course, these issues are just as relevant for the conventional cancer care as they are for complementary therapies and lifestyle factors. When it comes to the evidence, it is clear that the side effects reported from complementary therapies are far less in number and far less serious in nature when compared to the side effects reported from conventional cancer therapies.

Traditional Medicine

Traditional medicine includes well-documented or otherwise established medicine or therapies that are based upon the accumulated experience of many traditional health care practitioners over an extended period of time.

The Therapeutic Goods Administration (TGA) in Australia provides a specific definition: "Traditional use refers to documentary evidence that a substance has been used over three or more generations of recorded use for a specific health related or medicinal purpose."

Traditional therapies include traditional Chinese medicine (TCM), Ayurvedic medicine (from India), Tibetan medicine, western herbal medicine, homeopathic medicine, indigenous medicines, and aromatherapy. These traditional medical systems represent a different paradigm of health care when compared to conventional Western medicine.

Alternative Medicine

This is the domain of what is sometimes described as unorthodox or unconventional or unproven medicine or therapies. Alternative medicine generally describes medical interventions that are not widely taught at medical schools, not generally provided at hospitals, and are outside peer-accepted mainstream medicine and standards of care. The strong implication, or even fact, is that these therapies are not supported by a significant Western medical research base.

Examples could include aromatherapy, intravenous chelation and vitamin C, ozone therapy and psychic surgery. There are many of these therapies, and they are often difficult to evaluate and they need to be considered with due caution.

Lifestyle Medicine

Lifestyle medicine is defined rather formally as the application of environmental, behavioral, medical and motivational principles to the management of lifestyle-related health problems in the clinical setting.

In practice, lifestyle medicine is concerned with what a person can do for themselves in the context of their daily life. By contrast, there are all the things that could be done to or for you under the banner of conventional, complementary, traditional or alternative medicine. Lifestyle medicine focuses on what you can do for yourself. The other approaches involve either a therapy provided by a therapist (whether that be surgery, acupuncture or a massage) or a compound you take (that could include antibiotics, chemotherapy, supplements or herbs).

Lifestyle factors or therapies include physical factors such as nutrition (food, fluids and juices), exercise, exposure to sunlight and creative activities. They also utilize mind-body interventions that can include psychosocial activities, group therapy, mind training (positive thinking, affirmation, imagery), meditation, yoga, qigong, tai chi, healthy emotions (relationships, communication, laughter, forgiveness, etc.), personal development and transformation. Lifestyle factors also encompass spiritual pursuits such as exploring meaning and purpose in life, prayer, spiritual healing, religious practice and spiritual development.

Lifestyle medicine forms the substance of this book and a summary of recommendations makes up chapter 21.

INTEGRATIVE MEDICINE • Healing in the Balance

Let us be clear now. Conventional medicine, traditional medicine and CAM focus on things that are done to you or for you. Lifestyle medicine focuses on the things you do for yourself. While some may choose to do only one or the other, it has always been my contention that it is wise to bring together, to integrate, the best of all that is available. I am committed to using what works best. Integrative medicine is the answer.

Integrative medicine is defined as the blending of conventional, natural and complementary medicines and/or therapies with the aim of using the most appropriate of either or both modalities to care for the patient as a whole. Integrative medicine considers the person's body, emotions, mind and spirit. Integrative medicine is open to integrating the services of a wide range of health practitioners and modalities in a way that is often described as holistic medicine.

Integrative medicine, therefore, is an umbrella term. In fact, integrative medicine is what good medicine always was. It takes account of the health, healing and well-being of the whole person and it works cooperatively within an interdisciplinary environment to draw on all means possible to achieve the best results possible.

THE TRUE NATURE OF HEALING • A Personal View

How wonderful it would be to fully recover physically from cancer. My wish is that everyone diagnosed with cancer has this experience. How then do we best set about healing a diseased body? If disharmony is the root cause, obviously anything that re-creates harmony will have a healing effect. However, if there is obvious physical disease, the symptoms may be so severe and so physical, it may not be possible for those involved to normalize the situation using only the energies available through subtler avenues. Often it is necessary to alleviate the immediate situation with surgery and purely physical medicine, just to ensure a continuation of life.

This is a fine balance to strike. Physical treatments are tried and proven and will have a place for a long time, a fact often overlooked by overzealous advocates of alternative medicine. But it is important to remember that it *is* physical medicine and frequently does not go beyond the treatment of the physical symptoms. Once the physical situation is stabilized, it becomes important to turn the attention to the underlying causes and their correction to effect a complete cure. Is being physically well enough?

Surely, we all know people in good physical health who are otherwise miserable—grumpy, bitter, angry, resentful, unhappy relationships all around. There are plenty of people for whom emotional healing seems like a distant dream. For them, to be emotionally well would be wonderful and there is no denying that, but would it be enough just to have good emotional health?

Leading health authorities claim over 20 percent of the population in countries like Australia and the United States suffer from a diagnosable mental illness in any one year. Twenty percent! That is one in five. For those people who are perhaps dealing with anxiety, confusion, mood or personality disorders, depression and so on, to be well in their mind would be marvelous, and that too is true. But is even that, even being mentally well, enough?

Clearly it would be wonderful to have a fit body, healthy emotions and a sound mind, but there is more to life—more to being really well, more to being fully happy. There is the spiritual dimension to consider.

One way to consider this is to contemplate what does bring happiness and contentment into our lives. Many people rely on things outside of themselves or the people around them for their happiness. If the kids are happy, I am happy. If people are speaking well of me, are being kind to me, I am happy. If work is going well, if the bank balance is OK, I am happy. If I have the right house, the right car, the right partner, then of course I am happy. Or am I?

What we can observe is that the people and the things around us can change; often at times and in ways that are both unexpected and seriously inconvenient as it may seem. So relationships change, finances change, status changes—everything around us has the clear potential to change.

So while it is true that having nice things around us and being in the company of nice people is pleasant and a cause for some happiness, if we are solely dependent on the things outside of us and the people around us for our happiness, we will always be vulnerable. Life changes; people change, move on or die; fortunes fluctuate. Many diagnosed with cancer know this to be all too true. However, take heart. There is a deeply comforting answer. Lasting happiness, enduring happiness, is a very real possibility. Clearly, lasting happiness is a state of mind. The answer to real happiness is not to be found outside of us. The answer to real happiness resides within us. The quest for real happiness leads to the spiritual path.

SPIRITUAL HEALING • The Quest for True Happiness and Good Values

Many people I have worked with found their cancer diagnosis profoundly challenged their spiritual view. Many with an established conviction found that conviction deeply disturbed, while others of little conviction found their thoughts turning to their church once again. The Bible is very clear on this. There is no need for guilt, no need to hesitate. The Prodigal Son story is definite. Any time is a good time to return home. If disease and difficulty does take someone back to their spirituality, that gives added meaning and benefit to the initial suffering.

However, while many people are passionately interested in their spiritual life, not everyone is interested in a formal religion. There is a significant difference between spirituality and religion. Religion is how we express our spirituality within the context of a particular system of faith and worship. Spirituality is to do with finding inner peace, finding meaning in our life and developing good human values. One would always hope that spirituality played a major part in religion, but clearly, spirituality can exist outside of religion.

While the primary motivation for entering the spiritual path may be to seek real happiness, the primary outcomes from following the spiritual path are to enhance our human values, to make ourselves into better human beings and to serve humanity.

All the great religious traditions have at their core this quest to find true happiness, to find meaning in life, and the desire to cultivate positive human values. All share the potential to fulfill that quest. However, because people are different, it is natural that different religions, different paths toward this same end will fit with some people more closely than with others. The best religion for any one of us will be whatever religion takes us most directly, most reliably to that inner happiness and helps us to become kinder, more useful people.

Unfortunately, in modern times many are disenchanted with the answers and the direction they receive on these matters from formal religions. Many are looking deeply in their own way. Seeking more than dogma, they want logical and compelling answers. They want practical and effective techniques and prefer to pursue their spirituality in a general sense rather than through a religion specifically.

What is clear is that the practice of a given religion is not essential to being a good, honest and sincere person. Indeed, there is plenty of evidence that tells us the practice of a given religion does not always ensure being a good, honest and sincere person. By contrast, it is almost impossible to consciously pursue the spiritual path and to not become a better, more honest and more sincere person.

When we are ready, the task for each of us is to find and to follow our own spiritual path. Of course, this may or may not be focused via a religious path. What is clear is that many I speak to say that cancer provoked their spiritual inquiry and practice. They report that doing so helped to make sense of their cancer, and that their spiritual development became a major reason why they express some gratitude for the cancer. Many feel that their most significant healing actually took place in their spiritual lives.

So, aspiring to inner peace, happiness and good human values is easy to understand. What of meaning?

There are three big philosophical questions that need to be satisfied on the spiritual path. Where did I come from? Who am I? and Where am I going? As in, what was I, or what was going on before I was born, what meaning and purpose is there in this life I am experiencing now, and what will happen after I die?

To explore these questions, one way to begin is that we could say spirituality addresses the gap between how things appear to be and how they really are. So I could be described as the son of my parents, father of my children, husband to my wife. In some of my various daily activities I could be described as teacher, a student, a health educator, an entrepreneur, a researcher. There are so many designations or names that can be assigned to the many and varied roles I fulfill and are all summed up in my name, Ian Gawler. You might like to take a lighthearted pause and consider all the "titles" that you function under from time to time. However, if all these are stripped away, who are you, really? What is in your heart's essence? What is your true nature?

These questions have been active in my own mind since I can remember. The answers I had already came to informed the way I managed my leg being amputated and my health descending into the depths before I recovered. Courtesy of the intensity of that recovery process and then courtesy of working with thousands of others exploring the meaning and purpose of life, more insights followed. In the spirit of sharing human experience and gently provoking your own spiritual inquiry and development, my biography *The Dragon's Blessing* authored by Guy Allenby,[35] documents some of those insights, along with the life events they were associated with and their observable consequences.

RECOMMENDATIONS FOR THE SPIRITUAL PATH

Making progress along the spiritual path is like learning or progressing in any field of endeavor. It requires study and practice. This is like the wings of a bird. If a bird only has one wing, it flaps around in circles in a pretty unhappy state. To fly, a bird needs two functional wings.

To develop our spirituality, first we need to study. Many gain great benefit from reading and from attending lectures, conferences or retreats. When the time comes, an authentic teacher will deepen all this. But clearly we then need to practice. This book is full of directions, and here is a specific summary for the spiritual path.

Value Your Spiritual Life

- Recognize the importance of your inner life. I have known people who died profoundly healed. Their bodies may have been weak, but the strength of their spirit was extraordinary.
- Give time for your spiritual life. Be gentle on yourself. Allow time for reading, for reflection, for daydreaming, for formal contemplation and meditation. Make time for this.
- Consider how you can be supported on the spiritual path. Who are your spiritual friends? Who do you discuss these matters with? Is there a group

to attend that nourishes you spiritually? What about professionals like a counselor with a spiritual focus, or even a spiritual teacher?

- Aim to be authentic. More and more, seek consistency between your inner and outer lives.
- Do be aware that often there are more questions than answers, particularly as we first turn our thoughts inward. Be comfortable with the mysteries, hold the questions—be patient.

Be Ethical, Avoid Harm

As much as possible, take your spiritual values into daily life and reflect these values in what you do, how you speak and how you think. It is a fact that a well-developed spiritual view will lead to a healthy, healing lifestyle. This is something to delight in—the fact that being motivated by good ethics leads to healthy eating and drinking takes us away from smoking, drugs and excesses in life, and takes us toward a healthy sex life and satisfying work.

Train the Mind

Everything in this arena makes sense. Consider what is helpful and most immediate to meet your needs. Consider:

- Affirmations and imagery—based upon understanding how the mind works and how we can use it intelligently to good effect.
- Psychotherapy, CBT and counseling—for when more personal help is wise.
- Practicing and developing:
  - **Generosity:** Learn how to give and let go.
  - **Discipline:** This is the discipline of kindness, doing what is kind to you and to others.
  - **Patience:** This is the quality of not being upset by others; it is the quality of spiritual endurance.
  - **Diligence:** This is like discipline but is better described as finding joy or delight, being enthusiastic about doing what is good for you.
  - **Meditation:** Recognize the difference between therapeutic and spiritual meditation. Do some regular meditation with a spiritual focus.
  - **Wisdom:** Develop your spiritual view. Aim to see things as they really are.

Deepen Your View

The way to take a spiritual theory into practice and embody it in your life involves three steps.

LISTEN AND LEARN

This is how we acquire new knowledge. Maybe we read, or we listen to teachers; we take things in with our intellect and develop some understanding.

CONTEMPLATE

To advance a theory, to deepen our understanding, we benefit from sitting quietly, relaxing and then focusing our mind on the topic at hand. This helps us to think things through thoroughly, but then it leads to deeper understanding, insight and even revelation.

INTEGRATION

Contemplation takes a theory down from our head into our body. We come to embody what we know.

So we repeat this process; we listen and learn, we contemplate and we integrate. The more we do this, the more we become authentic, the more consistency there will be between our spiritual view and our worldly life. One very good measure of profound healing and true health is this measure of our authenticity.

Coming back to our old friend death, when we die what will be most important is what sort of life we lived and the state of our mind. Authenticity is one of the best gauges of all this.

My wish is that you lead an authentic life. My wish is that you live a long and happy life!

Oh, and if all else fails, you might like to do what my old friend Barry the ophthalmologist recommends. Barry says when all else fails it is time to reach for the Viagra eye drops. You know them? They are really good for when you need to take a long, hard look at yourself!

And there is a moral to his recommendation—lighten up. While all of this is extremely important, do remember your sense of humor.

A FINAL WORD ON HEALING

So balance in all things. Start with the immediate things. Define your medical treatment plan. Attend to your lifestyle right at the start and then, once there is some stability, consider the other options. Chapter 21 provides a summary of all the options and a suggested pathway, but first, the more radical side of healing.

CHAPTER 20

The Sealed Section

The Special Case of Subtle-Energy Medicine

THERE MAY BE VALUE IN TAKING SOMETHING OF A RISK AND SHARING SOME of the experiences I had with subtle-energy medicine, with paranormal healing phenomena, and particularly psychic surgery in the Philippines. First, it is widely known that I have benefited from such treatments and I am sure this needs clarifying. Second, psychic phenomena are most intriguing. If they can be shown to be genuine in just one instance, the implications are vast indeed. I find it a fascinating area.

Warning: If this field of endeavor or this type of conjecture is not to your taste, please do not be put off by it. Having had remarkable experiences, I seek to explain them. If I do not do so adequately, that is my shortcoming. The other more concrete things covered in the book to this point stand in their own right, and in my experience are fully justifiable. What follows is the product of experience, reading, conjecture and contemplation. It may shed some light on what to me is a truly wonderful area—the mysterious area of subtle energy healing. But if this is of no interest, simply move on to the next chapter.

It is interesting to note how many types of paranormal phenomena are cropping up today, and the interest they are producing. Debate on psychic surgery has been intense for quite a few years. Reports of miraculous cures have been countered with claims of quackery, sleight of hand and the use of chicken's blood and tissues of nonhuman origin. People like Uri Geller have bent spoons and started clocks. At the same time, the Russians experiment with psychokinesis, that is, moving objects using psychic energy alone without touching them. If these things are talked of openly, what experiments are going on in secret?

In the healing arena, Kirlian photography is being used to distinguish between healthy and diseased tissues. A sophisticated technique of photography, it reveals what is claimed to be the health aura. Clairvoyant healers now, and in ages gone by, have claimed to be able to see this subtle energy emanating from their patients. Acupuncture has been accepted into the conventional treatment repertoire despite there being no conventionally accepted explanation for its means of action.

We are getting a lot of hints, demonstrations of the possibilities. Frequently, patients in dire need are being drawn by such phenomena, sometimes turning their backs on conventional treatments. Patients can see that there are practical benefits to be gained. But there is a great need for balance—the ability to decide what to do and when.

So far we have been doing just this. We have been considering the patient's role in cancer and what they can do to help themselves back to health. While the principles of diet, positive thinking and nutrition break enough new ground for some, the area of psychic surgery introduces us to a whole new frontier.

A PERSONAL ACCOUNT

When my leg was amputated in 1975 with bone cancer (osteogenic sarcoma), there had been no other sign of the cancer. It reappeared, however, and secondary cancer was diagnosed later that year. I was told that the medical options of chemotherapy and radiation were not likely to improve my chances of living more than another three to six months and that they would have unpleasant side effects. No medical treatment was recommended, while at the same time I was told the cancers were likely to double in size every month.

Concentrating on meditation and diet, I saw no growth at all over the first three months. Then, through a combination of factors, mostly to do with my trying to do too much each day and so creating new stresses, I deteriorated rapidly. Initially the searing pain of sciatica running down my left side restricted my mobility. Then my weight fell away and I was confined to bed. Finally, it was confirmed that my right kidney was obstructed and severely swollen. I had reached my lowest point.

In desperation, my first wife, Grace, and I left for the Philippines in March 1976. I weighed a little more than 84 pounds, compared to my

normal 126 pounds (I was around 168 pounds before having my leg amputated). My color was likened to that of a jaundiced custard. Pain forced me
to lie down except when it was absolutely necessary to move.

We were motivated by the conviction I would still recover, but knew little
of what to expect. I had heard of the Filipino healers from several people,
notably an aunt and friends who had helped to introduce me to the dietary
regime some months earlier. They had provided the address of one healer,
one young Filipino boy whom they thought might be helpful, and one hotel.
While excited by the possibilities, and open to them, I was basically skeptical
and certainly critical in my approach to healers. The first thing I did in the
Philippines was to buy a movie camera. If I was to be tricked, I wanted to
record it.

Two days after arriving, I had my first operation performed by a small,
shy Filipino healer. Traveling to his house early in the morning, we were met
by his cousin who doubled as business manager. He told me that after the
treatment I was to return to my hotel and rest a few hours. For twenty-four
hours I was not to bathe or drink coffee, alcohol or carbonated drinks. He
also took twenty-two dollars from us, the amount this healer charged in
those days. It was the first and last time we were asked for money.

Most of the healers work on a donation-only system. Most are very simple people of peasant background with a strong Roman Catholic influence.
They are not used to handling large sums of money. They say they are using
a God-given power and accept what goods or money their patients can offer
in return. Those few who did charge large amounts seemed to have become
preoccupied with material things and found their healing powers had waned.
However, they were the exceptions, not the rule.

After the formalities, I was ushered into the operating theater. This was a
small bare room with a large wooden table to one side. The healer stood at its
center, flanked by two assistants. At his feet were two buckets. One was used
as a repository for the bits and pieces that were removed, the other contained
already bloodied water and was used for washing hands between operations.
There was no pretense of sterile technique. We later learned that the healers
have been shown to be able to destroy disease-causing organisms by merely
passing their hands over them.

This day, there was no preamble. I was asked to strip to my shorts, to lie
back down on the table, and to pray as best I knew. Under the circumstances,

it was easy! The healer moved forward and quickly entered my abdomen with his fingers. He held his hands together, with fingers outstretched and just overlapping a little. I felt a pop, as when you poke a finger through a stretched rubber balloon. Grace was called over for a better look. As the healer pulled his hands apart she could see the lining of my peritoneal cavity and the tumor inside my pelvis. He then continued by taking some fresh tissue, similar to loose connective tissue, from the area. Blood welled up from within the incision, while there did not seem to be any bleeding from the skin itself. He finished by withdrawing his fingers, leaving a small pool of blood on my skin. When this was wiped away there was no scar visible. The performance was repeated in several other places and then I was unceremoniously told to get dressed and to return the next day. It had all taken five minutes.

I was excitedly asking Grace what she had seen as we returned to our hotel where I reluctantly agreed to lie down for a short rest. I slept extremely heavily for the next three hours, and after lunch I had another unexpected reaction. All my joints began to ache, one after another. I felt nauseous and colicky, and my head began to spin. As these symptoms became more severe, I began thinking my surgeon's gloomy predictions about my death might prove correct after all.

However, the Filipino boy, who soon showed that he had wisdom far beyond his years, was familiar with the problem, and said this frequently occurred. He explained that the healers were able to mobilize the body's own defenses. Once this process was set in motion, it frequently produced a classic healing reaction with an intensification of some or all of the patient's symptoms. Chronic conditions are often brought to a head and after a short, acute episode, healing progresses.

After a very uncomfortable twelve hours and a good night's sleep, I did, in fact, feel a great deal better. Within two days I had flushed all my analgesics down the toilet. Pain relief is a common sequel to this type of treatment and I am sure this is due to both a physical and psychological benefit. The healers are very aware of the psychological impact of this visually dramatic procedure. They recognized that if a patient believes the disease they have is normally considered to be terminal, then it takes something quite out of the normal to change that belief system and replace it with positive healing thoughts. They happily admit that their healing relies on its psychological impact as well as its physical effects.

We stayed on for four weeks and visited five healers during our first trip. Some people seek help from just one healer—others, like me, go to more. There are no set rules and it is important for the patient to accept responsibility for their own decisions and be guided by their own thoughts and feelings. The effects must also be put into perspective.

I returned from the first trip about 13 pounds heavier in weight, with no pain and with good mobility. My surgeon was amazed by the improvement. While there was no decrease in the actual cancer, there was no doubt my general condition had improved dramatically. He said he could not understand it, and that there was no medical explanation to account for it.

I continued to meditate and develop my dietary program, as well as pursue any other avenue that might help keep this healing process going. Soon our movie films were back and they confirmed what we had seen with our own eyes. It appeared that I had been operated on without anesthetic or instrument. I had felt no pain, although I had bled and tissue had been removed. No scar remained as a visible sign of the procedures, but above all else, I had improved. *Something* had happened.

If just once a healer's hand, even a finger, had gone through my skin under these conditions, then my view of reality, my knowledge of physics and how surgery was possible, was quite inadequate to explain it.

SEEKING ANSWERS

There are three choices anyone faces when considering such an extraordinary phenomenon:

- It is a trick to be discounted.
- It is a miracle to be merely marveled at and thankful for.
- It is a genuine phenomenon that requires an explanation.

The history of physics is marked by the development of new theories that were required to justify previously unexplained phenomena. Whether it be Archimedes' "Eureka!" in his bath, or Einstein's theory of relativity, all of physics has been a product of our attempts to explain the world as we observe and experience it.

I feel sure that the current wave of interest in psychic phenomena is really prompting us to look again at the nature of the world around us. The real message of the Filipinos is to offer a psychic signpost to a new awareness. For, if it is genuine—as I have come to believe it is—then it forces us either to take the easy way out and dismiss it as a miracle, or be brave and reconsider the nature of matter and the power of the mind.

THE NATURE OF MATTER

Most of us accept matter as being solid and finite. We sit on a chair and it feels solid enough. It looks solid. We tap it and it reassures us further by sounding solid. No doubt it has a taste and smell to add to its claims to solidity. But is it? What is it made of, really?

For it is the evidence of our five senses that we are relying on to call the chair solid. These five senses of touch, sight, hearing, taste and smell are very helpful for us in day-to-day situations, but they have quite a limited range when compared to our modern precision instruments. If the wavelength of light our eyes registered was just a little wider, we would all have X-ray vision. Imagine the difference just that one small change would have. Our view of reality would be transformed! And how often do we "see" something, take it to be real, and only find out later we were mistaken?

So if we want to understand the nature of matter, we go to modern physics with all its marvelous technology. As the physicists analyze matter they look more closely at it, probing it with the aid of microscope, electron microscope and mathematical theory.

Most of us would be familiar with one of the results—the atomic concept of matter. The atom is a model for the ultimate building block. These building blocks are combined like pieces of a child's interlocking building game to form all the substances we know.

The atom is represented as having a central nucleus with electrons circling it in orbit, much like the planets as they orbit the sun. But, if we enlarge an atom to a size to which we can relate, we see just how "holey" matter really is. For, if we represent that central nucleus by a pea about one-quarter inch across, then, on that scale, the nearest electron would be the same pea-size; it would be 575 feet away and it would be going at the incredible speed of 1,242 miles per hour! Can there be all that space in what we consider to be solid? It has been calculated that if all the space was taken out of the atoms which make up the human body, the resulting mass would be smaller in size than a pin's head!

And it does not even stop there, for now the physicists have probed the atom still further. First they thought the nucleus and electrons were made of smaller and even smaller particles of solid matter. But now they say something even more startling. There is nothing solid there at all. The atom is merely the product of concentrated energy. *Matter is concentrated energy.*

We all know Einstein's famous equation, E=mc2. But we seem to fall short of grasping its implications. E stands for energy, m for mass, and c for the speed of light. The equation is saying that mass, or matter, is a product of energy and light—as esoteric a statement as formulated by any ancient sage.

This, to me, is the most remarkable thing of all. The modern physicists are becoming the New Age philosophers. For, as they probe deeper into the nature of matter, they are forced to investigate energy and so seek to understand it. For, if all matter is made of energy, what makes the difference? Why does one "block" of energy come together to build a rock, another a tree, and another me?

The brave few physicists in the vanguard, who once more are prepared to ask that most vital question, "Why?" Why does energy take the multitude of forms that it does? these physicists are forced to introduce another concept—that of consciousness. They say that it is consciousness that actually produces the energy we are talking of, and that it is then this energy which is interpreted by our five senses as the thing we call matter.

CONSCIOUSNESS, ENERGY AND MATTER

What a concept! Consciousness produces energy; energy produces matter. Thought precedes form. Thought produces form! It leaves me concluding that my physical form is the result of the sum total of my consciousness. I must presume, therefore, that I and all those around me are all essentially reflections of our overall consciousness. Further, given our highly ordered world, I must presume an all-pervading, interconnected consciousness to provide the basic framework in which it all happens.

Most humans have a similar view of reality—the world, as each one knows it, is basically similar. We interpret and respond to a basic universal energy pattern. Within this matrix we radiate our own sphere of influence—

project our own thoughts and energies and so adjust the picture. For those capable of generating novel thought and projecting it with power, the whole picture can change at will. Reality is limited by our ability to conceive its possibilities.

Can we then understand more of the true nature of man? How can we formulate a model that takes into account these ideas of matter being consciousness and which also accounts for the phenomenon of the familiar physical world?

Why does some vast, all-pervading consciousness create the energy patterns that combine to produce the things we call atoms, which in turn combine in varied ways to produce the many things we call matter? And what, then, sparks this matter to produce a living organism with consciousness in its own right? And given all that, why do we see so much disease? We are now getting to the basic questions to which healers and patients seek to find answers as they attempt to formulate a basic paradigm within which to approach disease and its treatment.

Presently, all forms of paranormal phenomena are coming under scrutiny in the West. Parapsychology is an emerging science wrestling with these questions, but as yet no unifying principles have been commonly accepted.

However, if we turn to Eastern thought and metaphysics, there is a recurring model that both makes sense of the phenomena and provides a framework in which to operate.

Most major civilizations have had a tradition of an esoteric science in their culture. Being esoteric, it was hidden from the mainstream of the people but used by those initiated into its secrets in a very practical way. Despite the diversity of cultures, there is a remarkable agreement on basic principles. Even more remarkably, these principles relate to the concepts now being put forward by the modern physicists.

In the esoteric lore of the Ancient Egyptians, Chinese and Greeks, the Indians of North America and the Incas of the South American continent, the Polynesian Kahunas and Filipino healers, the Vedic seers of India, the early Christians and, more recently, the medieval alchemists and mystics of Europe, we find this recurring vision of man. It is esoteric in nature but still it is used in a very practical way. All these people saw man's physical body as being the end result of a series of interrelated and interdependent subtle levels of consciousness.

LEVELS OF CONSCIOUSNESS

Basically, they saw man as being the sum total of seven levels of consciousness. To each level is assigned the form of an energy body. Only the energy of the physical body is dense enough to register immediately with the five senses and hence with the direct perception of another person. The other energy bodies can only be deduced by inference or perceived directly by clairvoyant or extrasensory perception. If we consider the emotional—or astral level, as it is frequently called—then I might think you are happy because I can see you smile and hear you laugh, but this does not mean I am appreciating your emotions directly or accurately. You may be putting on a front. A clairvoyant, however, might be able to see your emotional body directly, say in terms of subtle color emanations, and so have a better idea of how you really do feel. Similarly, healers often say they base their physical diagnosis on perception of the subtle energy of the health aura.

The seven levels of consciousness are given various names and I have used the following:

Divine or True Nature	Spiritual Essence
Spirit mind Spiritual-intuitional mind Higher intuitional mind	Higher self, soul or spirit
Mental-intellectual mind Emotional-astral mind Physical-etheric mind	Lower self, personality or ego

The levels of consciousness are represented on an ascending scale purely for convenience as in actuality, each is interrelated with the other.

The different kingdoms are also related in this scheme. Each kingdom is said to be concentrated in a different area of consciousness. The mineral kingdom is right in the physical level. A rock is a very physical thing! The vegetable kingdom is primarily in the physical but peaks into the emotional. Experiments with lie detectors have confirmed this ancient esoteric view by registering the emotional reactions of plants. This is well explained in *The Secret Life of Plants* by Tompkins and Bird.[36]

The animal kingdom is strongly involved with the physical and emotional levels and also has activity in the mental sphere.

Bringing Ego and Spirit Together

Next comes man, who has the most exciting prospects. We human beings are active on the physical, emotional and mental levels, and for us there is the possibility of making direct contact with higher levels of consciousness. For human beings there is this exciting distinction between our egos and our spirits, and the even more exciting prospect of uniting the two.

The ego is very similar to what we call our personality, as it includes our physical form, our emotions and our thoughts. The ego is that part of our self we tend to be most familiar with as well as being the most obvious part of our self that other people tend to know us by. The ego is the vehicle through which we project ourselves out to the world at large. But also we have what is often described as our spirit, the higher self or inner core of our being. Our spirit is the more permanent, purer, less complicated part of our being.

Many of us are aware of the nature of our ego or personality and work on this level. Only in moments of contemplation or inspiration do we make contract with our higher self or soul. The gap that links our ego with our soul is "the eye of the needle" spoken of in the Bible, and the mind acts as the fulcrum between physical and spiritual man. Intellect must be transmuted into intuition to bridge that gap.

Our life purpose is to make that leap. Our goal is to be freed of the limitations of personality, and soar free as spiritual beings.

Death plays its part in this process by providing new beginnings. At death, all of us that is the ego—our body, emotions and thinking mind—drops off, and our consciousness persists in the other states. Usually, our new functional body is our astral body, or it may be a higher body, depending on our stage of development. In this altered state of consciousness, we develop further, before reincarnating into a new physical body for the purpose of advancing toward the state of perfection intended for all of us.

Reincarnation is governed by the Law of Karma, which is basically the spiritual law of cause and effect. Just as physically for every action there is an equal and opposite reaction, so also spiritually, as you sow you shall reap.

Hence, good actions have their rewards and bad ones need to be compensated. The aim of the game is to progress beyond the law of karma. Then, free of the bonds of past activity, actions can be performed for their intrinsic "correctness," without any thought as to the benefits they might produce. This leads to a state of enlightenment in Eastern terminology, or to reunion with the Divine in the Christian view.

This concept helps to explain the seeming disparities around us and provides an incentive toward ethical, moral conduct in all situations.

SUBTLE-ENERGY HEALING

But back to healing. The etheric body is vital to our considerations. It is the counterpart of our physical body. It is composed of a very subtle energy that is visible to sensitive people such as clairvoyants, and known as the health aura. It is this vehicle through which the other levels of consciousness impinge on the physical.

This subtle energy is centered on seven chakras. "Chakra" is a Sanskrit word used to describe the concentrations of this subtle energy that is said to be located in seven different regions located along the spine and up into the head. Each chakra is a reflection of one level of consciousness and in turn relates most directly to one particular endocrine gland.

Chakras can be thought of as energy transformers in an electricity grid. They relay energy to a network of power lines, that are called meridians or nadis and which radiate throughout the physical body. The meridians correlate with the nervous system that in turn regulates the secretions from the endocrine glands. The hormones, so released, travel throughout the body via the blood and are instrumental in maintaining the body in its natural state of balance; hence the link from consciousness to matter. From the realm of consciousness, energy streams forth to vitalize etheric energy in the individual chakras. This energy then passes via the meridians to influence the nervous system's regulation of the endocrine glands. The hormones that then flow via the blood are vital in maintaining the physical body.

In this view, then, the physical body is the end result of formative energies as mediated by the etheric body that is in a state of dynamic flux. The characteristics of our etheric body will vary with the quality of the energies coming from the various formative levels of consciousness and with how its physical counterpart, the body, interacts with its own immediate physical environment.

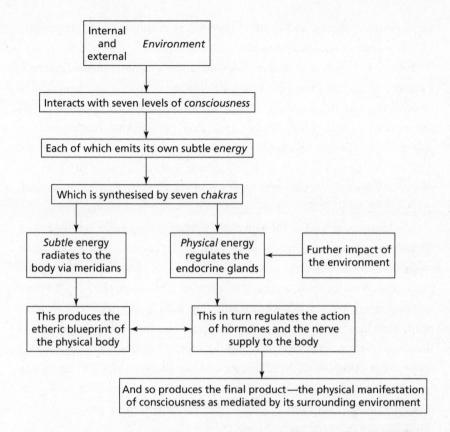

Disease can be due to purely physical causes such as diet and exercise or the rare case of a true accident. However, many current diseases relate to aberrations in our emotional world, while many others are centered in our mind. This fact is recognized by the growing attention being paid to psychosomatic disease and the role of tension and anxiety in the production of disease.

Accepting our basically spiritual nature, it is easy to see the spirit's overriding involvement and to consider disease in man as the end stage of disharmony between the spirit and the ego—or friction between the higher self's attitudes and the lower self's actions. When such disharmony is left unresolved, it manifests as a physical reality so that we are forced to confront it.

Disease then provides an opportunity to progress beyond our limitations. To gain the benefit of disease, to learn its real lessons, all aspects must be considered. Yet, in the immediate situation, it is often the physical condition that seems to be of prime importance. Most people living in the physical world do reject disease and death. They wish to continue here to experience and to progress as much as possible.

However, let us pause to reconsider the miracle of pure, physical surgery. Consider again the incredible trauma following a broken leg. It is easy to imagine the soft tissue damage, fragmented bones and then perhaps a steel pin inserted to hold things in place. Yet, after medical intervention and the passage of a relatively short period of time, function will return to normal and later X-rays will show little, if any, evidence of the damage. Just how can this be? What does initiate this truly wondrous healing that produces such magical effects?

We know quite a lot of the process, but what of the cause? We know a lot about how it happens. But why does it happen? I contend that a basic, relatively permanent blueprint of the body's form, as provided by the etheric body concept, does make sense of the situation. Although the physical form is traumatically altered in such accidents, the basic pattern, the etheric blueprint, remains. So, given the right conditions, healing will proceed so that the physical form once more matches the etheric, and normal function will return. It is a mistake to think that an outsider heals anything. A healer can be a most useful catalyst in the healing process, but the healer's role is to create the correct conditions whereby the patient's healing processes themselves can re-create the normal state.

Consideration of this subtle-energy model also accommodates the many other forms healing can take. Dietary considerations, for instance, act first on the physical level to purify the physical organism. But, as food has its own etheric energy, it can be a source of vitalization on this level also. This is one reason why many people advocate the use of pure foods raised in as natural a way as possible. The more natural, the fresher and more vital our food, the more subtle energy it has. Also, it is believed the subtle energy of food can be increased by being produced and prepared by a sensitive person, attuned to such ideas. On the other hand, the etheric value of much of the present-day mass-produced processed food must approach zero, or even have negative connotations.

Meditation acts to balance the higher and lower selves. In a state wherein the physical, emotional and mental levels are removed from one's direct awareness, the intrinsic purity of the higher self can operate to reharmonize the etheric blue print and so lead on to the re-creation of the normal physical situation. Dr. Ainslie Meares said that meditation produces a return to a state wherein the immune system is induced to function normally. This causes the body to recognize and reject the presence of cancerous cells. This, he said, is mediated via an influence on hormonal levels. You can see the similarities in concept, the explanations being to me a matter of degree.

The extraordinary Filipino healers are able to channel large amounts of direct healing energy. Sometimes they operate on a purely physical level. More often, however, they are operating on the precursive levels, notably the etheric and astral. Some are effective on the mental level, and a rare few heal on the spiritual level. Christ was a Divine Healer—capable of healing on any level.

This etheric energy of which we have been speaking has its global and universal counterpart, tied up with the all-pervading consciousness. It is on this energy that the psychic surgeons and other faith healers draw. Most of them merely accept their healing talents as God's gift of the Holy Spirit in action, and leave it at that. However, it is not too hard to use our model and to consider the possibility that what they are doing is drawing upon a universal energy, focusing it with their minds as a lens focuses the rays of the sun, and then emitting it through their fingers in a beam of energy that can be compared to a laser beam.

This beam of energy can then neutralize the positive and negative charges holding tissues together at the molecular level. In the absence of these forces, the tissues separate and can be entered. When the energy is withdrawn the body's etheric forces reassert their blueprint effect so that the physical structures resume their normal state, with no scarring.

Alternatively, some people believe psychic surgery is performed through the action of harmonics. They theorize that the healers are able to cause their hands to resonate in harmony with the tissue of their patients, so that the two can intersperse, much as two gases or two liquids can intersperse.

Regardless of how it is achieved, once the healers are inside the body, they utilize a magnetic faculty that enables them to draw together the diseased energies and remove them—a bit like a magnet can draw iron filings to itself. It is important to realize that such changes in phase do occur—a good example being how steam can be condensed to water. Maybe what the healers do is to concentrate the subtle, formative energies associated with a physical symptom of disease and actually precipitate them into physical form. Could this be a demonstration of energy giving rise to matter—a true materialization?

MY OWN INTEGRATION

In the Philippines I was told my bone tumors were too dense to be removed physically, but that the etheric energies associated with them could be taken away. My physical form would then return to match this normalized blueprint if I did not re-create the destructive etheric energies. So, after the initial boost, it became important to seek out the causes of disharmony within myself.

After the Philippines experience, I gained a remarkable and generalized healing boost. Yet the tumors kept growing, although slowly. It was obvious to me I had not made the necessary changes in myself. Only after many more efforts, culminating in meeting Sai Baba, a holy man of India, was I really able to get free of my cancer problems.

There still remains the ongoing process which faces each one of us—that of developing a system in which to maximize our potentials, correct our shortcomings, and live in accord with our principles.

These subtle energies we have been considering can be drawn upon and used in a positive, practical manner. All of us do radiate these subtle energies. They are colored by the quality of the "vehicle" through which they pass. Therefore, if we do want to use them more fully, it is vital that we seek to be as free as possible from complications within our own personalities or egos, and be open to allowing these subtle, but powerful, healing energies to flow freely.

SUBTLE-ENERGY MEDICINE • Recommendations

What to do? Times have changed. Few people I know these days go to the Philippines for healing. But many people continue to benefit from prayer, from Reiki, from visiting those who are regarded as having "healing gifts" and those who have some psychic awareness. There is no doubt in my experience some people have been helped greatly by subtle-energy medicine in one form or another.

This is another area where we need to be guided by our own sensibilities.

Maybe you regard all this as mumbo jumbo. No problem—just focus on what you find helpful. However, if you are curious, if you are interested, the best way to investigate is the way you would investigate anything. Find out what you can, check out the books, any references, the Internet; speak to your friends and seek word-of-mouth endorsements. Then if you do go to visit any practitioner of subtle-energy medicine, just like with a counselor, allow the first meeting to be like a job interview where the basic task is to decide whether or not you will go the second time. If you do decide to see a practitioner of this type, the best thing is to then commit. Do all you can to dispel any doubts, give yourself over to the treatment, and hope for a miracle. I know people who have been lucky!

Now it is time to pull all the pieces of the healing journey together, to summarize, and to formulate a plan.

CHAPTER 21

Recommendations

An Action Plan

SO OFTEN I HAVE MET PEOPLE WHO FEEL HOPELESS, AS IF THERE IS NOTHING they can do to help themselves. Then, presented with all the very real possibilities we have been discussing, they soon find themselves wondering where to begin, how to fit it all in, what to do. There is a great deal of information, a great many useful techniques, included in this book. The task now is to sort out the priorities and make a plan. While it is an obvious fact that individuals do vary, in general the following would be a reasonable order of priorities for those looking to help themselves toward maximizing their potential.

FOR PEOPLE RECENTLY DIAGNOSED AND BASICALLY WELL

Answer the four basic questions:
1. Do I really want to get well again?
2. Do I choose to accept responsibility for my situation? If taking responsibility, lifestyle medicine will always make sense; get started on that as soon as you can—meditation, positive thinking, diet and exercise being the immediate priorities.
3. How relevant is conventional medicine, traditional medicine and CAM?
4. Which particular external therapies shall I use?

(Details: The introduction and chapter 13.)

Assess each therapy according to the principles:
1. What are my expectations with no treatment?
2. What are the expectations for me if I have the proposed treatment?

3. Are there any side effects to the treatment and, if so, what might they be?

4. How will my own response to that treatment affect the outcome?

(Details: chapter 3.)

MEDICAL TREATMENT

If a specific therapy is suitable for you, and you decide to have it, commit yourself to it fully; work to minimize any potential side effects and maximize the benefits.

LIFESTYLE-BASED, SELF-HELP TECHNIQUES

Meditation

This is the ideal first step because it deals with stress, will help you to regain balance in body, mind and spirit, to think calmly and clearly, and to act appropriately.

If quality of life is your prime aim, begin with three sessions of ten to twenty minutes daily, and once it is working well, maintain one or two sessions of ten to twenty minutes daily.

If you want to gain maximum benefit from meditation, begin with three sessions daily of whatever period you feel comfortable with and build as rapidly as possible to three sessions of forty minutes, up to one hour each day.

(Details: chapters 4–6. Read *Meditation—An In-Depth Guide*. Consider using a CD to guide you or using my downloadable meditation program, Mind-Body Mastery.)

Dietary Considerations

Once the meditation is becoming integrated into your day, consider your dietary choices.

MAKE NO CHANGE

The average Western diet—high in fat, protein, salt, sugar, alcohol and refined foods, and low in fiber, vitamin and mineral intakes—may be inadequate. The "average" person would do well, therefore, to consider change. Recognize that change in this vital area has the potential to be stressful. Spend time to think the changes through, discuss them, and plan for them. Be clear on your aims and choices. Meditation makes change easier. Seek professional guidance. Get excited by the possibilities!

THE WELLNESS DIET (CHAPTER 13)

This is a good, sensible approach, as it avoids known risk factors and concentrates on foods that are known to carry preventative factors or actively promote health. Essentially, it is low in fat, protein and alcohol, avoids salt, sugar and refined foods, and has a high-fiber content. It is a plant-based, whole-food diet. Its primary constituents are the fruits, vegetables and grains. Ideally, the recommendations of the Wellness Diet then become a lifelong way of eating.

THE HEALING DIET (CHAPTER 14)

This is the more intense approach that is better suited to those who want to emphasize their dietary considerations. It includes consideration of an initial mono diet of three to ten days to provide an element of fasting, detoxification, transition and regeneration.

The recommendation is to continue with the Healing Diet until cancer-symptom free; or if you were symptom free when you started the Healing Diet, continue it for two months before gradually transferring to the ongoing Wellness Diet.

FOLLOW A SPECIFIC, FORMAL DIET

For example, the macrobiotic approach or the Gerson Therapy (see Appendix G). The last mentioned, particularly, is suited to a clinic situation and it is not recommended to be attempted at home without skilled guidance and the committed support of at least one permanent, full-time helper.

My personal experience, coupled with the feedback received from thousands of other people affected by cancers, leads me to believe that the suggestions summarized in (b) and (c) are the best way to proceed with your diet.

(Details: chapters 11–14.)

Positive Thinking

With meditation and dietary considerations, positive thinking completes the three basic ingredients of healing and well-being. Recognize the basic need to be positive, and to use the mind training techniques that you need in your particular situation.

If you do feel depressed or negative, start by working on exercise and a creative activity. By actually doing something physical and positive, you will set the whole process in motion. Gardening is my favorite activity. Exercise also warrants being a strong priority—aim for thirty minutes daily.

(Details: chapters 7–9.)

Spiritual Development

For most, this is another essential. Recognize that your endeavors in this area may be the most important of all.

RELIGION

Follow your own preferences here. Very few people change their religion through an experience with disease, but many find their convictions strengthened. This may well be a time to return to your religion.

REFLECTION, INTROSPECTION, CONTEMPLATION

Highly recommended as long as they are not associated with guilt or other negative emotions. Seek to understand your past, accept your present, and work "in the now" toward a happier, healthier tomorrow.

YOUR VIEW

Your view, or belief system, can limit your horizons or leave you free to soar above any situation with a smile on your face. Spend time reading, thinking, in contemplation, and in evolving your own theories. Open yourself to the possibilities.

SPIRITUAL HEALING

This may be catalyzed by others, but often comes with personal experience. Learning to love that part of your inner self, your spiritual essence, is an integral part of loving God, the universe, and your fellows. Once you can love yourself, you can recognize the inner truth in others. Then you can see that they too are seeking to be free of limitations and to express their inner perfection. Along with this, you will realize that it is not enough to dwell in spirit. The body is the temple of the soul and you need to give it due consideration.

Healing is complete when harmony is found in body, mind and spirit.
(Details: chapters 19–20.)

Healthy Emotions

Relationships frequently require as much healing as the physical body.

Make peace with as many as you can. Use the imagery technique of forgiveness once your meditation is working well.

The immediate family may need all these principles just as much as you do. Often it is the patient whose physical symptoms reflect a malaise involving one or several other closely associated people. Encourage your family to support you and to join you in as much of your program as possible, particularly the big three: meditation, diet and positive thinking.
(Details: chapters 16–17.)

Pain Control

Another essential life skill for all to learn at some stage. Do the recommended pain control exercises and be aware of the other possibilities.
(Details: chapter 10.)

Consideration of Death and Dying

This is another vitally important issue that is best acknowledged, contemplated, discussed and then used as motivation to live well, to live fully in the present moment.

Formulate your will and an enduring power of attorney.
Discuss your choices for end-of-life care.
Principles: Be brave enough to reflect and contemplate upon what you anticipate to happen. Look at your fears if any. Actively seek the opportunity to discuss the whole area with a good listener and especially, if possible, with your closest relatives. With the fears confronted and allayed, and with the benefit of regular meditation and contemplation, death can be genuinely seen as another very natural and positive part of life.

(Details: chapter 18.)

Healing

Be convinced that true healing lies within and work toward your own health and well-being. However, healers who can act as catalysts in the process may be very useful and appropriate. Be aware of the possibilities and use your own judgment. I certainly *do not* routinely recommend that anyone should jump on a plane and dash off to the Philippines, India or wherever; nor would I say it is unwise to consider doing so. However, if you do seek healing help from an extraordinary source, find out as much as you can about it before you begin. Having made your choice, strive to be open to the best possible outcome and commit yourself to the requirements of the healing technique involved.

(Details: chapters 19–20.)

Imagery

Imagery can be an "optional extra" to add to the meditation once the latter is going well. It does utilize the active, more willful side of the mind, whereas meditation relies on the stillness.

You could use the gentle, abstract methods such as the white light imagery or the healing journey.

If you choose to use more active and personalized images, you are advised to read and study my book on this subject, *The Mind That Changes Everything*.[37] This will add extra clarity. Also, you may benefit from seeking qualified guidance. If you use imagery regularly, do it for a few minutes three times daily. Then aim to continue on from the imagery, to let go and to experience moments of stillness whenever possible. Seek to be as relaxed as you can be.

Whether you do use imagery or not, do persevere with the meditation, as almost all people who persevere do establish an effective practice, and it has special benefits.

(Details: chapters 8–9.)

Remember: A journey of a thousand miles begins with just one step.

FOR PEOPLE IN A CRITICAL CONDITION

The same basic approach applies. You may feel quality of life issues are more important than efforts to overcome your physical symptoms. In this case, some medical and self-help techniques may be counterproductive. Changes in diet may just cause anguish, whereas meditation always leads to peace of mind and remains the priority. Most people who use all the principles find they apply to any life situation and so make for a good life—and a good death.

Faced with a crisis, your attitudes and beliefs assume paramount importance and peace of mind should be the main aim. So do seek to avoid or resolve situations of conflict as the calm that follows is enduring. I would never abandon hope of conquering disease, as it is my firm belief that healing is possible in any situation.

I am confident the techniques we have discussed in this book can work. However, they only have a chance to work if you apply them. Of course it is important to gather the best support around you that you can, but then it is up to you. You can greatly improve your situation. You can be confident of that. It is not reasonable, however, to expect that everyone will be freed of their physical symptoms. Some still die as a result of their cancer, but success or failure is not marked by death. Success is marked by poise and equanimity. The greatest successes I have seen have been in people who have developed a strong, stable and life-affirming "I choose to live to the full" stance but at the same time have been able to accept what life had to offer in return, even if it is dying. However, a great many have become well, and virtually all who have applied themselves to these principles have felt a great deal of benefit. Any effort will be rewarded.

FOR THOSE INTERESTED IN PREVENTION OR IN MAXIMUM HEALTH

Surprise! The same principles still apply. The degree to which you apply them depends on your priorities, beliefs and expectations.

As an ideal prevention program that would lead to maximum health, I confidently recommend:

1. **Meditation:** Ten to twenty minutes once or twice daily.
2. **Healthy Nutrition:** The basic Wellness Diet.
3. **Positive Thinking:** Keep developing this, using the techniques already summarized.

4. **Make time**—yes, *make* time—to dwell on and implement the recommendations for spiritual development, positive emotions, pain control, considerations of death and dying, and healing. Regular time for contemplation is highly recommended and imagery also may find a place in your life.

A SUMMARY

I am confident that these basic, self-help principles and techniques are worthy of application in virtually all conditions. They may be applied to other disease states besides those of cancer or merely used as aids to maximize health.

Make total health your goal. Make that elusive, ephemeral, wonderful, joyous state of harmony in body, mind and soul your life ambition. Seek to develop your potential to the full.

Be patient yet persevere, for the goal is real and within reach. Be gentle with yourself. Most have ups and downs along the way. Remember, it is your belief system that validates your actions. If your actions are not in line with your belief system, you are almost certain to produce disease. You may have pondered on boozing, smoking and shuffling old George, who probably thinks that his life is OK and so has no inner conflict. By doing so he accepts substandard health. But while he may have no obvious physical symptoms of disease, his version of health is a pale image of his potential.

Once you have a glimpse of *your* true potential you will realize that we all have the capacity, the potential to heal and to be really well. Accept that it can take time. Make a start. Just being on the path to true health in body, mind and spirit will transform your life and bring you peace. Life *was* meant to be good.

Happiness is to be found along the way, not just at the end of the path.

My wish for everyone is a long and happy life.

Appendices

How to Develop Effective Relationships with Your Doctors

FROM THE POINT OF VIEW OF A PERSON WITH CANCER, HAVING AT LEAST one doctor that you can trust and communicate with is a very important element in the healing process.

You need someone who can provide accurate and complete information, to the level it is known medically, and to the level you choose to know—someone who can be sensitive to the physical, psychological and spiritual state of both you and your family.

What is needed is a doctor who is focused on your welfare, who respects your thoughts and feelings, and who responds to them—a good communicator.

It is a sad fact, that with the thousands of people we have worked with over the years, it has been rare to find a patient who has not had at least one major medical complaint that had at its core poor communication. Many patients and partners are glowing in praise of the general care and attention they receive medically. Yet, it is unusual for these people not to have had at least one bad experience. Others are openly hostile about the way they have been treated and spoken to. Clearly, there is a need for good doctor/patient communications, better training for medical practitioners and more support for self-help techniques such as meditation and positive thinking.

Often it seems that the patient, the person with the illness, needs to take an active, gently assertive role in improving communication levels.

Communication is a two-way process. Your part as a patient/partner/support person is to express yourself and listen objectively to the doctor. Here are some points that build good relations.

Practice Gentle Assertion

This means expressing yourself clearly and accurately, ideally free of emotion, with the intention of informing the doctor of your needs and preferences. Inform your doctor of:

- The level of information you want provided;
- Who you want involved in major decision making—which professionals, family members and/or friends;
- Which doctor is to take the central coordinating role and be the focus of your decision making and treatment;
- Who you regard as a technician, who a counselor, communicator, adviser. Ideally, doctors will fill many of these roles but some may need to be regarded as one only.

Ideally, Seek a Medical Partner

A key medical person that you can trust, a good communicator. Someone who will do their best to give you as accurate and complete information as you ask for, who can speak in a language you can understand, who is sensitive to and responds to your state of mind, who respects your choices and supports you. A general practitioner or family physician is highly likely to fill this role and so a warning. Often people go to their family doctor with their early symptoms and are then referred to specialists for detailed investigation and treatment. Many then become caught up in the ambit of the specialists and do not return to the family doctor. The point is the GPs are generalists. They often have a broad, holistic or integrated view. They are usually good communicators, are great problem solvers and excellent advocates for their patients. They can be ideally suited to be the head of your healing team.

At Consultations

- Take a second person, preferably a partner. They will provide good moral support, remember questions and answers and be more stable, especially if emotional issues arise.
- Write your questions down before consultations and take them with you.
- Request extra time (in advance) for questions and discussion if necessary.

- Take notes during consultations or even ask if you can use a voice recorder. The amount of important information that can be forgotten in a consultation is great and you do need to retain it!
- Feel free to ask for explanations, elaborations, options, opinions.
- Be prepared to explain and justify your preferences.
- Inform the doctor what self-help options you are using—for the sake of information, education and inclusion.

Consider a Second Opinion

For major decisions, always give strong consideration to obtaining a second opinion. Go to someone outside the medical group, hospital or circle of the first opinion, so that it is, in fact, an independent opinion. Cancer medicine, like any other complicated field, is subject to personal experiences and preferences. It may be that a second opinion could provide a very different treatment option that warrants your consideration.

Be Prepared to Change Your Doctor If You Are Not Satisfied

Always try first to resolve problems by communicating with the doctor. Explain your situation if you do experience any difficulties or dissatisfaction. Often this will lead to resolution and healing of another sort—the healing of an important relationship. If not, there is no need to feel guilty—ask for a referral to someone more suited to your needs or make your own enquiries. A good doctor-patient relationship is vital to your health and well-being.

Aim to Be Confident of All Your Choices

Keep enquiring, listening, questioning and talking until you feel you are clear on the options and what is the best approach for you to follow.

Remember, it is unlikely that you can know or appreciate all the facts, all the options, all the fine details. It is likely there will come a point where you will have to say, "In the light of all I know and feel at this point in time, this is my very best option."

Do aim to clarify that option as clearly as possible, so you can confidently commit yourself to it. This is the first essential in positive thinking and will set you on the path toward achieving the best possible results.

Further suggestions on decision making are in chapters 1–3.

Recognize, Value and Use Your Own Resources

Remember that whatever treatment is available medically, as a human being you have emotions, a mind and a spirit. That makes you an incredibly powerful being. Add to that the support and love of well-directed family and friends and you can achieve exceptional results—peace of mind and the best possible physical outcome.

Commit to Your Decisions and Follow Through

Once you have clarified your options and made definite decisions, commit to what you plan to do. Better still, embrace all you do. Be enthusiastic. Welcome any treatments you do commit to. Do all possible to support yourself, your good intentions and those around you, including your health professionals.

What to Do to Enhance Surgery, Chemotherapy or Radiotherapy

General Recommendations to Support Medical Treatment

Step 1. Mental Preparation

1. Collect a team

  1. Decide who is on your team, who you consult, who you take advice from.
  2. Decide who will be your key medical adviser—maybe a GP interested in integrative medicine is best for this, maybe a nurse-practitioner? Maybe your oncologist or your surgeon? Who will it be?

2. Decide and commit

  1. The aim is to explore your options carefully, make an informed choice with a clear decision, then commit to it.
  2. In some situations the logical choice regarding what to do will be obvious, and sometimes it will not be so obvious. To ensure good decision making, as well as using your intellect, meditate so that your mind becomes calm and clear, and you have more direct access to your intuition and your wisdom. Put all this together and you will make good choices.
  3. Once you arrive at a decision, seek all the support you can and aim to embrace all that you do.

3. Prepare for the best

  1. Once you do make a choice and commit to a particular treatment regime, be really conscious of preparing yourself and consider all you can do to:

2. minimize any potential side effects
3. maximize the benefits
4. make the whole experience meaningful.

4. Study and apply the healing principles set out in this book!
5. Work hard to be confident and have faith in your decisions and your plans. Aim to create a healing environment, physically, emotionally, mentally and even spiritually around yourself.

Step 2. The Immediate Practicalities

1. Eat well—at least follow the Wellness Diet, but ideally use the Healing Diet.

1. Include in your diet anticancer foods such as raspberries or pomegranate; fresh turmeric; broccoli sprouts; cabbage; etc.
2. Use the nutritional principles of the Healing Diet to create a cancer-unfriendly environment in your body and to turn the tables metabolically on the cancer.
3. Consider organizing healthy "meals on wheels" for hospitalization if the hospital food is inadequate. Friends or family might drop off juices, nutritious meals and snacks.

2. Keep the fluids up. Remember to keep drinking—at least 68 ounces in total per day.

1. Include seven juices per day—These are particularly good around chemotherapy treatment times, as they provide a good source of easy to absorb nutrients in a balanced package, are gentle on the bowel and their nutrients are easily absorbed. Green juice especially is particularly useful during radiation and chemotherapy.
2. Smoothies are excellent if eating is difficult, appetite is down, or weight loss is an issue. Use any nondairy milk as a base, add banana, soy yogurt, plus a little honey and/or carob or cocoa powder.

3. Exercise regularly—at least three to four times each week for around thirty minutes, but ideally daily.
4. Meditate—ideally, three long sessions daily (forty to sixty minutes per session).

5. **Imagery**—consider using the white light healing journey or specific personal healing imagery, especially while receiving treatments.
6. **Massage can be very helpful**—once a week or as it suits.
   1. Be mindful during the massage so you experience the greatest benefits for your state of mind.

7. **Supplements** may well be useful and ideally you clarify these possibilities with a doctor trained in nutrition, or another suitably qualified health professional. Particular supplements to discuss include:
   1. Multivitamin/mineral supplements
   2. Vitamin C
   3. Magnesium, iron and zinc
   4. Floradix as a supplement or eat liver (organic calves liver) to aid blood quality, especially if you know your blood cells or platelets have dropped down.
   5. Strath tonic has been shown to minimize potential side effects of radiotherapy and may be helpful with chemotherapy. Green tea, turmeric, seaweeds, rooibos tea and spirulina are all thought to offset potential side effects of chemotherapy and radiotherapy and are worth considering.
   6. Consider using slippery elm powder three times a day or aloe vera juice to protect from an unsettled stomach and bowel while undergoing chemotherapy.

8. **Support your bowel.** Take regular probiotics supplementation or eat yogurt daily (natural, organic soy yogurt is best) to maintain healthy bowel flora.
9. **Check your vitamin D levels regularly.** They need to be between 100 and 150nmol/l. Use supplements if necessary, especially if out of the sun for extended periods. Buy the 5,000 IU capsules that can be purchased over the Internet.

Step 3. Emotional Preparation
1. **Be authentic.** Healthy emotions are authentic emotions. Read the chapters on emotional health and find the people in your life you can share your emotions with safely and authentically. It is natural to have emotions

surface from time to time; express them authentically and then get on with what you need to do to recover.

2. Communicate. Think about who you need to say things to, and what you want to say—and do it!

　1. With children repeat two things regularly (as well as the obvious telling them that you do love them):

　　• "It (as in the cancer) is not your fault" (offsets guilt).

　　• A major reason why you are doing this treatment (including all you are doing for yourself) is because you want to survive and to continue to be with them (offsets feelings of abandonment).

　2. Read *How to Help Children Through a Parent's Serious Illness* by Kathleen McCue.

　3. Get professional help if you are stuck.

3. Practice gratitude. Develop a sense of gratitude for the skill of your medical team and for the effectiveness and accessibility of the medical system. Be grateful for all the support you generate.

Step 4. Spiritual Preparation

1. Generate acceptance. Accept what is happening now and what has happened to you in the past. Adopt a relaxed mode, but one that also has a resolve for a good outcome. Commit to making the best of the situation you are in (e.g., combine acceptance and commitment). This will provide the clarity to do whatever the circumstances require, which may be doing nothing in particular, or it may require action. The clearer you are, the clearer your choices will become—this is one of meditation's major benefits.

2. Make time for the big questions. Maybe this is time to be contemplating the meaning and purpose of life, to be questioning what it is all about.

　1. It is certainly a good time to be making peace with those around you, anyone outstanding from the past, and to be reconciling your own inner life. Consider your own spiritual tradition and how you relate to it now. Is it time to be going to church, or to be hearing a great spiritual teacher speak somewhere? Give attention to seeking out the organizations, the people, the books that can help you with this.

2. Take time to sit quietly and to also discuss these matters with a spiritual friend.

3. Many find that it is the time they spend on the big questions that enriches their lives for the better, and that this becomes a happy side effect of the illness.

Preparing for Surgery Specifically

Step 1. Consider Collecting Blood

Preoperation, organizing collecting your own blood via your doctor may well be possible and may make sense for a possible retransfusion.

Step 2. Practice Inner Rehearsal

This is a valuable technique you can start as soon as surgery is booked in, and you can do it daily right up to the time of the surgery. Many people find this exercise really useful even as they go into theater and are being anesthetized.

Imagine:

- The physical reality of the cancer shrinking in the time leading up to the surgery (particularly around its outer margins), and that when the surgery is performed the cancer will be easy to remove—a bit like shelling a pea out of its pod.
- The whole construct that goes with the cancer being contained within the physical mass of the cancer itself. What this means is that you imagine all the causes and all the physical, emotional and psychological dynamic of the cancer being contained within the cancer itself. You imagine everything and anything to do with the cancer is contained within its mass. Then you imagine that when the actual physical lump is removed surgically, everything associated with the cancer is removed at the one time. This is a bit like an exorcism, a purge, that takes more than just the physical lump—it takes the spirit, the energy, everything associated with the cancer out of your system.
- Imagine during the operation the surgeons being pleased with the surgery and saying things like, "This is easier than we expected," "It's all going really well," "The operation went well."

- Imagine that you will experience a rapid and complete recovery—you are pleasantly surprised by the lack of pain, and there or no postoperative infections or any other side effects.
- Imagine yourself in the future, fit and well, looking back at the surgery and being grateful for a full recovery. You could imagine visiting the doctor when you are well and you are looking back on the time of your illness and discussing all you did to become well again.

Regard the Postoperative Period as a New Beginning

Consider that you need a time of convalescence. Try not to go back to work for some time and rest your body regularly.

The Traditional 5-Step Process of Meditation

TRADITIONALLY, ONE COMMON WAY TO DESCRIBE AND TO TEACH MEDITATION was to consider it as just one step in a five-step process. This process began with:

Concentration

A beginner would take up a set position, relax physically and then attempt to concentrate upon just one thing. It should be emphasized that the relaxation and the concentration were complementary and some of the techniques actually did place emphasis on the means of becoming relaxed. The more you relax, the easier it is to concentrate.

The focus for the concentration may have been on just about anything, but these are the most common:

- An activity—Breathing, in particular, has been widely used, as has dance and meditative movement such as the Chinese art of tai chi.
- An object (such as a candle or a painting)—Icons have been used for this, as have mandalas or complex, symbolic paintings.
- A sound—Usually such a sound would be repeated over and over. This could be done out loud as with chanting, or silently as with a repetitive prayer or a mantra. A mantra is a word or group of words repeated continuously as in the practice of transcendental meditation (TM).
- A thought—Generally a particular quality would be concentrated upon; truth, honesty, love and compassion are typical examples used. This particular practice is often called contemplation or analytical meditation.

Whatever the nature of the focus for concentration, the aim was to think of that focus and nothing else. This took people's attention away from random, distracting thoughts and helped to focus their attention. Once this was achieved, meditation was under way.

Meditation

Meditation in this context was defined as the ability to concentrate on one thing to the exclusion of other thoughts. It was an active process of the mind that required some effort. In this traditional sense, meditation was really undistracted concentration. When practiced long enough it led on to:

Contemplation

Contemplation could begin once the act of concentration had become automatic and effortless. Then, it was as if the mind slipped into overdrive. When this occurred, instead of the logical, thinking part of the mind being at work, a heightened state of awareness developed and the intuitive, creative, wisdom aspect came into play.

It is important to recognize that the mind does have these two distinctive ways of functioning—one rational and conscious, the other more abstract, intuitive and wisdom based. Most of us are very familiar with the day-to-day rational processes of the brain. All day our brain is thinking, analyzing, evaluating. We have a steady flow of thoughts from the time we first arise to the time when we lapse into sleep at night. This rational, mental activity is normally associated with the left half of the brain.

Normally, we would associate times of nonthinking with sleep or unconsciousness. However, we may have experienced fleeting moments of nonthinking consciousness in the pleasant reverie that sometimes descends just before sleep. This peace is similar to those wonderful moments when a glorious sunset or a major work of art touches our inner core and leaves us in rapturous silence. We are then involved with that more abstract, less rational brain activity which is predominately associated with the right side of the brain. Often in those moments of reverie or silence, we can experience useful, even profound insights.

Many of us then, could be laughingly referred to as half-wits because, being overly rational creatures, we only use half our brain's potential! Contemplation complements our rational thinking and is a way to exercise the other half of our brain. By doing so, fresh insights can be gained and new levels of meaning obtained.

The mind, however, is still active during this contemplative phase of the process. In contemplation it is just being used in a way with which we are not so commonly familiar.

Prolonged contemplation leads on to the experience of unification.

Unification

This is a still more abstract state. To explain, during our normal daily experience, when we become aware of an object, we have a sense of duality. Look again at this book you are reading. There is the book in front of you, and there is that part of you that is aware of the book. It is natural to feel the two are separate. There is you, and there is the book. There is also the process of being aware of the book.

Now, here is the interesting and exciting bit! Through contemplation, you the contemplator, the object of whatever you are contemplating, and even the act of contemplation itself, merge so that there is no sense of separation, no sense of duality. Just an abiding sense of unity. A sense of oneness. In our example, you no longer feel separate from the book, you feel at one with it.

This union, this sense of oneness that can be catalyzed by concentrating on any particular object in the manner described; this union is what the mystics of all ages have sought so earnestly and waxed poetic about when they found it. It led on to a final state, illumination.

Illumination

This has been described as "the knowing that passes all understanding." In this state, a totally new experience of reality would be revealed. This experience was direct, immediate and totally satisfying. It was the experience of truth, absolute truth in a way that was clearly and unmistakably revealed. In some traditions this experience is called enlightenment.

We can understand how this five-step process works if we use the example of concentrating upon a candle. Initially, concentration is required to sit still and to focus our attention on a candle. To begin with, the mind will almost certainly tend to wander—What is for dinner? What am I doing tomorrow? Should I scratch my nose? Etc.

Eventually, with persistence and effort, we can concentrate on the candle without being restless or without being interrupted by other thoughts. This is meditation. This is undistracted awareness. Soon contemplation will follow and it is as if another thought process begins. Abstract thoughts of the candle become apparent. The symbolism of the candle, its shape, its light, its fire, may be reflected upon and these qualities provide a new level of understanding. For example, you may feel as if the light of the candle is a symbol of the spiritual essence within you and feel enriched by this awareness.

As time goes on such thoughts gently fade and all awareness of activity and time are lost. Only in retrospect can you be aware that you were in a state in which you felt at one with the candle. This is unification. This sense of oneness may extend beyond the candle and your immediate environment to give a direct appreciation of your oneness with everything around you. This type of mystical experience puts a smile on people's lips that does not readily fade!

Finally, a new clarity may dawn. From contemplating the candle you may have sensed something of the nature of your own inner essence; now, in illumination, you may experience the truth of that inner essence, and come to realize that it is within yourself and every one of your fellows. This knowing is irrefutable. It is not the knowing gained through reading or listening to others. It is the knowing of direct experience. It may not even be justifiable in rational terms; no worry, you know it as truth.

Prayer, Hope and Science

MANY PEOPLE HAVE A POSITIVE PERSONAL EXPERIENCE OF PRAYER SIGNIFI-
cantly transforming some aspect of their own life or that of someone close to
them.

Prayer is defined in the *Oxford Dictionary* as "a solemn request to God or
an object of worship; a supplication, thanksgiving, or other mental act
addressed to God" and as "a formula or form of words used in praying"—so
in the literal English sense, God figures prominently in prayer.

Prayer in relation to healing falls into one of two categories: intercessory
prayer, which involves praying for the benefit of another person; or personal prayer, which involves praying for oneself.

When it comes to scientifically validating the healing potential of prayer,
nearly all the published research focuses upon intercessory prayer (IP).

Much excitement was created in the research and wider communities in
1988 when the cardiologist and committed Christian, Randolph Byrd published a landmark paper demonstrating the benefits of IP for people recovering in a coronary care unit (CCU). Working in the San Francisco General
Hospital, Dr. Byrd used a prospective, randomized, double-blind protocol
making the study quite sound from a scientific point of view.

Practicing "born again" Christians were assigned to pray for people they
never met, and who did not know if they were being prayed for or not. They
were instructed to pray daily for the rapid recovery of those assigned to them,
and for the prevention of any complications and death, in addition to other
areas of prayer they believed to be beneficial to the patient. The results
demonstrated that those prayed for had significantly fewer complications
and required less medication. Mortality was the same for those prayed for

and the controls. Byrd's often-quoted study attracted a good deal of support and criticism.

The Harris study in 1999, was another similarly well designed and well-conducted study that showed positive benefits in reducing complications in a CCU. However, the most recent Cochrane Review (Roberts 2007) on IP is not favorable. The Cochrane Reviews, which are given a good deal of weight in medical circles, aim to provide the evidence base on a particular subject and commonly use a process that selects for high-quality research while filtering out observational and population based studies. Roberts concluded that the current evidence base for IP was so unequivocal as to not warrant further research of the subject. This view is not shared by many other researchers, clinicians and members of the wider public for whom the topic of IP remains of great interest.

Personal prayer involves a spectrum of inner practices that range from prayer in the traditional sense, through to the repetition of a particular prayer or the use of a mantra, and on into the use of contemplation and sitting quietly in silence. Techniques in this spectrum include praying for oneself by appealing for divine intervention or praying that the best outcome possible will flow from the present circumstances and trusting in that outcome. But this type of prayer can also cover a range of inner practices that may produce significant cognitive shifts such as from despair to acceptance, and can include the use of visualization and contemplation that leads to insight, clarity and the development of particular traits such as compassion and happiness. It even may be that simply sitting quietly in silence is the most powerful healing practice of all.

Personal prayer has had very little specific research published on it. However, this form of practice overlaps with that of contemplation and meditation which have attracted a great deal of recent study. It is relatively easy to make the theoretical connections between the practices of personal prayer, contemplation and meditation. As such, it is reasonable conjecture that many of the positive health benefits associated with the practice of meditation are likely to be reproduced via personal prayer. Here it is worth noting that there are currently more than six thousand studies in the medical literature around the world attesting to the positive benefits of meditation in a wide range of physical and psychological conditions.

In summary, the existing research on the healing benefits of prayer are scant and include both positive and negative findings. Research in this field is challenging but, due to the huge public interest, warrants more attention. There may be particular benefits in examining the linkages between the practices of personal prayer, visualization, contemplation and meditation and the wealth of research available and continuing in the latter fields.

Definition of the Mind

THE MIND IS AN EMBODIED AND RELATIONAL PROCESS THAT REGULATES the flow of energy and information.

To fully understand this definition you may find it helpful if we attempt to explain the terms a little first, and then you contemplate the words as a whole.

Let us start with the meaning of "regulates the flow of energy and information." Of course "regulate" means to control; but what is being controlled? "The flow of energy and information." The mind regulates how we use energy—what comes in and what goes out. In crude terms, it decides what we eat and drink, it decides what exercise and activities we pursue. It regulates how we use our energy. The mind also has the capacity to gather, to store and to control the way we use information. It decides what we read, what we learn, even how we learn—and then it uses that information as it sees fit. The mind has the potential to change everything.

What then of "the mind is an embodied and relational process"? Embodied first: the mind exists in a manner that is intimately connected to our physical body. While it is concentrated in the brain, it is widely accepted that the mind is not confined to the brain. In fact it even extends beyond the nervous system generally and is to be found actively functional in all parts of the body. Yet you can pull the body apart and you will not find "the mind." "The mind" is to do with the body, but it is far more than a piece of the body.

Next, we need to be aware of one of the most important qualities of the mind. You can change it. We used to laugh at the old, somewhat sexist maxim, "It is a woman's prerogative to change her mind." Good news! We all can do it. In fact, the exciting new field of neurobiology that focuses on neuroplasticity clearly establishes the brain and the mind are far more flexible and malleable than ever we thought.

It is not so long ago neurobiologists taught that the brain actively developed up until the age of around five to eight years. This theory dictated that all was set in proverbial concrete around that age and the brain only deteriorated as we became older.

The concepts, knowledge and clinical experiments connected with neuroplasticity have changed all that. Neuroplasticity refers to the brain's ability to change its structure and function according to how we use it. Norman Doidge's groundbreaking book, *The Brain That Changes Itself*,[38] has eloquently described the advances in the current understanding that likens the brain more to our muscles than our bones. Even our bones do change a little over time but our muscles respond rapidly to whether we use them or not. Importantly, when we choose to, we can train our muscles—and they respond.

Neuroplasticity tells us that we can learn how our mind works, train it, and have it function more effectively. When we train our mind, we can rely upon it to bring us better health, more effective healing and profound happiness.

But now, back to the definition. The mind is "a relational process"; it exists within the context of relationships. All that we do depends upon our relationships—those we have with our environment, other living things and ourselves. Because we have a relationship with our self, we look after it. Depending on the quality of that relationship we look after our body better or worse. Not many people self-harm by actually cutting their bodies; some do, but many self-harm by eating badly or not exercising. Many trash the environment and treat other creatures or people badly because they have a poor relationship with them. So the mind is a process that is affected by relationships.

That leaves "process" to consider.

Process: The *Oxford Dictionary*: "a continuous and regular action or succession of actions occurring or performed in a definite manner." Take a moment to consider this and be prepared to become a little excited. The mind being defined as a process means that it is an active "doing," not a sedentary object.

When all this is put together, these words define the mind not as a passive noun but as an active verb!

Viewed this way, the mind is well described as an emergent property. This means it is fluid, active, constantly changing. The mind exists in close relationship to our body, but is not our body, not even just the brain. The mind functions in relationship to all around us. It is affected by the environment we are in, the animals and the people we interact with. The mind regulates all our vital functions. It collects, stores, retrieves and uses information. It controls the energy that flows through us—the physical energy, emotional, mental and spiritual energy.

It is well worth taking the time to sit quietly and contemplate this definition. Sit quietly, learn the definition, close your eyes, and reflect on its meaning. Whenever your mind wanders onto other things or spaces out, notice you are off track as soon as you can, be gentle with yourself, and simply return to your contemplation. Practicing active reflection like this takes a thought from being nebulous and fleeting to something you anchor firmly in your understanding.

When you do this, you will have even more clarity regarding why we say, "It is all in the mind." It is the mind that regulates and changes everything.

Adapted from *The Mind that Changes Everything* by Ian Gawler, Brolga Publishing, Melbourne, 2011

Coffee or Caffeine Enemas

1. Use fresh ground coffee.
2. Add 2 tablespoons of ground coffee to 500mls (1 pint) of water, bring to the boil and simmer for ten minutes. Many people find half the quantity of coffee and half the quantity of water (250mls) has a very positive effect and is enough.
3. Cool to body temperature and pour through a fine filter into the enema bag. Use a gravity-fed type of bag.
4. Go to the toilet first if necessary. When first using enemas you may benefit from a washout enema of plain water to evacuate the bowel before the coffee enema is administered, but this is not necessary routinely.
5. If insecure, lie on a plastic sheet. Most people learn to retain an enema quite easily, especially if they relax.
6. Lie on your right side with your legs tucked up a little. Consciously relax.
7. Insert the enema tube's lubricated nozzle through the anus and gently allow the liquid to flow in.
8. Switch off the flow and remove the nozzle.
9. Relax for ten to fifteen minutes while retaining the enema. Reading is a good distraction if you need it.
10. Go to the toilet and evacuate the bowel.
11. Be sure to wash your enema equipment thoroughly after every use.

The Gerson Therapy and
My Own Nutritional Path

MY INTEREST IN NUTRITIONAL THERAPY FOR PEOPLE AFFECTED BY CANCER was kindled when my own cancer reappeared after the initial surgery. At that time I was told that the conventional medical treatments offered no prospect of a cure. By a happy chain of events, I was taken to a lecture on the Gerson Therapy. I was amazed to find that Dr. Max Gerson had an exciting, comprehensive and novel theory on cancer and its nutritional treatment. Even better, he had documented cases of restoring terminal patients to health in his book, *A Cancer Therapy: Results of Fifty Cases*.

Gerson was a medical practitioner who as a young man used a dietary regime to relieve his own otherwise untreatable migraine attacks. He then developed this regime and documented good results treating tuberculosis patients. He treated his first cancer patient, reluctantly and with little optimism, in 1928. She had a complete remission.

Winston Churchill said, "Men occasionally stumble over the Truth, but most pick themselves up and hurry off as if nothing had happened."

No doubt Gerson did stumble across this treatment. However, he spent the next thirty years attempting to validate his results while modifying and improving the diet according to clinical experience.

My feeling from reading Gerson's work is that he had a great faith in nature. He believed that cancer was a multifactorial, degenerative disease. He regarded it as the product of our food and environment being too far removed from nature. He believed that we have exceeded the body's ability to cope with unnatural products. Like me, Gerson saw cancer as a disease of society, a disease of lifestyle. He listed the overuse of artificial fertilizers and chemicals in the soil, the overrefining and adulteration of food with toxic additives, the poor preparation of food and the pollution of our environment generally as being individual factors that combined to adversely affect the body's function as a whole. He postulated that over a period of time these factors weakened the body's resistance. Then, when one final trigger factor produced the localized symptoms, the depleted defenses of the body were unable to eliminate or even contain it. Cancer was the localized sign of a generalized condition—a multifactorial, chronic, degenerative condition.

Gerson had developed these views way back in the 1930s! He was one of the first to suggest that cancer involved the impairment of the body's natural defenses—the immune system—in this generalized way. He was stating way back then that cancer involved a problem of immune deficiency. It is only recently that the medical mainstream has begun to explore this avenue and to share this basic concept. Gerson was way ahead of his time. He recognized that once the symptoms of cancer appeared, there was a problem that included more than just the localized lumps and bumps. The whole body was diseased. Often, however, cancer is treated as a localized problem as if it is only the lumps and bumps that are the disease and the rest of the patient's body is fine. Gerson's hypothesis was that if the rest of the body can be returned to a healthy condition, then it would react to and eliminate any cancer, anywhere in the body.

This, then, was Gerson's aim—to restore the normal function of the body.

Gerson recognized the theory he worked with, the nutritional basis of his diet and the supplements he used, were subject to medical argument. He was very pragmatic, however. His saw results with his methods and so he preferred to work toward a fully acceptable medical explanation as he continued treating his patients. He claimed a high recovery rate, even of terminal cases. There is evidence that he did achieve remarkable results, made more remarkable by considering that most of his patients had been through the conventional treatments first and gained no success.

Gerson's is a very strict and involved regime to follow, and it certainly calls for professional guidance. I certainly recommend *against* anyone trying Gerson's diet on their own. It needs to be described as a therapy rather than a diet. As well as the need for supervision and monitoring, there is a need for at least one person to assist with preparation. My first wife was involved for about twelve hours each day helping me with it. Obviously, the level of commitment needs to be very high on everyone's part. It would not be possible to live a normal life, let alone go to work, while following the diet intensively. It is really a regime best conducted in a live-in clinic situation. Full details of the regime are best studied via the books he or his daughter, Charlotte Gerson, has written.

So, there are plenty of reservations regarding Gerson's therapy. However, it is well worth mentioning, as his ideas stand on their merits. Also, for those interested in intensive diets, Gerson's is the soundest and best to my knowledge. Most others are adaptations of his.

The main benefits I gained from the three months I did on the Gerson Therapy is that it certainly helped me to detoxify and to purify my system. As a consequence of this, along with the intense meditation I continued with, I found myself to be very sensitive to what new foods I could add and eat reliably, and those I continued to need to avoid. For example, for me, dairy products and eggs were two of the things I needed to avoid.

Using an ongoing process of experimentation, trying foods and observing their reactions, I steadily developed a new way of eating that stood me in good stead for the healing phase of my recovery—the Healing Diet. Once I was free of cancer, I continued to experiment and fairly soon arrived at what could be described as a maintenance diet—the Wellness Diet. Over the years, based on current research and particularly the feedback from thousands of people with cancer who have given serious attention their nutritional management and therapy, the Healing Diet and then the Wellness Diet have evolved to where they are today.

Fishing for Answers:
Sustainable, Healthy Fish

FOR NONVEGETARIANS, FISH HAVE HEALTH BENEFITS COURTESY MOSTLY OF their omega-3 fatty acids. Also, they are a good source of protein. However, most of us are alert to the vexed issue of contamination of our fish by pollution, as well as the sustainability and environmental problems of overfishing and damaging fishing practices.

It is claimed that currently 70 percent of the world's fish species are fully exploited, overexploited, depleted or recovering from depletion. It is a scary thought to know the best estimates are that if current trends of overfishing continue, stocks of all fish currently being commercially fished will have collapsed by 2048. The question, then, is what fish are best to eat? What to do?

Say No to Farmed Fish

The trend toward increasing aquaculture, the farming of fish, makes sense in theory but does not seem to have the right answers as yet in practice. Most people are unaware that commercially farmed salmon are genetically modified to become what are called tetraploids—that is, they have a double set of genes so they grow faster. Then they are fed on other fish, a practice that is very inefficient and damaging to other fish stocks. It takes 4½ to 9 pounds of wild fish to produce 2 pounds of farmed salmon. While increasingly vegetable proteins are being used for feed, these result in lower levels of the valuable omega-3 fatty acids in the salmon. Seaweed may be a more viable food source for fish farming, but that remains to be seen. Also, disease is emerging as a major issue among intensively reared fish. Increasingly, significant amounts of antibiotics are being used to manage infections (as happens continually in the intensive rearing of chicken).

So wild-caught fish are preferable, but which ones?

Know Where Your Fish Came From—The Further out to Sea and the Less Polluted the Waters, the Better

Fish that are caught in more remote areas away from built-up, polluted areas are obviously preferable. So choose fish that live further out to sea, that are the deeper sea varieties, and come from less-polluted areas and countries.

Choose the Smaller Species Rather Than the Big Predator Fish

Pollutants accumulate as you go up the food chain. For example, it is well known sharks accumulate heavy metals and the mercury levels in big fish can be very toxic.

Check Out What the Sustainable Fish Are in Your Area

This is a regional as well as international issue and the need is to check your local conditions. In Australia, a good guide is found on the Australian Marine Conservation Society's website: marineconservation.org.com.

The international Marine Stewardship Council has developed a certification system that mostly shows up on packaged seafood and features a distinctive blue MSC label. See their website: msc.org.

Goodfishbadfish.com.au has a very user-friendly list of sustainable seafoods, with reasons for the various listings and practical preparation tips.

Avoid the Unsustainable Fish That May Also Have Health Issues

Again, say no to farmed fish.

Say no to wild caught barramundi, blue grenadier, cods, garfish, gemfish (hake), groupers, Murray cod, orange roughy (deep-sea perch), shark, snapper, marlin, swordfish, toothfish and tuna (unless the tuna is troll, pole or line caught).

Fish That Are Best to Avoid, but Not So Bad

Blue-eye trevalla, coral trout, flathead, gunard, John Dory, kingfish, ling, mulloway, red emperor, red mullet, red snapper (redfish) and silver trevally.

Fish That Are OK to Consider

Wild-caught bonito, bream, eel, King George whiting, leatherjacket, mackerel, mahi mahi, mullet, tailor, trevally and whiting.

Imported canned salmon and sardines are usually acceptable.

Avoid Scallops from the Wild
Seafood That Is Best to Avoid, but Not So Bad

Lobster and prawns (farmed prawns are likely to be better environmentally).

Seafood That Is Acceptable to Consider

Farmed: abalone, oysters, scallops and blue mussels.
Wild: blue swimmer crabs, mud crabs, squid, calamari and octopus.

All this information may seem a little imposing at first, but it is like many things. Take your time to think it through. If you are planning to eat fish, find out what is available locally, where you can get healthy, sustainable seafood, develop a good relationship with your supplier, and then it is easy and satisfying.

Relative Levels of Caffeine

THE LEVEL OF CAFFEINE IN INDIVIDUAL DRINKS VARIES ACCORDING TO THE source and the method of preparation. What follows are general indications only.

Product	Approximate Levels of Caffeine per 100 ml—in mgs
Percolated coffee	38–65
Drip coffee	55–85
Espresso	170–225
Decaffeinated coffee	2–7
Black tea	28
Green tea	17
Coca-Cola	10
Red Bull	32

Dark chocolate tends to have around three times more caffeine than milk chocolate. The more cocoa in the chocolate, the more caffeine.

The average block of chocolate weighs around 100 grams (3.5 ounces) and 100 grams of dark chocolate contains around 70 milligrams of caffeine, compared to 21 milligrams in 100 grams of milk chocolate.

Approximate Alcohol Content in Various Drinks

THE LEVEL OF ALCOHOL IN INDIVIDUAL DRINKS VARIES ACCORDING TO THE manufacturer and other factors. What follows are general indications only.

Product	Approximate % of Alcohol in Various Drinks
Fruit juice	Less than .1%
"Nonalcoholic" beer	Around .5% or less
Light beer	Around 3%
Standard beer	4%–5%
Stout	5%–10%
Cider	4%–8%
Wine	10%–15%
Sparkling wines	8%–12%
Port	20%
Liquors	15%–55%
Spirits	Around 40%
Rum	35%–50%
Whisky	50%–60%

The Preparation of Sprouts

ADD A LITTLE LESS THAN ONE-QUARTER INCH OF ALFALFA SEEDS TO THE bottom of a 2-pound jar.

Cover well with water and leave soaking for eight hours.

Cover the jar with chicken wire or any screen, holding it on with a rubber band. Invert the jar, pouring off the water.

Rinse and drain twice.

Store upside down, ensuring good drainage and air circulation. You can obtain racks for the purpose. Sit them on the kitchen bench, away from direct sunlight.

Rinse the developing sprouts thoroughly with water twice daily, both morning and evening (three times in hot weather).

In four to five days the seeds will have sprouted and be nearly an inch long with little green heads. It is best to have four jars at various stages of development, as a family can easily devour the contents of one each day.

Sprouts are an ideal source of fresh, vital food, especially in winter. They are claimed to be one of the highest sources of vegetable protein and are packed with vitamins and minerals. Highly recommended and something young children often enjoy participating in producing. However, if you prefer, they are readily available for purchase.

Food Combining

THIS IS LIKE FINE-TUNING WHERE THE INTENTION IS TO EAT COMBINATIONS of foods that are most easily digested together.

To determine how well or how badly two groups of foods combine, refer to the following chart. Identify the first food in the left-hand column and follow it across until you reach the vertical column under the name of the second food. Where the two columns meet, provides the answer.

For example, starches (third down on the left-hand column) combined with fats (third from the left in the top column) equals a fair combination.

Acid fruits (bottom of the left-hand column) combined with sweet fruits (third from the right, top column) equals a poor combination.

Primary proteins: almonds, Brazil nuts, cashew nuts, hazelnuts, pine nuts, pistachios, walnuts, pepitas, sunflower seeds, sesame seeds, wheat germ, lecithin, soyabean.

Secondary proteins: peanuts, cheese, eggs, yogurt, poultry, meat, fish.

Fats: avocados, oils, macadamia nuts, pecans, coconut, olives.

Starches: oats, rice, wheat, corn, rye, millet, buckwheat, lima beans, red beans, navy beans, mung beans, broad beans, garbanzos, lentils, chestnuts, breadfruit, jackfruit, sweet potato, Jerusalem artichokes, pumpkin, taro yams.

Melons: cantaloupe, watermelon, honeydew.

Vegetables: globe artichokes, fresh sprouts, beetroot, carrot, peppers, rutabaga, parsley, Brussels sprouts, cauliflower, cabbage, celery, lettuce, turnips, fresh beans, fresh peas, zucchini, chayote, marrows, squash, broccoli, asparagus, eggplant, silver beet, spinach, tomatoes, onions (best cooked).

Sweet fruits: bananas, figs, custard apples, Monstera deliciosa, persimmon, all dried fruits.

Food Groups	Primary Proteins	Secondary Proteins	Fats	Starches	Melons	Vegetables	Sweet Fruits	Sub-Acid Fruits	Acid Fruits
PRIMARY PROTEINS	Good	Poor	Poor	Poor	Poor	Good	Poor	Fair	Good
SECONDARY PROTEINS	Poor	Fair	Poor	Poor	Poor	Good	Poor	Poor	Fair
FATS	Poor	Poor	Good	Fair	Poor	Good	Fair	Fair	Fair
STARCHES	Poor	Poor	Fair	Good	Poor	Good	Fair	Fair	Fair
MELONS	Poor	Poor	Poor	Poor	Good	Poor	Fair	Fair	Poor
VEGETABLES	Good	Good	Good	Good	Poor	Good	Poor	Poor	Poor
SWEET FRUITS	Poor	Poor	Fair	Fair	Fair	Poor	Good	Good	Poor
SUB-ACID FRUITS	Fair	Poor	Fair	Fair	Fair	Poor	Good	Good	Good
ACID FRUITS	Good	Fair	Fair	Poor	Poor	Poor	Poor	Good	Good

Sub-acid fruits: mulberry, raspberry, blackberry, blueberry, grapes, pears, apples, cherries, apricots, peaches, plums, nectarines, pawpaw (papaya), mangos, guava.

Acid fruits: grapefruit, lemon, orange, lime, mandarin, pineapple, strawberry, kiwifruit (gooseberry), passionfruit.

Prepare your food with love and joy. It is good stuff.

Dietary Analysis

THE NUTRIENT CONTENT OF THE DIETS SUGGESTED IN THIS BOOK WERE analyzed by Dietary Analysis (Australia). They used a computer model based on the Australian Food Exchange Tables. Where no Australian values were available, they used British tables. They then based comparisons on the recommended daily allowances set down for nutrients by the USDA. There were some problems. We found that there were some things that are normally used in this diet for which the computer did not have values. Also, the bread figures used were based on salted breads that, therefore, dramatically raised their sodium levels. But, overall, this was the best analysis available.

Samples were analyzed of the Wellness Diet as being used by:

1. A 110-pound female with light activity.
2. The same diet with the addition of six juices.
3. The Gerson Diet as applied to a 155-pound male with light activity.

The results are summarized and show a supplement of vitamins E, B_{12} and zinc may be useful. Perhaps this is another indication for a multivitamin formula that assures an adequate supply of all these vital nutrients.

The Wellness Diet came out low in energy. This was an expected finding based on our clinical experience. While we certainly see people lose excess weight in this diet, our experience is that people's weight very commonly stabilizes at a lean, fit level. If lack of energy was experienced or weight loss continued, it could be easily rectified by eating more carbohydrates. Also, you can see from the charts that follow, that adding six juices leads to a predicted weight gain. However, again in our experience, weight does again stabilize for most people at a lean, fit level.

It should be noted that the figures given are the result of examining a three-day sample diet.

Legend

PROT	= Protein
CHO	= Carbohydrate (sugars & starch)
ENGY	= Energy
Ca	= Calcium
P	= Phosphorus
Fe	= Iron
Na	= Sodium (constituent of ordinary salt)
K	= Potassium
B-CRT	= Beta-carotene (orange plant pigment)
RETIN*	= Retinal (vitamin A)
B_1	= Vitamin B_1 (thiamine)
gm	= gram weight
mg	= milligram weight
mcg	= microgram weight
B_2	= Vitamin B_2 (riboflavin)
NIACIN **	= Vitamin B_3 (niacin)
VIT-C	= Vitamin C
VIT-E	= Vitamin E
B_6	= Vitamin B_6 (pyridoxine)
B_{12}	= Vitamin B_{12}
Zn	= Zinc
FIBER	= Dietary fiber
CHOL	= Cholesterol
FOLIC	= Folic acid
Mg	= Magnesium
kJ	= kilojoules
CAL	= 1 calorie (4.2kj)
RDA	= Recommended daily allowance

  * Includes RETINAL produced in the body from B-CAROTENE
** Includes NIACIN produced in the body from TRYPTOPHAN

Wellness Diet—110-Pound Female

		Supplied by Diet	Recommended % of RDA (RDA)	
WATER	gm	1535.88	***	
PROT	gm	62.02	55.11	113
FAT	gm	52.36	***	
CHO	gm	325.71	***	
ENGY	kJ	8080.74	9184.80	88
ENGY	Cal	1930.42	2194.17	
Ca	mg	870.64	400.00	218
P	mg	1298.73	**	
Fe	mg	20.44	12.00	170
Na	mg	2418.24	***	
K	mg	5493.97	***	
B-CRT	mcg	21330.11	***	
RETIN	mcg	112.83		
RETIN*	mcg	3667.85	750.00	489
B1	mcg	1577.20	918.48	172
B2	mcg	1661.87	1102.18	151
NIACIN	mg	14.97		
NIACIN**	mg	24.90	14.70	169
VIT-C	mg	274.39	30.00	915
VIT-E	mg	11.33	12.00	94
VIT-B_6	mcg	2837.73	2000.00	142
VIT-B_{12}	mcg	.80	2.00	40
Zn	mg	10.51	15.00	70
FIBER	gm	62.88	20.00	314
CHOL	mg	123.00	300.00	41
FOLIC	mcg	627.67	200.00	314
Mg	mg	629.50	300.00	210

*** RDAs have not been set for these nutrients. However, dietary goals do exist for some of them.

% of Total Energy in the diet provided by:	
1. PROTEIN	= 12.3 (Recommended = 10%–12%)
2. FAT	= 23.3 (Recommended = 30%–35%)
3. CHO	= 64.4 (Recommended = 55%–60%)
Energy (DIET)	= 8,081 kJ (1,930 Cals)
Energy (RDA)	= 9185 kJ (2,194 Cals)
Difference (DIET—RDA):	= 1104 kJ (264 Cals)

If the diet record is accurate and is typical of the patient's diet for the rest of the week, then the above energy difference would result in the patient LOSING .2kg (.5 lbs) per week.

Wellness Diet and Juices—110-Pound Female

		Supplied by Diet	Recommended % of RDA (RDA)	
WATER	gm	2795.93	***	
PROT	gm	75.08	55.11	136
FAT	gm	54.98	***	
CHO	gm	499.33	***	
ENGY	kJ	11001.48	9184.80	120
ENGY	Cal	2628.16	2194.17	
Ca	mg	1387.75	400.00	347
P	mg	1745.93	***	
Fe	mg	30.94	12.00	258
Na	mg	3043.75	***	
K	mg	9475.91	***	
B-CRT	mcg	75950.76	***	
RETIN	mcg	52.83		
RETIN*	mcg	12911.29	750.00	1722
B1	mcg	2505.44	1100.15	228
B2	mcg	2467.31	1320.18	187
NIACIN	mg	21.97		
NIACIN**	mg	33.99	17.60	193
VITAMIN C	mg	561.56	30.00	1872
VITAMIN E	mg	12.63	12.00	105
VITAMIN B$_6$	mcg	3226.73	2000.00	161
VITAMIN B$_{12}$	mcg	80	2.00	40
Zn	mg	11.67	15.00	78
FIBER	gm	69.18	20.00	346
CHOL	mg	123.00	300.00	41
FOLIC	mcg	915.67	200.00	458
Mg	mg	792.00	300.00	264

*** RDAs have not been set for these nutrients. However, dietary goals do exist for some of them.

% of Total Energy in the diet provided by:	
1. PROTEIN	= 10.8 (Recommended = 10%–12%)
2. FAT	= 17.7 (Recommended = 30%–35%)
3. CHO	= 71.5 (Recommended = 55%–60%)
Energy (DIET)	= 11,001 kJ (2,628 Cals)
Energy (RDA)	= 9,185 kJ (2,194 Cals)
Difference (DIET—RDA):	= 1,817 kJ (434 Cals)

If the diet record is accurate and is typical of the patient's diet for the rest of the week, then the above energy difference would result in the patient GAINING .4kg (.9 lbs) per week.

Gerson Diet—155-Pound Male

		Supplied by Diet	Recommended	% of RDA (RDA)
WATER	gm	4,121.97	***	
PROT	gm	164.90	69.90	236
FAT	gm	95.00	***	
CHO	gm	642.35	***	
ENGY	kJ	16,312.35	11,650.00	140
ENGY	Cal	3,896.88	2,783.09	
Ca	mg	1,659.12	400.00	415
P	mg	3,743.34	***	
Fe	mg	86.09	10.00	861
Na	mg	4,091.26	***	
K	mg	15,108.84	***	
B-CRT	mcg	99,999 Plus		
RETIN	mcg	41,914.20		
RETIN*	mcg	69,373.41	750.00	9,250
B1	mcg	4,852.52	1,631.24	297
B2	mcg	1,7875.20	1,957.48	913
NIACIN	mg	105.20		
NIACIN**	mg	131.58	26.10	504
VITAMIN C	mg	927.28	30.00	3,091
VITAMIN E	mg	13.20	05.00	88
VITAMIN B_6	mcg	6,073.00	2,000.00	304
VITAMIN B_{12}	mcg	500.00	2.00	9,999 Plus
Zn	mg	50.27	15.00	335
FIBER	gm	62.14	20.00	311
CHOL	mg	1,850.00	300.00	617
FOLIC	mcg	2,268.37	200.00	1134
Mg	mg	969.68	350.00	277

*** RDAs have not been set for these nutrients. However, dietary goals do exist for some of them.

% of Total Energy in the diet provided by:	
1. PROTEIN	= 16.2 (Recommended = 10%–12%)
2. FAT	= 20.9 (Recommended = 30%–35%)
3. CHO	= 62.9 (Recommended = 55%–60%)
Energy (DIET)	= 16,312 kJ (3,897 Cals)
Energy (RDA)	= 11,650 kJ (2,783 Cals)
Difference (DIET—RDA):	= 4662 kJ (1,114 Cals)

If the diet record is accurate and is typical of the patient's diet for the rest of the week, then the above energy difference would result in the patient GAINING 1.0 kg (2.2 lbs) per week.

Dietary Regime for Small Animals with Cancer

THIS ARTICLE WAS FIRST PUBLISHED IN THE "CONTROL AND THERAPY" ARTI-cles of the Post Graduate Committee in Veterinary Science *publication, University of Sydney, and has since been slightly revised.*

Does this sound familiar? "Your dog has cancer, there is nothing we can do. Shall we euthanase him now or later?"

This is a précis of an often repeated, if more gently expressed, diagnosis and sentence. It leaves the animal and owner without professional support, and likely to prematurely terminate a loved pet's life or to seek help from unqualified alternative sources. It leaves the practitioner missing out on an opportunity to follow through a stimulating and helpful exercise in disease management.

Having been through it myself with osteogenic sarcoma and having felt the benefits that dietary considerations offer, I have developed a dietary regime that I am confident offers help to animals with cancer. I present it on the basis of clinical experimentation with the knowledge that it does improve the quality of the animal's life. It has not cured anything as yet, although it has been instrumental in several remissions. I do feel, however, that it has prolonged life in many cases and am certain it has made the most of many difficult situations. It has also eased many people's minds when they want to do something constructive instead of just watching their animals die. Many owners comment on how fit and active their animals became on this nutritional package, despite the presence of tumors. Also, when the diet is followed, it is frequently noted that the animal's demise, when it comes, is rapid. Rather than the drawn-out, steady deterioration frequently associated with cancer, the animal remains well, often fitter than usual, until there is a sudden collapse. Then, if a decision regarding euthanasia is required, it is usually easily made.

Overall, the diet has many positive attributes. The principles are to detoxify the body, correct mineral imbalances, restore the digestion, and feed a well-balanced diet. I have included several supplements including Vitamin C, as I believe there is good evidence to do so.

The diet recognizes that we are dealing with carnivores, but that protein intake is better restricted a little.

Here it is.

Basic Components

Meat 40% by volume—stewing steak type; lean is preferable.

Vegetables 40% volume—concentrate on yellow ones (e.g., pumpkin, carrot) and green ones cooked minimally.

Brown Rice 20% volume—well cooked.

Presented as a stew; meat and vegetables should be cooked as little as acceptance dictates (e.g., generally well cooked to begin with and less as the pet's palate adapts). It is useful if carrot and greens especially are given raw— just grate finely. If all except the grains will be eaten raw, so much the better.

Fed to appetite demands, once daily.

Fast one day per week.

Additives: for 33-pound dog (adjust according to the pet's weight.)

- 1 teaspoon cold-pressed flaxseed oil—added after cooking.
- ¼ teaspoon kelp powder or granules—presoaked or cooked with rice.
- 1 tablespoon brewer's yeast—not a bitter variety—add to stew.
- 3 drops Lugol's iodine (can be made up by a pharmacist on request)— add to stew or drinking water.
- 200mg Potassium Orotate—crumble onto stew.
- 2 pancreatic enzyme tables, give by mouth (dogs usually eat these like treats).
- ½ Oroxine (thyroxine sodium) 100 mcgm tablet Welcome Aust.—give by mouth.
- ½ teaspoon Sodium ascorbate powder—available in small packs from health food shops or chemists—sprinkle onto stew—generally well accepted. If not, use coated 1,000mg tablets and give 2 tablets.

Dogs generally accept the diet readily, cats more reluctantly. Implementation obviously requires the owner's participation and tends to lead to the veterinarian becoming intimately involved in the whole procedure. This diet can be used as an adjunct in the treatment of any chronic degenerative disease.

Ian Gawler's 1978 Case History

THE FOLLOWING REPORT IS REPRINTED FROM THE *MEDICAL JOURNAL OF Australia*, 1978, 2:433.

The patient, aged 25, underwent a mid-thigh amputation for osteogenic sarcoma 11 months before he first saw me two-and-a-half years ago. He had visible bony lumps of about 2cm in diameter growing from the ribs, sternum and the crest of the ilium, and was coughing up small quantities of blood in which, he said, he could feel small spicules of bone. There were gross opacities in the X-ray films of his lungs. The patient had been told by a specialist that he had only two or three weeks to live, but in virtue of his profession he was already well aware of the pathology and prognosis of his condition. Now two-and-a-half years later, he has moved to another state to resume his former occupation.

This young man has shown an extraordinary will to live and has sought help from all the alternatives to orthodox medicine which were available to him. These have included acupuncture, massage, several sessions with Philippine faith healers, laying on of hands and yoga in an Indian ashram. He had short sessions of radiation therapy, and chemotherapy, but declined to continue treatment. He has also persisted with the dietary and enema treatment prescribed by Max Gerson, the German physician, who gained some notoriety for this type of treatment in America in the 1940s. However, in addition to all these measures to gain relief, the patient has consistently maintained a rigorous discipline of intensive meditation as described previously. He has in fact, consistently meditated from one to three hours daily.

Two other factors seem to be important. He has had extraordinary help and support from his girlfriend, who more recently became his wife. She is extremely sensitive to his feelings and needs, and has spent hours in aiding his meditation and healing with massage and laying on of hands.

The other important factor would seem to be the patient's own state of mind. He has developed a degree of calm about him which I have rarely observed in anyone, even in oriental mystics with whom I have had some considerable experience. When asked to what he attributes the regression of metastases, he answers in some such terms as: "I really think it is our life, the way we experience our life." In other words, it would seem that the patient has let the effects of the intense and prolonged meditation enter into his whole experience of life. His extraordinarily low level of anxiety is obvious to the most casual observer. It is suggested that this has enhanced the activity of his immune system by reducing his level of cortisone.

Ainslie Meares, MD, DPM

[Since this report was written the patient has been declared free of active neoplastic disease. —AM]

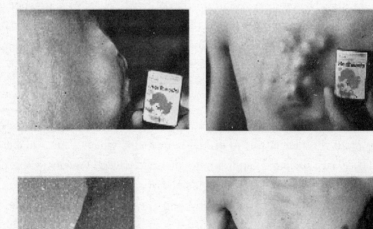

Important note. In the original article, the date for the top two photographs was incorrectly recorded. The photographs were taken in October 1976 (and have Kodak dates imprinted on their reverse), while the bottom two were taken on the April 25, 1978.

Ian Gawler—30-Year Follow-Up—2008 Case History

THIS ARTICLE APPEARED IN THE *MEDICAL JOURNAL OF AUSTRALIA*, 15 December 2008: 189 11/12663–665.

Thirty-year follow-up at pneumonectomy of a 58-year-old survivor of disseminated osteosarcoma

George A Jelinek and Ruth H Gawler

A 1978 case report in the Journal described a 25-year-old man with disseminated osteogenic sarcoma whose metastases regressed after treatment with diet and intensive meditation. Thirty years later, there has been no recurrence of his cancer, and a recent pneumonectomy for chronic bronchiectasis revealed mature cancellous bone in the resected lung. The man is otherwise well. (MJA 2008; 189: 663–665) MJA • Volume 189 Number 11/12 • 1/15 December 2008

Clinical Record

A man who is now 58 years old was diagnosed in 1974, at the age of 24, with histologically confirmed high-grade osteogenic sarcoma of the right femur (Figure, A). His right leg was amputated in January 1975. Histopathologically, the tumor was described (in a 1994 review of the case) as follows: "The tissue is replaced by a cellular malignant spindle cell tumor forming osteoid and bone and having a disorganized pattern of proliferation . . . confirming the diagnosis of a high grade endosteal osteosarcoma (osteogenic sarcoma)."

In December 1975, widespread bony and pulmonary metastases were diagnosed. Despite being told in March 1976 that he had only 2–3 weeks to live, the man survived until September that year, when he underwent three cycles of palliative chemotherapy with vincristine, adriamycin, cyclophosphamide and dacarbazine, as well as brief palliative radiation therapy. He elected to discontinue these therapies as his condition deteriorated further.

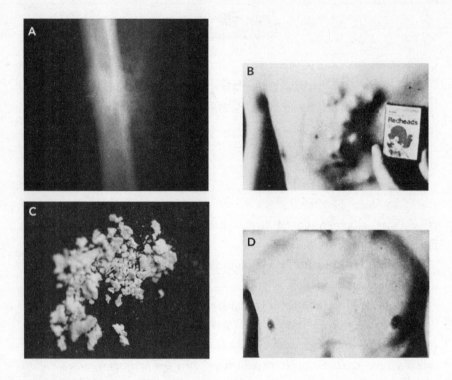

The patient then consulted prominent psychiatrist and hypnotherapist Dr. Ainslie Meares, who reported his case and his subsequent remarkable recovery in the Medical Journal of Australia in 1978.[1] When Meares first saw the patient, he had visible bony tumors protruding from his ribs, sternum (Figure B) and iliac crest, and was coughing up blood containing small spicules of bone (Figure C). Meares taught him how to meditate, and both he and the patient felt this was a key component in recovery, although he also adhered faithfully to a vegan diet and tried many alternative therapies, including massage, acupuncture, faith healing and others.

The patient recovered and returned to full time work, founding and running self-help groups for people with cancer, but had persistent reminders of the original illness. Presumably related to immune suppression from chemotherapy, he developed pulmonary tuberculosis in June 1978, and was treated for this condition for 12 months. This progressed to cavitation and severe bronchiectasis, causing repeated bouts of pneumonia and persistently elevated erythrocyte sedimentation rate (ESR).

Chest x-rays in November 1989, 15 years after the patient's diagnosis and subsequent recovery, showed evidence of previous tuberculosis and ongoing bronchiectasis, with a left hilar mass compressing the left upper lobe bronchus by 50%. Views of the lumbar spine and pelvis, taken at the same time to investigate ongoing back pain, showed abnormalities initially thought to represent progressive metastatic disease. The report noted "progressive metastatic disease with large osteoblastic deposit right ilium, sacrum, and invasion into L5." That report was amended 4 days later, after comparison with films from 1978, to state "The appearances in the body of L5 . . . are those of metastatic disease but this appearance is essentially unchanged." A thoracic computed tomography scan performed a few days later showed evidence of previous left lung tuberculosis.

With no further treatment, the patient's condition remained stable. X-ray images of the chest, pelvis and lumbar spine in 1993 were unchanged from 1989. Lung function testing in 1996 and 1999 showed satisfactory function, with an FEV1/FVC (forced expiratory volume in 1 second/forced vital capacity) ratio of 2.56 L/3.40 L. Indeed, the patient was well enough to go trekking in Nepal for three weeks in 1999 to a height of about 16,000 feet above sea level.

However, two episodes of left lower lobe pneumonia in 2004 and chronic bronchiectasis resulted in referral to a thoracic surgeon with a view to pneumonectomy. Noting the patient's chronically elevated ESR, indicating ongoing sepsis, and recurrent chest infections, the surgeon recommended left pneumonectomy while the patient was still young enough to tolerate the surgery.

In December 2004, pneumonectomy was performed. As the patient had relied on elbow crutches since the original leg amputation, it was hoped that a minimally invasive approach might preserve chest wall skeletal structure and musculature, but because of widespread adhesions and tuberculous scarring, this was not possible. A complicated 5-hour pleuropneumonectomy was performed, with the pericardium being opened to enable access to the pulmonary veins, precipitating a short period of intraoperative ventricular fibrillation.

Macroscopic pathological examination showed a small, collapsed, scarred left lung. The lung parenchyma was abnormal, and bronchiectasis, cavitation and scarring were widespread, but there was no obvious tumor. Microscopic examination showed severe bronchiectasis, but there was no evidence of mycobacterial infection. The report noted that "palpation of lung parenchyma deep to the hilum reveals a rock-hard consistency, impossible to section with a knife. Using a saw, horizontal cuts . . . reveal a centrally located bony mass 35–30mm about, surrounding the bifurcation of the left main bronchus." Histopathological examination of decalcified sections showed "a bony mass surrounding and incorporating large central bronchi and neurovascular structures. Much of the bone has a mature cancellous appearance with normal appearing osteocytes, and mature fat within the intertrabecular spaces. In addition there are foci of coarse sclerotic and heavily calcified bone which are devoid of viable osteocytes. No viable tumor is present."

After steady postoperative recovery, the patient returned to fulltime work and remains well.

Discussion

Osteosarcomas are rare malignant tumors of the skeleton characterized by formation of immature bone by tumor cells. At the time of this patient's diagnosis, osteosarcoma was a devastating disease with very low survival rates.[2] Most patients died within a year of diagnosis. Management centered around limb amputation, with palliative chemotherapy and radiation therapy for recurrences. Over the past 30 years, management has improved dramatically. With the use of limb-sparing surgery, induction and adjuvant chemotherapy, and surgical excision of metastases, survival rates of around 60% can now be expected for patients presenting with localized disease.[3-5]

There are limited data examining long-term outcomes among patients recovering from osteosarcoma. A few articles have reported long-term follow-up, including surveillance for recurrence,[6] the development of other cancers,[7] and cardiac toxicity from chemotherapy agents.[8] Metastases have been known to develop as long as 14 years after diagnosis.[6] While there is a report of spontaneous regression of a pulmonary metastasis that developed 5 years after treatment for osteosarcoma,[9] the fate of regressed secondaries has not been well documented.

Today, pulmonary metastases are often resected, but this is while the tumor is active. In this patient's case, the lung was resected, for other reasons, 30 years after the original diagnosis, and incidentally, a large piece of mature cancellous bone was found surrounding the left main bronchus. This presumably represented bone formation by a long-since regressed secondary tumor, similar to the bone found in the primary tumor at the time of amputation.

It is clear from the 1978 report that large sections of the externally visible osteogenic secondaries were resorbed as the cancer regressed. This was most obvious on the patient's chest wall (Figure D). However, some spinal and pelvic bone formed by the secondaries appears to have remained intact after tumor disappearance, as illustrated by the fact that x-rays taken of the spine and pelvis 15 years after diagnosis and recovery were identical with films of 11 years earlier and by the presence of bone in the resected lung.

It is interesting to consider the possible factors involved in this man's remarkable recovery. Spontaneous remission is a possibility, although exceedingly unlikely at such an advanced stage of disease, and its coincident timing with a wide range of self-help measures adopted by the patient makes this explanation even more improbable. Certainly, the patient had widespread disease from which recovery, even today, would be very unlikely. Although the patient received a short course of palliative chemotherapy and radiotherapy to his lumbar spine, it is unlikely that this would have been curative with such widespread metastatic disease. Meares and the patient attributed the remarkable recovery to intensive meditation,[1] and it is true that the patient meditated from 3 to 5 hours daily after developing secondaries. He still regularly meditates and teaches others with cancer to do so. His fastidious adoption of the Gerson diet[10] for 3 months, followed by adherence to a plant-based wholefood vegan diet may also have played some part. Such a lifestyle approach, incorporating meditation and vegan diet, has recently been shown to cause significant modulation of gene expression and biological processes associated with tumor growth.[11]

Apart from illustrating the value of maintaining hope in the face of apparent hopelessness, this case shows that, long after tumor regression, metastatic lesions from osteosarcoma may contain significant amounts of residual bone. Even in the absence of tumor, these bony deposits may cause health problems in their own right, depending on their location. Our understanding of such unlikely survival continues to improve with the recent demonstration that modifiable lifestyle factors affect gene expression in patients with cancer.[11]

ACKNOWLEDGMENTS

We are grateful to Professor Peter Clarke, who performed the pneumonectomy, and Mr. John Doyle, who undertook the amputation, for their assistance with the provision of past records and review of the manuscript, and to Dr. Sandra Neate for her critical review and helpful suggestions.

Competing Interests

Professor Jelinek is a friend and colleague of the patient, and Dr. Ruth Gawler is related to the patient.

Author Details

George A. Jelinek, MD, FACEM, DipDHM, Professorial Fellow1,2

Ruth H. Gawler, MB BS, MGPPsych, FACPsyMed, General Practitioner and Therapist3

1 Department of Medicine, University of Melbourne, St. Vincent's Hospital, Melbourne, VIC.
2 Department of Emergency Medicine, St. Vincent's Hospital, Melbourne, VIC.
3 The Gawler Foundation, Yarra Junction, VIC.

Correspondence: George.Jelinek@svhm.org.au

References

1 Meares, A. Regression of osteogenic sarcoma metastases associated with intensive meditation. *Med J Aust*, 1978; 2:433.
2 Picci, P. Osteosarcoma (osteogenic sarcoma). Orphanet *J Rare Dis*, 2007; 2:6.
3 Jaffe, N., Carrasco, H., Raymond K., et al. Can cure in patients with osteosarcoma be achieved exclusively with chemotherapy and abrogation of surgery? *Cancer*, 2002; 95: 2,202–2,210.
4 Wittig, J. C., Bickels, J., Priebat, D., et al. Osteosarcoma: a multidisciplinary approach to diagnosis and treatment. *Am Fam Physician* 2002; 65: 1,123–1,132.
5 Tan, J. Z., Schlicht, S. M., Powell, G. J., et al. Multidisciplinary approach to diagnosis and management of osteosarcoma—a review of the St. Vincent's Hospital experience. *Int Semin Surg Oncol* 2006; 3:38.
6 Strauss, S. J., McTiernan, A., Whelan, J. S. Late relapse of osteosarcoma: implications for follow-up and screening. *Pediatr Blood Cancer* 2004; 43:692–697.

7 Kim, M. S., Sim, Y. S., Lee, S. Y., Jeon, D. G. Secondary thyroid papillary carcinoma in osteosarcoma patients: report of two cases. *J Korean Med Sci* 2008; 23:149–152.

8 Longhi, A., Ferrari, S., Bacci, G., Specchia, S. Long-term follow-up of patients with doxorubicin-induced cardiac toxicity after chemotherapy for osteosarcoma. *Anticancer Drugs* 2007; 18:737–744.

9 Bacci, G., Palmerini, E., Staals, E. L., et al. Spontaneous regression of lung metastasis from osteosarcoma: a case report. *J Pediatr Hematol Oncol* 2008; 30:90–92.

10 Gerson, M. *A Cancer Therapy: Results of Fifty Cases.* New York: Station Hill Press, 1995.

11 Ornish, D., Magbanua, M. J., Weidner, G., et al. Changes in prostate gene expression in men undergoing an intensive nutrition and lifestyle intervention. *Proc Natl Acad Sci USA* 2008; 105: 8,369–8,374.

Ian Gawler's History—A Summary

AS THIS HISTORY IS LONG AND COMPLEX, IT HAS OFTEN BEEN MISQUOTED. What follows is a chronology of key events in Ian's recovery from cancer and his ongoing life.

February 25, 1950: Born in Melbourne, Australia.

1972: Graduated in Veterinary Science—Melbourne University.

1973–1975: Leased veterinary practice at Bacchus Marsh, Victoria, at first in partnership, then as principal. Large practice with the focus on stud and performance horses and companion animals.

December 1974: Reported swelling in right thigh to local GP and referred to surgeon, Dr. John Doyle.

January 1975: Full anesthetic and open biopsy confirmed osteogenic sarcoma in right leg. Told prognosis was 5 percent chance of survival after five years. Five days later, on January 8, right leg was amputated through the hip. Postsurgical histology confirmed the diagnosis. Independent review of all pathology in 1994 confirmed the original diagnosis.

Found prosthesis less practical than crutches. Began to wear kaftans for comfort and esthetics. Began to meditate daily, improved the diet, and reflected deeply on the meaning and purpose of life.

November 1975: Rock-hard swelling detected inside right groin. Based upon the clinical picture, definitive X-rays and bone scans, Doyle diagnosed secondary osteogenic sarcoma in the right sacroiliac area and suspected more secondaries centrally in the chest. Advised medical treatment ineffective and not recommended. Advised prognosis was three to six months.

Ian reasoned that healing may be possible if the immune system could be activated. Began intensive meditation (initially three to five hours, then three) with Dr. Ainslie Meares (Melbourne psychiatrist and author of *Relief Without Drugs*). Began the Gerson Diet.

February 1976: No growth in cancer but complications began through weight loss and period of a couple weeks of severe back pain and sciatica. Confined to bed. Following more extensive investigations at Peter Mac-Callum Hospital, three palliative radiotherapy treatments to lower lumbar spine were administered, but were ineffective for pain relief. Chiropractic, megavitamin therapy and acupuncture gave slight relief but not persisted with. Medically directed injections of Plenisol, a mistletoe extract, relieved pain and increased mobility.

Married Gail Kerr (later Gail changed her name to Gayle, then Grace) who had been Ian's veterinary nurse and who continued to support him throughout his illness and recovery.

March 1976: Hydronephrosis developed, pain reintensified, severe night sweats, jaundiced, cachexia with marked weight loss.

March/April 1976: Travelled to Philippines. Over four weeks, psychic surgery received from five traditional Filipino shamanistic healers. Marked pain relief, weight gain and general health turn around, although cancer unchanged.

April–October 1976: Continued with meditation, diet, and explored wide range of natural therapies aimed at stimulating the immune system and healing. This was a period of intense reading, introspection and personal development. However, the cancer continued to progress, with large masses slowly enlarging inside pelvis, mediastinum and through left lung, plus large eruptions of cancer on the exterior of the sternum.

October 1976: Cancer progressed to its largest size (as seen in photos in this book. This photo has been regularly mislabelled as being taken in October 1977, but the original has the Kodak print date on its back and it forms one in a sequence of over a dozen photos that are dated by Kodak). Otherwise, health very good.

Concerned by cancer growth, consulted oncologist. After more investigations and confirmation of the diagnosis, advised of experimental chemotherapy that could be attempted with uncertain results and probably significant side effects (transient nausea, short-term hair loss, high probability of sterility, possible heart muscle and eyesight damage). Two-year course of treatment recommended with Adriamycin, vincristine, cyclophosphamide and dacarbazine. After two weeks deliberation, commenced treatment while intensifying the diet, the meditation and other supportive, self-help procedures.

After ten weeks treatment, felt whatever benefits the chemotherapy had to offer had been received. However, the cancer had only slightly diminished in size over the period of treatment (as confirmed by the regular photos taken and the oncologist's written reports); and warned of the very real possibilities of rapid rebound growth if the treatment was ceased. Against medical advice, elected to discontinue treatment.

January 1977: Returned to the Philippines seeking more healing for the cancer, any side effects from the treatment, and in an attempt to understand psychic surgery. Rented a flat in Baguio and spent three months being treated, filming, talking and studying with healers. After a visit to Manila that was very polluted, began coughing up blood for the first time. This may have marked the onset of the TB that would not be diagnosed until June 1978.

April 1977: Journeyed on to India. Met with Sai Baba, who is regarded as an avatar (a divine incarnation) in India. He said, "You are already healed, don't worry"—another turning point. Cancer began to recede markedly.

May/June 1977: Journeyed to Cairo; England—Glastonbury, Findhorn, Iona; Europe. Cancer continued to recede and began coughing up spicules of bone from the cancer breaking down in lungs.

June–December 1977: Back in Torquay, Victoria. Maintained the diet, meditation, positive attitude, natural therapies and personal development.

December 1977: Moved to Surfers Paradise, Queensland. Recommenced veterinary work.

December 1977–February 1978: Employed in companion animal practice, Surfers Paradise, Queensland.

April 1978: All visible cancer cleared. Returned to India for three weeks and then moved to Adelaide, South Australia, to take up companion animal veterinary practice at Morphett Vale, living at Old Noarlunga.

July 1978: Rosemary, first child born. Following extensive tests, cancer pronounced all clear, but tuberculosis diagnosed. Treatment commenced. Doctors advised given the medical history that recovery is likely to take around one year. Intensified the diet, meditation, etc. TB cleared in three weeks.

September 1978: Case reported by Dr. Ainslie Meares in *Medical Journal of Australia* (MJA) (see full report earlier). Media attention led to increased enquiries from other cancer patients and families.

1980: Moved to country property at Yarra Junction, Victoria, and established a mixed veterinary practice. Lived in small shed, while building own house over a four-year period. Three home births in shed: David, August 1980; Peter, March 1982; Alice, November 1983.

1981: Ian and Grace initiated the Melbourne Cancer Support Group (MCSG). This innovative twelve-week program had the specific aim of helping people to learn and put into practice those things they could do for themselves. The intention was to actively support people as they set about increasing their quality of life and their chances of experiencing long-term survival. The first meeting was held on September 16, 1981. The meetings lasted two and a half hours each week and on average over thirty people attended each program. Each session had a theme and time was provided for discussion and mutual support. This was the first group of its type in Australia, and one of the very first in the world; a lifestyle-based self-help program that focused upon therapeutic nutrition, attitudes, positive thinking and healthy emotions, meditation and peace of mind. This program continues to be presented and continues to evolve based upon clinical experience and research.

1983: In December, a nonprofit, nondenominational, registered charity was established to support and extend the MCSG. As the years progressed, the Gawler Foundation developed an additional emphasis on the prevention of disease, lifestyle counseling and the generation of well-being and peace of mind for symptom-free people. The programs, having been based upon Ian's recovery to begin with, continued to evolve in line with feedback from the participants and with the latest research findings.

1984: The veterinary practice was sold to focus on the newly established foundation. Ian has done very little formal veterinary work since.

1984: *You Can Conquer Cancer* was first published by Hill of Content (the book was based on MCSG program) and launched by Sir Edward "Weary" Dunlop, patron of the Anti-Cancer Council and long-term advocate for Ian's work.

ABC TV presented a landmark, mind-body medicine documentary featuring the work of Ian Gawler and Dr. Ainslie Meares called *Mind the Healer, Mind the Slayer.*

1985: The first residential program was conducted for cancer patients and their families in December 1985 at Monash University. These were the first residential programs for people with cancer in Australia.

1987: Australia Day Honors: Ian was awarded the Order of Australia Medal for services to the community.

1987: *Peace of Mind* published by Hill of Content (now published by Michelle Anderson Publishing Pty. Ltd.)

1991: First phase of the Gawler Foundation's (TGF) residential center at Yarra Junction opened.

1992: Second phase of TGF's residential center at Yarra Junction opened.

1995–99: Ian founded and convened Mind, Immunity and Health, the first Australian conference designed specifically for doctors and allied health professionals interested in mind-body medicine. This conference continues as the Holistic Health conference, the annual conference of the Australasian Integrative Medical Association.

1996: *Meditation—Pure and Simple* published by Hill of Content (now published by Michelle Anderson Publishing Pty Ltd.).

Grace ceased working at the Gawler Foundation.

1997: In November, Ian and Grace separated, then divorced in mid-1999.

The Creative Power of Imagery published by Hill of Content.

1999: Ian co-led a meditation-based trek for three weeks in the Himalayas to altitudes of 16,000.

2000: Ian remarried, to Dr. Ruth Berlin—now Dr. Ruth Gawler, a GP with a master's in general practice psychiatry.

2002: Dr. Ruth Gawler began working at the Gawler Foundation.

Ian and Ruth initiated lifestyle-based, self-help programs for people with MS—in collaboration with Professor George Jelinek, MS survivor, professor of emergency medicine, author of *Overcoming Multiple Sclerosis.*[39]

2004: Ian's left lung was removed following ongoing complications from bronchiectasis and scarring resultant from the TB. Histology confirmed there was a boney lesion removed with the lung that was consistent with osteogenic sarcoma treated with chemotherapy.

Health is now very good.

2005: Senate Inquiry into Cancer Services in Australia made a bipartisan recommendation that Gawler Foundation programs receive Medicare rebates. This is yet to happen.

2006: First endorsed training conducted for Cancer, Healing & Well-being— the twelve-week lifestyle-based cancer self-help group. (Ian first began annual trainings for people who wanted to lead cancer groups or teach meditation back in 1988). A network of the groups began across Australia, New Zealand and overseas.

2007: Endorsed training program commenced for teachers of meditation.

2008: Biography *The Dragon's Blessing* published by Allen & Unwin; author Guy Allenby.

Ian's medical case—a thirty-year follow-up of Dr. Ainslie Meares' report in 1978 written by Professor George Jelinek and Dr. Ruth Gawler—was published in the *MJA* in December (see full report earlier).

2009: Ian was featured on ABC TV in *Compass: A Good Life.*

Ian retired from the Gawler Foundation at the end of the year.

2010: *Meditation—An In-Depth Guide* is published by Allen & Unwin.

Grace Gawler challenged some of the timelines and reasons postulated for Ian's recovery in the *Medical Journal of Australia.* These claims were answered by George Jelinek and Ruth Gawler in the *MJA.*

2011: *The Mind That Changes Everything* was released by Brolga Publishing.

2012: Ian launched *Mind-Body Mastery*, a downloadable meditation program with an innovative support package to enhance learning and increase frequency of practice.

Haines and Lowenthal, writing in the *Internal Medicine Journal* (IMJ), disputed Ian's diagnosis of secondary cancer and hypothesized he only had TB. They did this without checking the facts with Ian or his treating doctors and without Ian's permission. These claims were refuted as being incorrect by Ian and Ruth Gawler in separate letters to the IMJ that were accompanied by details of the original medical reports from the time of his diagnosis along with statements from his original doctors.

You Can Conquer Cancer—a completely revised and rewritten version—was released by Michelle Anderson Publishing.

References

1. Meares, A. *Relief without Drugs,* 1968, Souvenir Press, London.
2. Sogyal, R. *The Tibetan Book of Living and Dying,* 1992, Ryder, London.
3. Gawler, I. J. ed. *Inspiring People,* 1995, The Gawler Foundation, Yarra Junction.
4. Kraus, P. *Surviving Cancer,* 2008, The Gawler Foundation, Yarra Junction.
5. Doll, R., and Peto, R. *The Causes of Cancer,* 1981, Oxford University Press, New York.
6. Kune, G. Edited Proceedings, The First Slezak Cancer Symposium, *"The Psyche and Cancer,"* 1992, Melbourne,
7. Gawler, I., and Bedson, P. *Meditation—an In-Depth Guide*, 2008, Allen & Unwin, Sydney.
8. Kraus, P. Op cit.
9. Kabat-Zinn, J. *Full Catastrophe Living,* 1990, Delta Books, Bantam Doubleday Dell Publishing Group, New York.
10. Frankl, V. *Man's Search for Meaning,* 1963, Pocket Books, New York.
11. Gawler, I. *The Mind that Changes Everything*, 2011, Brolga Publishing, Melbourne.
12. Coué, E. *Self-Mastery Through Conscious Auto-Suggestion,* First published 1922, this edition, 2007, Cosimo, New York.
13. Simonton, O. C., and Matthew, S. *Getting Well Again,* 1978, Bantam, New York.
14. Dossey, L. *Healing Words—The Power of Prayer and the Power of Medicine,* 1994, Harper Collins, New York.
15. Sackett, D.L.R., et al. "Evidence Based Medicine: what it is and what it isn't," *BMJ* 1996; 312: 71–2.
16. Yogananda. *Autobiography of a Yogi*, First published 1946, this edition, 2007, Sterling Publishers, New Delhi.
17. Gerson, M. *A Cancer Therapy: Results of Fifty Cases,* 1958, Totality Books, California, USA.
18. Ornish, D., et al. *Journal of Urology* 2005; 74: 1065–1070.

19. *The New Gawler Foundation Cookbook*, 2012, The Gawler Foundation, Yarra Junction.

20. Pauling, Dr. L., and Cameron, E. *Cancer and Vitamin C,* 1979, Linus Pauling Institute of Science and Medicine, New York.

21. Pert, C. *Molecules of Emotion,* 1998, Simon & Schuster, London.

22. Brandt, J. *The Grape Cure,* 1996, Health Research, Pomeroy, USA.

23. Kune, G. *The Home Health Guide to a Cancer-Free Family,* 2005, Michelle Anderson Publishing, Melbourne.

24. Doll, R., and Peto, R. Op cit.

25. Le Shan, L. *You Can Fight for Your Life,* 1978, Jove Publishing.

26. Simonton and Matthews. Op cit.

27. Temoshok, L. and Dreher, H. *The Type C Connection: The Behavioral Links to Cancer and Your Health,* 1999, Collingdale.

28. Miller, M. and Rahe, R. H. *Life Changes Scaling for the 1990s,* 1997, *Journal of Psychosomatic Research*: 43:279.

29. Kübler-Ross, E. *On Death and Dying,* 1969, Macmillan, New York.

30. McCue, K. *How to Help Children Through a Parent's Serious Illness,* 2011, St. Martin's Press, New York.

31. Kübler-Ross, E. Op cit.

32. Moody, R. *Life After Life,* 1979, Bantam, New York.

33. Morgan, G. et al. *Clin Oncol,* 2004; 16:549–60.

34. Gawler, I. *Cancer, Chemotherapy and Lifestyle,* available via the research section on the website www.iangawler.com.

35. Allenby, G. *The Dragon's Blessing,* 2008, Allen & Unwin, Sydney.

36. Tompkins, P. and Bird, C. *The Secret Life of Plants,* 1974, Penguin, Melbourne.

37. Gawler, I. *The Mind That Changes Everything,* 2011, Brolga Publishing, Melbourne.

38. Doidge, N. *The Brain That Changes Itself,* 2008, Scribe, Carlton North.

39. Jelinek, G. *Overcoming Multiple Sclerosis,* 2009, Allen & Unwin, Crow's Nest.
   The Australian Concise Oxford Dictionary, Melbourne, Oxford University Press, 1987.

The Holy Bible, Revised Standard Edition, New York, Thomas Nelson, 1972.

More Information on Ian Gawler

Book

Meditation: Pure and Simple

Downloadable Meditation Program

Mind-Body Mastery—with ongoing online support:
www.mindbodymastery.net

Ian's Website

www.iangawler.com

Ian's Blog

gawlerblog.com

To contact the Gawler Foundation:

PO Box 77, Yarra Junction, Victoria 3797, Australia
Phone: (03) 5967 1730, or Fax: (03) 5967 1715
International Dialing: +61 3 5967 1730
E-mail: info@gawler.org
Website: www.gawler.org

Index

Page numbers in *italics* refer to photos, illustrations, figures, and charts.

Clackamas County Library
13793 SE Sieben Park Way
Clackamas, OR 97015

WITHDRAWN

FEB 05